The Myth of the Perfect Pregnancy

The Myth of the Perfect Pregnancy

A History of Miscarriage in America

Lara Freidenfelds

OXFORD
UNIVERSITY PRESS

Oxford University Press is a department of the University of Oxford. It furthers
the University's objective of excellence in research, scholarship, and education
by publishing worldwide. Oxford is a registered trade mark of Oxford University
Press in the UK and certain other countries.

Published in the United States of America by Oxford University Press
198 Madison Avenue, New York, NY 10016, United States of America.

CIP data is on file at the Library of Congress
ISBN 978–0–19–086981–6

1 3 5 7 9 8 6 4 2

Printed by Sheridan Books, Inc., United States of America

For my family

CONTENTS

ACKNOWLEDGMENTS

Books may have single authors, and yet they emerge from communities. I thank the many communities who have supported my efforts, pushed my thinking, and produced the marvelous scholarship I have built my work upon.

Thank you to the Mellon Foundation, the Newhouse Center for the Humanities, and the Department of Women's and Gender Studies at Wellesley College for the postdoctoral fellowship that grounded my research, and the warm and stimulating collegiality of faculty and fellows, especially Susan Reverby, Rosanna Hertz, Charlene Galarneau, Tim Peltason, John Burt, Sarah Bishop, Nathaniel Scheidley, Sarah Wall-Randall, and the members of Feminist Inquiry. Thank you to the Hagley Museum and Archive, especially Erik Rau, Roger Horowitz, and Carol Lockman, for a Hagley Exploratory Grant that allowed me sustained access to their wonderful collection. I am grateful to archivists David Rose at the March of Dimes archive; Russell Johnson at the University of California at Los Angeles Biomedical Sciences Library archive; and Alison Kotch at Meredith Publishing, for facilitating my access to the *American Baby* magazine archive. Thank you to the Princeton Research Forum for the support of a Frances C. Hunter Presentation Grant and sustained moral and intellectual support for independent scholarhood, and thanks especially to my PRF indy scholar mentor, Karen Reeds, who has been generous with clever and insightful ideas, good humor, and lunch dates. Thanks to the Chatham Public Library staff for graciously filling many years' worth of ILL requests, and to Chatham, Morris County, and the state of New Jersey for supporting a robust and research-worthy library system. Thank you to research assistants extraordinaire Wei-Ying Wang and Alexandra Pollock.

I thank my colleagues all over the country who invited me to speak and gave me thoughtful and well-informed feedback without fail: the University of California at Los Angeles History of Science, Technology and Medicine Colloquium; the University of California at Berkeley Gender and Science Program; the Yale University History of Science and Medicine Colloquium; University of Pennsylvania's symposium in honor of Ruth Schwartz Cowan; Rutgers University's Symposium on Maternal and Fetal Bodies; Kansas University Medical Center's Don Carlos Peete Lecture; the Bates Nursing History Center at the University of Pennsylvania; the Hagley Museum Research Seminar (especially commentator Amy Bentley); The Hastings Center; the Schlesinger Library at the Radcliffe Institute, Harvard University; and the University of Nebraska at Lincoln Linda and Charles Wilson Humanities in Medicine Lecture. Thank you to the American Association of the History of Medicine, my scholarly home base, whose members have provided brilliant scholarship, camaraderie, and many years' feedback on my work in formal presentations and hallway conversations alike. Thank you also to my colleagues at the Society for the History of Technology and the Berkshire Conference on the History of Women for their helpful feedback on conference papers.

A huge thanks to the people who read part or all of my manuscript and generously shared critiques and ideas. The Independent Women Scholars' Salon has been the center of my intellectual and writing life for over a decade and a constant source of good cheer, smart ideas, careful critiques, and pushes to think bigger. I thank these amazing IWSS swashbucklers: Joy Harvey, Rachael Rosner, Kara Swanson, Conevery Bolton Valencius, Kate Viens, Nadine Weidman, Ilyon Woo, Susan Lanzoni, Deborah Weinstein, Martha Gardner, and Monique Tello. Cara Kiernan Fallon is my NYC writing and lunch buddy, and I am grateful for her perceptive insights and cogent edits on the entire manuscript. I thank journalist and historian Randi Epstein for her helpful feedback on the whole manuscript and many fun and collegial lunches. Thank you also to Laurel Thatcher Ulrich, Katharine Park, Charis Thompson, Johanna Schoen, Chris Crenner, Ziv Eisenberg, Shannon Wythecombe, Allan Brandt, Erik Parens, Rose Holz, Emily Abel, John Freidenfelds, Kelly Freidenfelds, Lucy Freidenfelds, Jason Freidenfelds, and Sabrina Freidenfelds for crucial feedback on part or all of the manuscript and key, insightful conversations that shaped my arguments. Thank you to my agent, Lisa Adams, and my editor, Susan Ferber, for tweaking my words in just the right ways and advocating for my research and my message, and the peer reviewers at Oxford University Press for their clarifying questions and generous feedback.

Thank you to my playground communities at the Child Study Center at Wellesley College, Sprout House in Chatham, New Jersey, Washington Avenue School, and my Moms' Group in Berkeley. There are a lot of wise parents out there, and I was privileged to spend many hours learning from them while we watched our kids together. Thanks especially to Victoria

Budson, who inspired me with her example of how feminist work and caring for family go together and who taught me how to shape my own narrative. Thank you also to the teachers and babysitters who helped me balance writing and child care and loved and educated my children in equal measure, especially Renee Blanchard, Julia Friedman, Claire Thoma, and Caitlin McGlynn.

This book is dedicated to my family. My parents, John and Lucy Freidenfelds, my in-laws, Amy and Andy Wu, my siblings and siblings-in-law, Kelly Freidenfelds, David Brown, Jason and Sabrina Freidenfelds, Fran Wu-Giarratano and Paul Giarratano: you are my treasured parenting companions and role models. I am so lucky to have you. My spouse, Felix Wu: you are my partner in everything, the love of my life, and I can't imagine doing any of it without you. The kiddos—all my wonderful nieces and nephews, and my dear children Sebastian and Oliver—you are the reason for it all, and you make the effort worthwhile. I am so glad to be a part of your growing up.

The Myth of the Perfect Pregnancy

Introduction

"AHHHH!!! Congratulations!! I was wondering when you guys were going to start having kids!! So excited for you guys!!!" Michelle was thrilled to read food and lifestyle writer Emily Malone's pregnancy announcement on her blog, *The Daily Garnish*, in 2011. Hundreds of regular readers chimed in with their good wishes. "That is so exciting! Congratulations, and best wishes for a smooth pregnancy!" wrote Deanna. Yena gushed, "Oh my goodness, I gasped when I read 'baby'! How exciting—congrats to you both, sooo happy for you!" Another reader urged Malone to "Treasure every moment of this exciting time. I look forward to reading about your experiences. So excited for you!"[1]

Posted about two months into her pregnancy, Malone's announcement was a sweet thumbnail romance. Lovingly illustrated, it began with childhood photos of her and her husband, a Little League–playing Indiana boy destined from birth to meet a sparkly dress–wearing girl from Ohio. "Twenty-something years later—they met, fell madly in love, and got married." Tongue in cheek, Malone described "a happy family of four," above a picture of her and her husband with the dogs they each brought to the marriage. "And now sometime around October 15th, 2011—that family of four will become a family of five. No, we're not getting another dog (lord help us)—we're having a **BABY!**"[2]

Malone used her blog as a sort of pregnancy journal to share her real-time experiences with her readers and also to document her pregnancy for posterity. She modeled her blog posts on one of the many websites that send developmental updates. In her "Week 9" blog post, for example, she published a photo of herself holding up a grape to represent her baby. As

she explained, "I am a total sucker for the 'your baby is as big as a ____'
emails that I get every week. What can I say? I like progress, and I love food
analogies." Another photo showed Malone in profile. "As you can see, there
is no baby bump at all yet, and I don't imagine there will be one for a long
time. But it's still fun to take progress pictures, right?" Malone followed
the lead of bloggers inspired by the pictures in pregnancy advice books to
create a personalized series of "baby bump" photos, starting from the beginning of the pregnancy, meant to culminate in a pictorial time-lapse illustration of the entire pregnancy.[3]

Like many Americans today, Malone monitored, documented, and cared
for her pregnancy in its early weeks in a way that would have been un-
imaginable only a few generations earlier. Before she conceived, she had
been recording her menstrual cycles to try and facilitate conception, and
she took a pregnancy test within a day or two of her missed period (about
two weeks after conception). As soon as she got the positive result, she
read obsessively about pregnancy on the Internet. She called her doctor's
office immediately to make a prenatal appointment and was dismayed to
learn she would have to wait until eight weeks' gestation (four weeks after
her missed period) to see her practitioner.[4]

Malone shared her pregnancy announcement on her blog shortly before her first prenatal appointment, during which her obstetrician would
take a sonogram to confirm the pregnancy. She awaited the exam with
excitement, anticipating that "while the idea of being pregnant already
feels very real, I know that seeing and hearing this little miracle in person
will take it to a whole new level."[5] She and her husband indeed found it
thrilling. She wrote afterwards, "it was so incredible—I'll never forget
it!. . . We have both been smiling all day!"[6] Two months into pregnancy, at
a stage when women in the not-so-distant past would have been just beginning to trust their suspicions and intuitions that they might be pregnant, and waiting cautiously for the confirmation provided by a second
missed menstrual period, women in America today have often already
spent weeks celebrating, caring for, and growing attached to their expected children.

This twenty-first-century experience of the early months of pregnancy
differs dramatically from the pregnancy experiences taken for granted
by women of earlier generations. This book explores the momentous social, medical, and technological transformations that have reconfigured
the experience of pregnancy. There is much to celebrate in these historical transformations: women today have safer, healthier pregnancies and
babies and more control over their fertility than ever before. The pleasures
of parenthood begin earlier and with more intensity.

There is a dark side to this reconfiguration of the pregnancy experience, however. Many pregnancies miscarry, mostly in the early months. Emily Malone had two smooth pregnancies and births, resulting in two sweet little boys. Her next two pregnancies, equally anticipated and equally cared for, did not have the same happy result. Malone's third pregnancy began to miscarry at six weeks. She endured two weeks of constant doctor appointments, with multiple rounds of blood work to confirm the pregnancy was really ending, and when the miscarriage did not complete promptly on its own, she was prescribed the drug Misoprostol to self-administer at home. In the end she needed a dilation and curettage surgery (D&C) to clear her uterus. She managed all of it through a haze of sadness, while trying to more or less carry on at home with her two young children.[7]

A fourth pregnancy, confirmed with a home pregnancy test before she even missed her period, once again began to miscarry at six weeks. Despite some bleeding, an initial ultrasound seemed to bear good tidings. "I didn't have to wait for the ultrasound tech to tell me, I saw it the minute she turned on the screen. A tiny, beating heart. A little flicker. A sign of hope. I was completely and totally shocked. I met with the midwives afterward who had no explanation for the spotting, but told me, 'Congratulations mom, you're having another baby!'" They sent her home with reassurances and the ultrasound printout. But the midwives were too hasty with their benediction. Four days later, Malone began to miscarry in earnest. "I went back to the doctor, did more blood work and more ultrasounds, and what I saw this time was as heartbreaking as it comes—a tiny little heart, still struggling to beat along, but a little bit slower this time. There was nothing medically we could do, as I technically still had a living baby inside of me, although we all knew it was only a matter of time. I was sent home to watch and wait." A few days later, Malone returned for more testing, and ultimately another D&C.[8]

The same social practices and medical care that made Malone's first pregnancies so special in their early months—the anticipation of carefully planned conceptions, the early confirmation of conception with home pregnancy tests, the careful monitoring, the ultrasounds—made Malone's miscarriages especially painful. Malone took months to grieve before telling many of her family and friends about her losses:

> I knew how painful it was for me, and I didn't want to share that feeling with anyone. I prided myself on being strong and capable, and I couldn't handle what I knew would feel like pity. I think it was my last desperate attempt to maintain some sense of control over a situation that was so far beyond anything I could comprehend.

She made it clear that her delay did not stem from a reluctance to acknowledge what had happened. "It took me a long time to talk about it, but it's not something I'm ashamed of or hiding from." To Malone, not "hiding" meant acknowledging that she had lost two children. "The two babies we lost are as much a part of me as the two that I wrestle into rain boots each morning."[9]

In earlier generations, it was exceptional for a woman to consider a pregnancy loss at six weeks to be a lost child, rather than a lost opportunity or possibility, or a fleeting hope of pregnancy reversed by a late period.[10] Early miscarriages were not generally regarded as grave losses unless they were part of a pattern of infertility, signaling that a woman might not ever be able to have children. If a woman had reason to believe that she would soon have a successful pregnancy, an early miscarriage was regarded as little more than a temporary setback. Some women today continue to feel this way about early miscarriages, but they are far more likely to be censured than validated if they say so aloud.

As much as she yearned for another child, Malone found her losses traumatic enough that she was not sure she would try for another pregnancy. In the comments on Malone's blog post about her miscarriages, a reader named Katie offered empathy and the possibility of another ending yet to come:

> After two healthy babies, I also lost two babies. One with a confirmed heartbeat, the other too fleeting. Not knowing if I could take another loss, we tried again. I'm now typing this with our hard-won third sleeping in my arms. As deeply grateful as I am to mother my three healthy children, part of my heart will always miss those two lost. Thank you for sharing your story, so beautifully written and such a tribute to the village of womanhood.[11]

Malone and her readers described a peculiarly modern, and acutely emotionally painful, experience of early pregnancy loss.

THE COMMONNESS OF MISCARRIAGE

As much as a miscarriage can feel like a disastrous ending to a pregnancy, it is far from unusual. When a fertilized egg implants in a woman's uterus, about a week after conception, the resulting pregnancy is not remotely a sure thing: about 30 percent of implanted (and therefore detectable) pregnancies are lost, mostly in the early weeks. The chance of miscarrying goes down substantially with each passing week (see Figure I.1).[12] It

Chance of Miscarrying by Week of Pregnancy

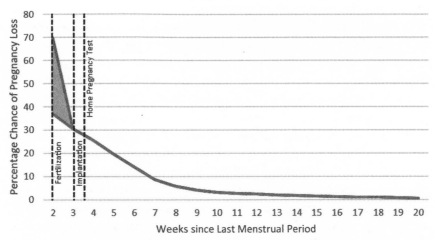

Figure I.1 The chance of miscarrying is high during early pregnancy and drops dramatically by week ten of gestation. Data from Sarah Tyler, "Datayze," https://datayze.com/miscarriage-chart.php?mode=graph; Gavin Jarvis, "Estimating Limits for Natural Human Embryo Mortality," *F1000Research* 5, no. 2083 (2016).

is commonly estimated that approximately 20 percent of confirmed pregnancies miscarry, reflecting an assumption that women typically take home pregnancy tests when their periods are a week or two late.

Many conceptions are lost before implantation as well. These losses cannot be measured directly. Laboratory and over-the-counter tests detect pregnancy by measuring human chorionic gonadotrophin (hCG), a pregnancy-supporting hormone secreted by the fertilized egg once it implants in the uterine lining, about a week or so after fertilization. In the days between fertilization and implantation, a pregnancy will not produce symptoms, and a loss at this early stage will not delay the following menstrual period. Scientists' estimates of the rate of pregnancy loss before implantation, based on the triangulation of data from studies of fertility and of *in vitro* fertilization procedures, range from a low of 10 percent to a high of 90 percent. Mainstream scientific consensus has been that probably about half of fertilized eggs do not implant.[13] If we assume about half of conceptions do not implant, the total loss of conceptions and early implanted pregnancies adds up to about 70 percent.

Miscarriages often take days or weeks to become evident. Early pregnancy losses often show up as "missed" miscarriages: it can take a few weeks for the body's hormonal signals to register the demise of an embryo and stop sustaining the gestational sac. Because a woman's body often reabsorbs an embryo at such an early stage, the pregnancy may appear on an ultrasound as an empty embryonic sac.

In pregnancies with multiple gestations, around 40 percent of the time one of the embryos miscarries while the other is carried to term. In the days before ultrasound, this type of miscarriage appeared to be very rare, but we now know that they are a common first-trimester occurrence. Outside of ultrasound evidence, these miscarriages are nearly undetectable, since they generally result in a healthy singleton birth.[14]

The majority of miscarriages are caused by chromosomal abnormalities that render the embryo incompatible with life. They are largely random and unpredictable. A woman who has had a miscarriage or two has no greater chance of miscarrying her next pregnancy than a woman who has never miscarried. Only about 1 percent of women have recurrent pregnancy losses (three miscarriages in a row), and of those, three-quarters eventually have healthy babies.[15] Around a third of women who have had two children have also had a miscarriage. Physicians understand early pregnancy losses to be a natural and normal part of healthy women's childbearing.

The rate of miscarriage does go up significantly for women in their late thirties; their eggs begin to lose chromosomal integrity. It can still be possible for a woman to have a healthy pregnancy in her early forties, but fertility gradually wanes over several years, first via more frequent early pregnancy losses and later as the hormonal triggers for ovulation cease to operate. Infertility due to the natural process of aging shows up first as unviable pregnancies and only later as lack of ovulation.[16]

All in all, early pregnancy losses are part and parcel of childbearing. However we think about pregnancy, we need to take miscarriage into account.

THE HISTORY

This book describes how a diverse array of social, medical, and technological innovations came together to reshape pregnancy and thereby create a new experience of miscarriage. The medicine and technology that most visibly structure modern pregnancy experiences are innovations of the twentieth century: ultrasound, pregnancy tests, hormonal birth control, modern prenatal care. But this book begins much earlier, because major cultural shifts in attitudes and practices relating to fertility and parenting started in the late eighteenth century, long before the advent of modern medical technology. Those fundamental shifts provided the impetus for modern pregnancy care and continue to underpin the stream of scientific and technical innovations that shape modern pregnancy.

To capture what childbearing was like before it became modern, chapter 1 describes how colonial American women experienced pregnancy in an era when life was always uncertain, the faithful were expected to trust God and submit to fate, and women were celebrated and respected for the bounty of their wombs. Childbearing could be exhausting and difficult, but children came when they came, and the process was largely regarded as inevitable and simply part of the natural and religious order of things. Early and abrupt endings, too, were part of the God-given order. Pregnancies came frequently and were regarded as tenuous until late in gestation. In an era when families frequently lost infants and children to infectious disease, early pregnancy losses received little attention.

The revolutionary years brought with them not just a visionary new form of government but also the radical new sensibility that individuals might reasonably strive to have control over their fate. Women began to imagine smaller families and to make explicit plans to limit the size of their families. This shift in intention came long before any meaningful innovations in contraceptive technology or knowledge. During the nineteenth century, couples used crude means—withdrawal, douching, abortion, and abstinence—to carry out their newfound intentions to become the masters of their reproductive destiny. In the twentieth century, modern birth control made fine-grained control of fertility more practical, and couples' expectations and intentions ramped up accordingly. Chapter 2 describes how this new intention to control fertility, realized with ever-greater precision using sophisticated new modes of contraception, eventually resulted in an unrealistic expectation of near-perfect control of conception and pregnancy outcomes.

At the same time that Americans began to envision controlling their reproductive destiny, they began to rethink their role as parents. Chapter 3 describes how over the course of the nineteenth century and into the twentieth, parents gradually focused less on the patriarchal, religious, and economic duties and benefits of parenthood and more on developing loving relationships with children. Like the shift in ideas about control of reproduction, this change in sentiment took place before modern medicine and public health would seem to justify it. Infants continued to perish at appalling rates even as parents came to mourn their losses with more evident anguish and less fatalistic resignation. Public health and medicine finally caught up during the twentieth century, as infant mortality rates decreased substantially. Over the generations, traditional economic and religious justifications for parenting diminished, and parents focused increasingly on their emotional relationship with their children. In the late twentieth and twenty-first century, the emotional focus of parenting continued to intensify. It also expanded into the months before birth, where it would clash with the biological reality of frequent early pregnancy loss.

These long-term and large-scale changes in sentiment and intention— the cultural consensus that fertility should be subject to individual control and planning, and that parenting should be primarily a matter of affection and attachment—gave force and shape to medical, technological, and social innovations in pregnancy care during the twentieth century. Chapter 4 describes the rise of prenatal care, and the ways in which obstetric care and educational materials advocating self-care during pregnancy made women newly self-conscious about their pregnancies and encouraged them to feel responsible for their pregnancy outcomes. Chapter 5 addresses the ways in which marketers encouraged pregnant women to take pleasure in the responsibilities of making purchases for the baby earlier and earlier in gestation, in the context of a blossoming consumer culture. Chapter 6 looks at the ways in which the abortion debates beginning in the 1960s fostered a rhetoric of "choice" and "life" that did not make room for the reality of the frequent miscarriage of wanted pregnancies.

In the late twentieth and early twenty-first centuries, new rituals emerged around the novel technologies of obstetric ultrasound and home pregnancy tests—rituals informed by the shifts in sentiment around fertility control and parenting solidified over the previous two centuries. These rituals diffused quickly through the culture and were cemented and elaborated in the twenty-first century as they were shared on social media and via pregnancy websites and smartphone apps. Chapter 7 documents the emergence of an ultrasound ritual involving "seeing the baby," and the extension of that ritual from a mid-pregnancy ultrasound to a much earlier exam at eight weeks, a point at which a pregnancy may not, in fact, have been successfully established. Chapter 8 looks at the ways in which home pregnancy testing has made the very earliest weeks of pregnancy feel more certain, and the baby more "real," than rates of early pregnancy loss might justify. In both cases, technological rituals further fed the expectation that careful planning and loving care ought to produce perfect pregnancies, an expectation belied by the miscarriages that were often confirmed in heartbreaking ways by these same technologies.

This book draws on extensive research, traditional and online, as well as a wide-ranging reading of historical and social science scholarship, to interpret contemporary childbearing culture, and the hopes, fears, and efforts that led us to it. At a time when much of the American cultural conversation about pregnancy is taking shape on line, pregnancy websites and apps and their associated discussion forums provide key insights into pregnancy experiences.[17] This book breaks new ground in the history of reproduction by weaving together contemporary voices from on line sources with historical voices from paper archives of women's letters and diaries, old pregnancy manuals and medical textbooks, unpublished market research and consulting reports, radio transcripts, television commercials, court testimony, women's magazine articles and advertisements, plaster models of embryos, and more. It also incorporates and extends insights from rich historical scholarship about pregnancy, childbirth, and the family.[18] It takes a contemporary dilemma—how did early pregnancy loss become an experience that many women find devastating?—and investigates the interwoven strands of history that help explain this present-day phenomenon.

As the contemporary stories in this book show, dominant norms surrounding childbearing cut across race, ethnicity, age, sexual orientation, and region of the country. They encompass a broadly construed middle class and those who aspire to it, and they set the standards against which even those with the fewest resources are judged.[19] Because middle-class women pioneered the innovations in birth control, parenting, prenatal care, and consumerism that shaped modern pregnancy, the history described in this book focuses on the American middle class. Today, affluent women like Emily Malone continue to have the resources to pursue these pregnancy and parenting ideals most fully, while a much broader swath of women participates in whatever ways they can.

The intentions and expectations that shape today's miscarriage experiences infuse the entirety of modern childbearing and parenting, far beyond the early weeks of pregnancy. The book's insights apply not just to pregnancies that happen to miscarry; nor are they limited to early pregnancy. Accordingly, this book illuminates the history of modern childbearing more broadly. It focuses on miscarriage, but the historical forces it describes have similarly reshaped a whole spectrum of childbearing and parenting experiences, from infertility treatment, to cesarean section, to helicopter parenting. A wide range of contemporary childbearing experiences are animated by the modern expectation of control and an emphasis on loving attachment, amplified and reinforced by modern technological and medical innovations. As with early pregnancy, childbearing and parenting have undoubtedly benefited from modern striving for perfect outcomes. But the striving has come at a cost, as inevitable imperfections spawn anxiety, guilt, and sadness. This book shows how we came to expect we might achieve childbearing and parenting perfection, if we only plan carefully enough, try hard enough, and love ardently enough. Understanding this history is a first step toward shaping a more realistic, forgiving, and ultimately more satisfying culture of childbearing for future parents and their children.

CHAPTER 1

꙳

Childbearing in Colonial America

"Sept. 14. My Daughter Mary born." Mary Vial Holyoke, the wife of prominent Salem physician Edward Holyoke, recorded the birth of her first child in 1760. Over the following twenty-two years, she recorded eleven more of her own births in her diary, as well as scores of children born to her relatives, friends, and neighbors. Many of the entries were similarly laconic one-liners. Sometimes she included a little more detail. A week after she was "Brought to bed of Peggy" in 1763, she wrote that she "[ate] meat for the first time," marking her convalescence. A week after that, she spent several days receiving a steady stream of female visitors who came to congratulate her on the birth. A well-to-do woman, she could afford to spend a month resting and recovering. She marked the end of her lying-in on "April 6. I rode out [with] Molly Appleton, my first getting out."[1]

Holyoke sometimes added more detail when something out of the ordinary happened, whether at her own birth or those of her family and neighbors. A few days before her eighth birth in 1771, she recorded that she was "Very poorly," a term she used interchangeably for illness and for labor pains, and that she "Put up bed." Despite her protracted illness the birth itself appears to have come upon her unexpectedly. "Very ill. Brought to Bed quite alone 11 A.M. of a Daughter." It must have been frightening to give birth without a birth attendant or her female friends around her. She added thankfully, "Child very well."[2]

It is easier to perceive the worry and relief in these terse entries with some knowledge of Holyoke's previous births, which did not always end well. In 1766, a month after her fourth birth, her newborn was "taken with a sort of fit, lay very bad for 8 or 9 hours." For six weeks the baby continued to have bouts of illness, until Holyoke sadly recorded, "My Dear Child Buried." Her next birth was the only one she covertly signaled ahead of time in her diary, noting that on August 23, 1767, she "First staid [sic] from Meeting," skipping church because she knew the birth was imminent. Perhaps it was already a problematic pregnancy. Normally the first Holyoke mentioned of her condition in her diary was when she reported being "taken very poorly" or "taken very ill," meaning that she had gone into labor. The baby was born on September 5 and baptized the very next day, unlike her previous babies, who were typically baptized about a week after the birth. The newborn was, indeed, frail. On September 7, "The Baby very well till ten o'Clock in the evening & then taken with fits." On September 8, "The Baby remained very ill all day." On the ninth, "It Died about 8 o'clock in the morning." On the tenth, "Was buried." Her diary entries, even briefer than usual and devoid of overt emotional expression, suggest she was trying to keep some emotional distance from an infant she knew might not live.[3]

In the end, Holyoke had four more babies who died shortly after birth, interspersed with several more that lived. Of her twelve children, six died shortly after birth, and three more died young. Only three outlived her. While Holyoke suffered significantly more losses than average for her time, there were few colonial American women who did not share the experience of losing babies to stillbirth, neonatal frailty, or childhood illness. Holyoke's diary reveals at least a small sense of the experience of the continuous cycle of pregnancies and the uncertainty of their outcomes in this era.

The early stages of conception and pregnancy, though, are much harder to locate in colonial American women's records of their experiences. Holyoke almost certainly suffered some miscarriages, but she never mentioned them. Nor did she record her missed menstrual periods, or her experience of "quickening," feeling the baby move in the womb in mid-pregnancy. Colonial Americans rarely wrote about anything having to do with sex, were circumspect about their pregnancies, and made brief records of births, obscuring attempts to understand how they experienced childbearing more broadly.[4] In addition to analyzing letters and diaries like Holyoke's, women's historians have cleverly extracted shards of evidence from religious sermons, medical advice books, court testimony, probate inventories, and material objects (e.g., cradles, clothing, and houses) to build a compelling picture of women's daily intimate lives in early America.[5] The experience of early pregnancy in colonial America was embedded in a broader culture of childbearing radically different from our own, one that drew on medical beliefs and practices that were widely shared across Europe and the New World.

A LIFE FILLED WITH CHILDBEARING

Colonial American women's lives, like those of their contemporaries in much of the early modern world, revolved around childbearing. Like Mary Vail Holyoke, most women spent the bulk of their fertile years pregnant or breastfeeding.[6] Women typically maintained approximately two-year spacing between the births of their children, likely through extended breastfeeding, which can suppress ovulation. Sexual traditions may also have contributed; it was believed that intercourse affected mothers' milk for the worse, and that breastfeeding was not appropriate during pregnancy, as the process of pregnancy tainted the milk and the demands of breastfeeding weakened the pregnant woman. Many couples may have abstained, or at least severely limited their sexual activities, while the wife was lactating.[7] This helped women space their pregnancies enough to avoid complete exhaustion, but it meant that particularly fertile women could have twelve or more children.[8]

Colonial American households were bustling places, full of children and of work. As historian Laurel Thatcher Ulrich has shown, early modern mothering was extensive rather than intensive. Mothers were praised for their fruitfulness in bearing many children more than for the magnitude of care they took in raising each one. And the reality of early modern households, particularly in the American colonies, was that there were many children to be looked after, on top of backbreaking household work.[9] Free women cared for their husbands' households; enslaved women faced the burden of working for their enslavers in addition to caring for their own children.[10]

Traditions for caring for babies and children gave mothers practical ways to take care of young ones while they worked. A newborn typically spent her first three months in the world swaddled from head to toe, carefully wrapped and pinned so that, it was believed, her limbs would grow straight, the soft spot on her skull would close, and she would develop into the shape of a well-formed child. Early modern parents had little faith in natural development and assumed that unswaddled children risked developing rickets and other deformities. Swaddling was also convenient. A mother could carry her baby around and lay her near whatever work she was doing at the moment. She could also leave the baby in the care of an older child, trusting the swaddling to protect a newborn from her own floppy frailty.[11] Older babies, both girls and boys, wore long petticoats and supportive corsets. Mothers sometimes put an older baby in a standing stool, resembling a modern-day walker but without sitting support. As a baby became more capable, she might be put in a go-cart, a standing stool with wheels that allowed her to scoot around the room, at least when someone could keep her from rolling her way into the kitchen hearth.[12]

Early modern parents did all they could to discourage their children from crawling, putting them in bulky skirts and propping them in a standing position whenever possible. Besides the dangers of open fires and rough, dirty floors, parents feared the animalistic appearance of crawling. As with swaddling, parents believed they needed to teach their children to stand and walk like humans. Otherwise they risked having children who permanently moved on all fours like animals. Babies were not regarded as fully realized humans at birth, but needed first physical, and later spiritual, guidance and nurture to become fully human.[13]

THE REWARDS AND DANGERS OF CHILDBEARING

In early modern societies, families and communities gave married women appreciation, respect, and authority when they had babies. Pregnant women were "lusty," in a "thriving way," "flourishing" and "fruitful."[14] Grateful families wrote gravestone epitaphs that celebrated prolific women's childbearing feats.[15]

In giving birth, a woman not only became a mother but was welcomed into the informal but influential community of matrons. When she went into labor, her married women friends and neighbors took care of her. They turned the parlor, with its master bed, into a lying-in chamber. They closed curtains and blocked keyholes, warmed the room with a larger fire in the hearth, and sometimes made the bed with special childbed linen handed down from mother to daughter. They brewed a special drink for the laboring woman, offered moral support, and traded stories about neighbors and friends, a tradition that gave a new meaning to "god-sibs," or godparents, and turned them into "gossips." The men were left to work, wait, and pray in the hall. The women's community consolidated in birth rooms gave mothers support and social structure.[16]

Free women with children took on important public and community roles. They attended other women in childbirth, creating a women's community that operated with substantial, if informal, authority in broader society. Judges appointed them to serve on committees to inspect female criminals or victims in cases that involved intimate knowledge of women's bodies, such as suspected rape or infanticide. A married woman with children was a full adult member of her community and was treated with respect as a source of authority on matters relating to reproduction.[17]

Children were a source of material and spiritual wealth as well, and for free women, they were a source of security in old age. Children could begin to work in the household and on the farm as soon as they were old enough to walk and follow directions. In enslaved families, children assisted their parents in ways that helped the family survive.[18] Free adult children were expected to help support elderly parents and were a crucial source of support for widows. Women and other dependents were expected to reside in a "family" under the supervision of a male head of household. Widows risked ending up in an almshouse or living under the grudging protection of a charitable neighbor if they did not have sons or sons-in-law to take them in.[19] Barrenness was dreaded and feared, and barren women were ridiculed and blamed for their condition.[20] An enslaved woman who found herself childless faced the possibility of having her marriage broken up by her enslaver.[21] Infertile women, white or black, were seen as unnatural and deficient and were usually blamed for the couple's infertility. A woman's sense of self-worth and purpose came centrally from her childbearing role.

At the same time, childbearing was exhausting and sometimes dangerous. Women thought of pregnancy as a sickly time and worried about the pregnancy's health if they did not feel sick.[22] Childbirth was viewed with apprehension. Approximately one in thirty women could expect to die in childbirth or as a result of postpartum complications. And others suffered injury from the birth process, living with serious discomfort from uteruses that would not stay in place or pelvic floor damage that left them incontinent.[23] As Mary Vail Holyoke experienced, frail babies often did not survive their early weeks. Stillbirths were more common than they are today, because midwives and physicians had few safe options for intervening effectively in dangerously prolonged births.

Women who were literate sometimes expressed their fears in their letters to their mothers and sisters. Ministers urged women to accept God's will and asked them to accept the risks of childbirth as a test of faith. Cotton Mather believed that women became full members of the church more often than men because childbirth inspired the kind of fear and vulnerability that opened one's heart to Christ.[24] In 1688 Martha Coit, a wife and mother from a prominent New London, Connecticut family, wrote a long and harrowing account of her sixth through tenth births, several of which ended in stillbirth. She recorded her story "for memory unto my own Speritual Comfort and for edefiecation and incoragement of my offspring to trust in the lord att all times: of gods gracious dealings with me in the times of sharp travil in Childe bareing."[25] Childbearing gave women's lives meaning, purpose, satisfaction, and respect, while simultaneously bringing life's biggest challenges.

TAKING PREGNANCY IN STRIDE

While colonial American women were often apprehensive about births, pregnancies were generally subsumed into the rhythms and needs of the household. Even elite women mostly treated pregnancy like a part of regular life. After all, a woman could expect to be pregnant or breastfeeding for the majority of her days until menopause. Pregnancy was understood as an inevitable and substantial part of being a married woman. Most women, apart from the very rich, continued to run their households; they cooked, cleaned, spun, tended a garden, milked cows, and preserved food. In mid-pregnancy, a woman might take the opportunity to travel by horse and by wagon to visit friends and relatives, since it was impractical with a nursing infant and the time between weaning one child and conceiving the next was often only a few months. She let out her regular skirts to accommodate a pregnant belly and continued more or less as usual.[26]

Women did, however, expect extra solicitude from their husbands. A good husband did his best to accommodate his wife's pregnancy cravings, since it was believed that her longing could mark the child if it was not satisfied. If an expectant mother was refused some enticing strawberries, for example, she might think of them with such longing that her child would be born with birthmarks the shape and color of strawberries. In the last months, a respectful husband made sure she did not need to lift anything too heavy or too high, since it was commonly believed that a woman who lifted her arms above her head risked wrapping the umbilical cord around the baby's neck, a recognized cause of stillbirth. What has come down to us as "old wives' tales" made sense in a context of daily, intense manual labor. Colonial women did plenty of hard physical work during their pregnancies in the course of normal housekeeping, but they were generally given special respect and protection from the most backbreaking physical tasks.[27]

Women who could not set aside even the heaviest work suffered the consequences during pregnancy, and colonial Americans drew a line between the acceptable substantial daily labor of a married "goodwife" and the overwork of women who survived without a husband's support. In one colonial court case, neighbors of Margaret Prince, who had a difficult delivery and a stillborn baby, blamed Margaret's troubles on the work she had done a few weeks earlier repairing her house in the absence of her irresponsible husband. Margaret had carried several loads of heavy clay in a bucket on her head to serve as daubing and repaired her house herself. When work was truly too strenuous, it was deemed inappropriate for pregnant women.[28] Slaveholders recognized that the heavy fieldwork they demanded from slaves caused miscarriages, stillbirths, and postpartum injury, and they grudgingly allocated somewhat lighter work to enslaved women in their last months of pregnancy and for a few weeks after birth. And yet because they wanted to believe that African women could work throughout pregnancy without injury, they often ignored pregnant women's suffering, prioritizing the short-term gain of a pregnant woman's long hours in the field over her and her children's long-term health and survival.[29]

At the other end of the economic spectrum, the high-society London physicians who wrote the bulk of the medical advice books imported into the colonies observed that their elite English patients sometimes tried to protect their pregnancies by remaining as sedentary as possible during early pregnancy to ward off the possibility of miscarriage. These physicians mostly dismissed their elite patients' precautions, idealizing a romanticized rural lifestyle. Physician-authors could see that rural, working women did not pamper themselves, and they were under the misimpression that those women seldom miscarried. They believed that rural women who worked outdoors, went to bed early, and ate a simple diet had many fewer miscarriages and other pregnancy mishaps than did coddled, sedentary wealthy women. Advice book writers blamed miscarriages on tightly laced corsets, late nights spent dancing, high heels, and rich foods, in addition to the traditional culprits of working to exhaustion or suffering chance frights. The lives of women like Mary Vial Holyoke and her neighbors were more like what these physicians pictured as an ideal.[30]

To the degree that medical writers advised their upper-class readers to take action to protect their pregnancies, they took popular explanations for losses and turned them into recommendations that pregnant women avoid all sources of possible disruption. Their advice, to keep a moderate, calm, and regular lifestyle, was of a piece with their medical advice in general. Whether a woman was pregnant, menstruating, or suffering from a chronic condition such as consumption (tuberculosis), she was advised to avoid strong "passions," stay cheerful, eat, sleep, and exercise in moderate and sensible ways and do what she could to coax her body into balanced regularity. Whenever the body was out of equilibrium or seemed vulnerable to becoming imbalanced, physicians gave similar advice: determine if the problem was that the body was too stimulated, in which case it needed calming foods and environment, or if it was that the body was weak, in which case it needed stimulating and supportive food and activities.[31]

In the colonies, even elite women's diaries do not show evidence of any extraordinary precautions taken to protect pregnancies, though Holyoke and others did record an extended period of rest after births. Physicians seemed to largely assume that this approach was for the best, ignoring the discrepancy between their romantic vision of rural life and the reality of its physical challenges that might cause miscarriages and birth problems.

THE AMBIGUITY OF PREGNANCY

After a colonial American woman married, she could expect pregnancy quickly and often. Mary Vial Holyoke had her first child ten months after her wedding.[32] Still, expecting to become pregnant and actually knowing that one was pregnant were not the same thing.

Obstetrics texts and popular reference manuals of the time printed long lists of pregnancy signs, which likely reflected common lore. For example, a little book called *Aristotle's Masterpiece* (not in fact authored by Aristotle, and more a haphazard compendium than a "masterpiece") taught readers all about sex, ways to enhance fertility, and how babies were born. A key source of information for virtuous housekeepers and curious schoolboys alike, it was reprinted hundreds of times between the late seventeenth century and the early twentieth century. The anonymous author spent three paragraphs describing the signs and symptoms of conception in detail. The book told readers to look for swollen veins under the woman's eyes and in her breasts; discolored eyes and face; reddened nipples; a flat belly; swollen, hard and sore breasts; "loss of appetite to victuals, sour belchings, and exceeding weakness of the stomach"; painful bowel movements; "wringing or griping pains, like the cramp. . . in the belly above the navel," unusual food cravings, and "a coldness and chillness of the outward parts after copulation, the heat being retired to make the conception." It also detailed two urine tests that were supposed to detect pregnancy, one by seeing whether the woman's urine grew small living creatures when it was kept in a bottle for three days, and the other by testing its effect on a green nettle.[33]

More sophisticated texts elaborated even further. One obstetric treatise added that at conception the pregnant woman would have felt a little shiver at intercourse, and the tight closure of the cervix afterward, as the woman's womb held tight to the man's seed.[34] Famed midwife Louise Bourgeois, attendant to Henri IV's wife Marie de Medici, also mentioned emotional changes in her widely distributed writings on midwifery: "They [pregnant women] feel more angry and easy to annoy than usual."[35] While most colonial women did not read obstetric treatises, the same cultural tradition produced the texts and the word-of-mouth advice women would have received from female friends and relatives. A woman with a reasonably supportive social network or access to a book like *Aristotle's Masterpiece* would have been aware of a host of possible signs of pregnancy.

Still, pregnancy could be difficult to discern and to distinguish from minor illness. First pregnancies were especially tricky. Seventeenth-century English midwife Jane Sharp wrote that "not one in twenty" women detected and recorded their first pregnancies accurately.[36] Perhaps many women did not have friends and relatives who freely gave advice on such an intimate matter. But it also appears that it took some personal experience with pregnancy to be able to accurately distinguish pregnancy from illness, or even from a normal state of health.[37]

Women gained confidence diagnosing their pregnancies as they weathered more pregnancies and learned how pregnancy signs manifested in their own bodies. They might take note of personal, idiosyncratic signs of pregnancy. For example, a German doctor who wrote up a number of his cases in the 1730s described a patient who always knew she was pregnant because she had a characteristic cough. Her neighbors even recognized it and spontaneously congratulated her on her condition when they heard her coughing.[38]

Women were more sophisticated and nuanced in their interpretations of a wide range of bodily signs and symptoms of pregnancy than most women are today. But without reliable pregnancy testing, early pregnancy could look a lot like minor or chronic illness. Only prior experience gave a woman the background she needed to have a good idea of when she was or was not pregnant.

A missed period was an obvious first sign of pregnancy but by no means a sure indicator. Women missed periods occasionally when they were working especially hard, had a moment of excitement or upheaval in their lives, or were ill. A newly married woman who had only recently left her childhood home to set up housekeeping with her new husband could easily miss a period from stress and strain.

While women waited and watched to see if a missed period was due to pregnancy, they sometimes worried. During early pregnancy, women could be apprehensive that their amenorrhea might be related to illness. Early modern women and their physicians interpreted bodily changes and treated illness within a humoral medical system, derived from ancient Greek medicine. They regarded the body as a system of flows, whose obstruction or diversion caused illness. Women's menstrual periods were regarded as an important component of healthy bodily flow, and a late period signaled some kind of obstruction. If it turned out to be a pregnancy, it was a healthy type of obstruction, but it could just as easily be a dangerous, illness-causing stoppage. If a woman were unmarried, she might take an emmenagogue, an herbal preparation expected to bring on the menses, to ensure that old blood did not gather in her body and make her sick. All a married woman could do was wait and see.[39]

Because of this uncertainty, women did not make public announcements of their pregnancies at least until "quickening," when they began to feel movement, around four months, though they might share their suspicions with close family members. One such private conversation was recorded by Samuel Pepys, a seventeenth-century English gentleman diarist. Pepys and his wife longed for a child for many years to no avail, so they likely discussed her menstrual cycles more than most couples. In one 1660 entry Pepys recorded that "My wife after the absence of her terms for seven weeks gave me hopes of her being with child."[40] Mostly, women waited for their pregnancies to announce themselves, with skirts taken out to accommodate a belly full with child.

It was not only newly married women who faced uncertainty in early pregnancy; even women who had already borne several children sometimes found it difficult to tell the difference between a pregnancy and an illness. Within the period's humoral understanding of the body, early miscarriages could easily be interpreted as healthful purgings of the body. Physicians treated acute illness such as high fever by encouraging the body to release its fluids and restore flow. They bled and vomited their patients and prescribed a variety of emetics and cathartics. Today, if a doctor saw a woman who suspected she had been pregnant, had a bout of acute illness with a prolonged high fever, and then had an extra-heavy and crampy period, he would suspect that she had miscarried, perhaps due to the illness. Early modern doctors and their patients would have seen these symptoms as an illness caused by stopped-up menstrual blood, which the body finally resolved through an extra-heavy period.[41]

A single episode of acute illness could cause confusion between illness and pregnancy even for someone who was generally healthy; various chronic health problems muddied the picture still further. Uterine and ovarian cysts and cancers could cause amenorrhea and irregular bleeding. Tuberculosis caused amenorrhea. Women missed periods because of poor nutrition as well, particularly during wintertime shortages. Food poisoning was a regular occurrence, and intestinal worms were almost seasonal in many places with warmer climates. An uneasy stomach or upset bowels was a run-of-the-mill, if highly unpleasant, health issue. Sexually transmitted diseases caused chronic leucorrhea, or "whites," in many women. In southern parts of the colonies, malaria was endemic. Seasonally, everyone infected was exhausted and suffered from periodic high fevers, headaches, muscle pain, and sometimes nausea. It could be hard to detect pregnancy signs amidst chronic illness, and early miscarriages could easily be missed or interpreted as late menstrual periods or illness-related bleeding.[42]

Physicians could be as hard pressed to differentiate between pregnancy and illness as the women who consulted them. Even later in pregnancy, women with chronic intestinal problems could be confused as to whether they were feeling kicks or gas, and their physicians were often equally stymied. In medical journals, physicians offered each other cautionary tales of women who appeared merely ill, but turned out to be pregnant instead, or pregnant in addition to being ill. It was important to differentiate because the same drugs that were meant to expel intestinal worms could expel a fetus, and extreme versions of the standard bleeding and purging treatments were not considered appropriate for pregnant women. Pregnancy could never be completely confirmed until a child was actually born or close to it, so a potentially pregnant woman had to be treated with caution.[43]

EARLY PREGNANCY FAILURE

If a woman was generally in good health, and she missed two menstrual periods and felt some other pregnancy symptoms, she might then call the heavy, crampy return of a period a "mishap": what we would call a miscarriage. Or she might call it a "miss," an "accident," a "slip," or an "abortion," all common terms for a spontaneous miscarriage.[44]

How might a colonial American woman have understood this experience? What might she feel she had lost? And what concerns might she have had? Sources for this kind of history are sparse: just a few firsthand accounts, primarily from personal letters, and some from husbands' diaries. But important clues appear in doctors' writings and patient records, legal statutes and testimony, and ecclesiastical laws and decisions.

First, she and her family might be concerned about her immediate health. Miscarriages could turn into hemorrhages, and while this was unusual at an early stage of pregnancy, such occurrences could be dangerous. Spontaneous miscarriages sometimes did not expel all of the material in the womb, which could generate serious infections. An apparently healthy woman could suddenly grow alarmingly feverish and succumb to sepsis a few weeks after a miscarriage.

Historian Linda Pollock has suggested that early modern physicians and women may have had an exaggerated sense of the dangers of early miscarriage because they did not distinguish between spontaneous and induced miscarriage (now called abortion). Miscarriages that had been induced were likely to have more dangerous symptoms because the herbal remedies that were used to induce them had profound effects on a woman's body. Because women did not publicize their abortive attempts, it was hard to know whether a patient's or a neighbor's miscarriage was particularly difficult because of drugs she had taken to induce it. Interrupted pregnancies appeared to carry immediate and frightening health risks.[45]

A woman and her family might also worry about the potential for this miscarriage to initiate a pattern of habitual miscarriage. In early modern medical theory, bodies developed habitual patterns of flow. Like regular menstruation, these flows could keep the body healthy and prevent stoppages and stagnations that led to illness. Physicians sometimes created weeping wounds and artificially kept them open to promote a healthy habit of flow. When it came to pregnancy, however, having the body habitually open up and release the contents of the womb was a disaster. Women and their physicians observed that some women seemed to have one miscarriage after another, rarely or never bringing a pregnancy to term, and they feared that having a miscarriage or two prepared the path for future miscarriages. Any particular loss early in pregnancy was not significant, but the prospect of a series of losses and few or no children was deeply worrisome.[46]

A woman who miscarried would also likely have wondered what she did to disrupt or corrupt the pregnancy. Early pregnancies were considered insecure, fragile, and unformed, and medical and popular texts almost always attributed failed pregnancies to something the pregnant woman had done. She might have eaten spicy food; had a fit of anger; had too much sex with her husband; lifted something heavy; encountered nauseating smells, or been startled, or sneezed too hard. Medical texts always suggested that the miscarriage had happened for a reason, not entirely as a matter of chance or because of an inherent flaw in the pregnancy itself.[47]

A modern reader would find these lists highly guilt inducing, because she would infer from them that she ought to have done more to avoid or prevent the cause of the miscarriage. An early modern reader might have read these lists differently, seeing in them the possibility of an explanation that lay outside some inherent weakness of her body. Or she might have found them so broad and exhaustive as to induce fatalism. In any case, they suggest curiosity and concern about the myriad reasons why one pregnancy might develop properly and another fall away.[48]

WHAT DID EARLY AMERICANS SEE IN A MISCARRIAGE?

How would a colonial American woman have thought about what she had lost? What would she have seen in the materials that emerged from her body? It is important to consider what the visual evidence would have indicated to someone looking at it without the intellectual framework of modern embryology, the confirmation of a hormonal pregnancy test, or a modern dilation and curettage operation. At an early stage of pregnancy, a miscarriage emerges as lots of blood and some bits of flesh. When a pregnancy ends abruptly, a woman may find an intact, round object the size of an olive, with the appearance of stubby limbs, amidst the blood and other tissue. However, in the majority of miscarriages, the embryo perishes weeks before it is expelled, and it is difficult or impossible to recognize anything like a formed fetus in it.

The visual appearance of a miscarriage would have been unlikely to surprise a colonial American woman and the people she might have consulted about it—her family, her trusted women friends, or her doctor. In evidence from letters and court records, medieval and early modern lay people described early pregnancy metaphorically in terms of the coagulation of milk, or the curdling of cheese.[49] Seed, or ejaculate, from the man was understood to combine with seed from the woman to create the liquid material for the initiation of pregnancy. It was understood to be nourished by the woman's menstrual blood, which therefore would not be released from her body during her pregnancy. A pregnancy that failed to coagulate properly into a fetus could easily look like mostly blood with bits of flesh.

She and her family would have been unsurprised that the process could have gone wrong. The development of seed into a child was understood to be a precarious and unpredictable process. It could easily be ruined by too much heat or cold in the womb. It could be jarred loose by jolting about in a carriage. Adding more semen through intercourse could make the womb too slippery, and the fetus could slide out. Sex during menstruation could trick the womb into trying to use menstrual blood rather than seed to produce a fetus, and it would produce a monster rather than a child. The womb might endeavor to produce a fetus in poor conditions and wind up producing a mola, or lump of undifferentiated flesh, instead. According to the medical theory of the time, a woman's womb could produce many things from seed and blood, of which a child was only one possibility.[50]

Whether a lost pregnancy was regarded as a child depended a lot on whether it looked like a child. Learned treatises in natural philosophy put the completed development of the form of the child, and its subsequent ensoulment, at between thirty and ninety days after conception.

In the seventeenth century, new embryological research was beginning to challenge this ancient wisdom dating back to Hippocrates, but old assumptions still dominated medical and popular literature. Folk wisdom equated ensoulment with quickening, or the movement of the fetus as felt by the pregnant woman, around four months of pregnancy. While these two timelines varied somewhat, neither learned nor folk theories granted the status of an ensouled human to a fetus until it had the physical form of a child.[51]

At what point did eighteenth-century women see the physical form of a child in their miscarriages? Women and their attendants examined the expelled contents and occasionally described them, in a few cases preserved in letters and court testimony. For example, in seventeenth- and eighteenth-century England, young single women who hid their deliveries and were subsequently prosecuted for infanticide sometimes testified that what had emerged from them did not have the form of a baby. While this testimony was obviously self-serving, it gives a sense of what could plausibly be understood to emerge in the place of a baby at delivery. Women explained that they had delivered "only blood," or "something like bloud of the bigness of her Hand," or "delivered of or Miscarried of . . . a hard substance" that "had not the form of a Child," or "a lump of Flesh," or "a false Conception."[52]

This perspective is confirmed in private correspondence as well. In sixteenth- century Germany, a young aristocrat with a sad history of repeated late miscarriages and stillbirths without any living children wrote to her mother to describe yet another failed pregnancy.

> [M]ost beloved mother, as I wrote to Your Grace last, I believed myself to be going pregnant. As Your Grace's child I cannot keep from you that I went like that until the nineteenth week and then I started [bleeding] and two pieces/ lumps came from me. One was rather large the other not so large, I allowed people to see them, also a midwife, they all agree that no child was with it [and] for that I thank the dear God.[53]

Physicians made the same kinds of interpretations. French physician Francois Mauriceau recorded his examination of two women patients who were disturbed at having miscarried but were then reassured when he told them they had expelled molas, or tumors, not children.[54] Letters and doctors' records show that it was not necessarily a simple or obvious judgment as to whether the products of conception had the form of a child, but the form provided the basic measure of whether a woman had actually lost a child and shaped medical and emotional reactions to the loss.[55]

Early modern women and medical practitioners may have actually been looking for the form of a fully developed newborn child in a miscarried fetus. Even a well-formed fetus was potentially regarded as a monster, or at least as questionably human. As historian Barbara Duden has pointed out, until the late eighteenth century, anatomical depictions of the unborn always showed either a picture of a little man dancing in the womb, or a naturalistic depiction of an infant ready to be born, rather than fetuses in earlier stages of development. Measured against the standard of a full-term infant, an intact fetus could look ill-formed and alien.[56] In 1799, when German anatomist Thomas Soemmerring published a series of drawings of embryos and fetuses arranged to illustrate the sequence of development, he had to argue against tradition and contemporary sensibility that they ought to be regarded as normal, even beautiful. "Seduced by old wives' tales, not only lay people who are ignorant in physiology, but also artists. . . perceive the form of the human embryo as repulsive, nay disgusting or monstrous."[57]

This is not to say that people never saw fetuses as children. Over the course of the Middle Ages, as the church increasingly emphasized infant baptism as necessary to salvation, there is evidence that parents increasingly worried about the status of miscarried and stillborn children. Archeologists investigating a church in southern France have demonstrated that between the sixth century and the eleventh century, the burial of late miscarriages and stillbirths moved from special areas far from the church to a cluster of graves against the east end of the church. Water from this most sacred part of the church, sheltering the altar, ran off the gutters onto the graves, a substitute for the baptism that could not be granted children who were not born alive. This placement of the graves must have mattered to parents, because they had to defy ecclesiastical prohibitions to bury the unbaptized within church grounds.[58]

When women had premature births and stillborn children because they were assaulted, they could, and sometimes did, prosecute for homicide. These suits seldom succeeded, but they were allowed by statute, and evidence suggests that they were taken seriously by juries.[59] The legal and religious status of fully formed, late-term fetuses could be complicated. But there is evidence that in many circumstances, by the late Middle Ages, they could potentially be regarded as children and, if they were, given legal and spiritual consideration.

One more clue helps to clarify the distinction between the fully formed, late-term fetus, which had at least the potential to be regarded as a person, from an early pregnancy, which was not seen as yet a person. In early modern France, following Roman law, pregnant women past quickening who had been condemned to death could not be executed until after the birth. Midwives were assigned to examine a woman who pleaded "benefit of the belly" and confirm whether she was actually pregnant. A woman who was "young with child" or "barely with child," meaning that she was pregnant but had not yet quickened, was not exempt from execution.

The language used can be confusing to modern readers. In early modern English, being "with child" meant being pregnant, but did not necessarily signal the presence of a baby. A woman needed to be "with quick child" to be understood to be pregnant with an actual baby and to be temporarily reprieved from execution in order to protect the life of her baby. If the examiners were uncertain, the execution might be postponed. The uncertainty was not over whether or not a woman was pregnant, but whether or not the pregnancy had proceeded past quickening, and therefore had been ensouled. A pregnancy before quickening was given no special consideration.[60]

Similar legal boundaries were drawn in other kinds of cases. Causing the termination of a pregnancy before quickening was not cause for prosecution, whereas it could be after quickening.[61] Women who procured abortions before quickening (and the practitioners who helped them) might be seen as morally questionable, but they could not be prosecuted for infanticide. When a pregnant woman was assaulted and miscarried as a result, the assailant could not be prosecuted for homicide unless she had already quickened.

It would be possible to read these latter cases as evidence not so much that early pregnancy was given a different moral status from late pregnancy, as that the aborter or assailant had to be given the benefit of the doubt. A woman who took abortifacient drugs before quickening might simply be trying to restore her menses, not realizing she was pregnant. An assailant could be prosecuted for his attack on the woman but not have realized that he was also attacking a child in the womb. The legal status of pregnant condemned criminals suggests, though, that early pregnancy was regarded differently than late pregnancy and that the same moral calculus was being used in all of these legal situations.

BRINGING DOWN THE MENSES

Married women used this same moral calculus when they occasionally used herbal remedies to "bring down the menses." Women, their families, and their doctors understood that closely spaced pregnancies were exhausting and potentially dangerous. Mary Vail Holyoke experienced the distressingly common problem that when a woman had a stillbirth or her newborn died, she began ovulating again right away and conceived while her body was still depleted from the previous pregnancy. This could trigger a string of bad outcomes in a vicious cycle.[62] Holyoke does not appear to have taken steps to prevent tightly spaced births, but a woman in her position who did would have been understood to have been acting honorably. When a woman who was already run down from illness or a recent birth believed that she might be pregnant again, she might try to do what she could to restore her menstrual cycle so that she could regain her strength before her next pregnancy. While abortion to cover the sexual sin of extramarital intercourse was seen as sinful and shameful, ending a pregnancy to preserve a woman's health was acceptable if not generally publicized. The goal was not so much to limit births as to space them in service of a woman's long-term fertility and her own and her children's survival.[63]

Like early modern treatments for many kinds of illness, herbal remedies worked to restore the menstrual cycle by making a woman so ill that it would provoke "evacuations" of all kinds. The way we would see it today, these remedies made women so ill that they lost their pregnancies. The dosage required to be certain of a result was undoubtedly dangerous. One eighteenth-century Connecticut court case described the increasingly aggressive and desperate abortive attempts of an unmarried woman and her lover, which led to the woman's eventual death.[64] Women balanced their desire to not be pregnant with the risks that increased with the dosage.[65] Since many pregnancies miscarry even without intervention, and a woman could mistake a simple missed period for a pregnancy, it could be that women gave these drugs more credit than they deserved, at least when used at lower dosages. Still, they were clearly effective at least in high dosages, and they were a well-documented part of a widely shared and long-standing materia medica.

The knowledge necessary to produce a miscarriage was a reasonably accessible and important part of legitimate medicine. There were circumstances in which evacuating the uterus could save a woman's life. Sometimes a fetus died but was not expelled, and the woman's womb became infected. Sometimes miscarriages were incomplete, and the womb needed to be stimulated to expel the remainder to prevent hemorrhage and infection. And sometimes, a woman had seizures that were recognized to be inevitably fatal if labor was not immediately induced.[66] The life and health of the mother, and her future fertility, were prioritized over the preservation of any given pregnancy.

LOSING A CHILD VERSUS LOSING A PREGNANCY

The reality of early modern life was that parents lost some of their children to the infectious illnesses that regularly swept through communities; children were also lost to accidents and to birth anomalies they had no way to treat.[67] Elizabeth Drinker, a prominent Philadelphia Quaker who was a contemporary of Mary Vial Holyoke's, wrote movingly of the death of her youngest child in 1784. This son, who she referred to a couple of weeks before his death as "our dear little Baby," passed away suddenly and unexpectedly.

> [O]ur dear little one after dilegint nursing had out grown most of his weekness and promised fiar to be a fine Boy, became much oppress'd with phlegm, insomuch that Docr. Redmans opinion was that unless we could promote some evacuation he could not live, he ordred what he thought might prove a gentle vomit, agitated him much, but did not work, and in little more than 20 minits from the time he took it, he expired aged 2 years 7 months and one day—about a week before he was fat, fresh and hearty—he cut a tooth a day before he dyed—thus was I suddenly depried of my dear little Companion over whome, I had almost constantly watchd, from the time of his birth, and his late thriving state seem'd to promise a [reward] to all my pains—he dy'd the 17 march, fourth day.[68]

Children were especially susceptible to infectious diseases that regularly attacked their communities, to seasonal bacterial infections from tainted water supplies, and to dangerous childhood illnesses, and they were all too often taken abruptly from their families.

Parents called upon their Christian faith to try to cultivate an acceptance of their children's deaths. In 1739 Massachusetts minister Ebenezer Parkman recorded the passing of his infant daughter. "About 10 she ceas'd to breathe. The will of the Lord be done! . . .O that we might have a due sense of the divine Mind concerning us!" Elizabeth Porter Phelps, a wealthy rural New Englander, reminded herself after her baby crawled to a boiling pot and scalded her hands, "Lord what a great mercy twas no worse. thou are our constant benefactor, O may this providence serve to put me upon consideration that the Child is thine. Let me never forget it."[69] Parents loved their children, but their faith required that they try to relinquish them willingly to God when He called them.

Knowing how vulnerable newborns were, mothers were sometimes cautious about becoming too attached right away. Esther de Beert Reed, a prominent Philadelphian remembered for her leadership in women's relief efforts for soldiers during the Revolutionary War, indicated such feelings in a letter to her relatives in England after she gave birth to her first child, a delicate girl, in 1771: "I believe I shall make a good nurse, and I think I shall like my little girl very well by and by. If she lives, it will make me more anxious than ever to return to dear England, as the education of girls is very indifferent here."[70]

Parents' caution extended to the months before the birth as well. Abigail Adams, who bore five children before she became First Lady, mused on her feelings after she gave birth to her last child, a stillborn daughter. "The loss occasions very different Sensation[s] from those I once before experienced," when her one-year-old daughter had died, "but still I found I had a tenderness and an affection greater than I imagined could have possess'd my Heart for one who was not endear'd to me by its smiles and its graces." It was a sad time for her and her husband John, and their twelve-year-old daughter Nabby had trouble accepting the loss. Abigail and John, as sad as they were, found their grief balanced by their great relief that Abigail came through the birth safely. As Abigail put it, "I have so much cause for thankfullness amidst my sorrow, that I would not entertain a repining thought."[71]

If a stillbirth was not quite the same as the death of a baby, a miscarriage was different still. Most women who kept diaries did not record their miscarriages at all. One of the few who did was Elizabeth Drinker. In contrast to her moving description of her child's death, a miscarriage was noted simply, "May 26. 1768. ED miscarried." Because Drinker never wrote about her pregnancies, it is impossible to tell precisely at what stage this pregnancy miscarried, though other evidence from her diary is suggestive. Drinker weaned her son Billy on February 6, about three and a half months before the miscarriage. Billy was almost exactly one year old, and medical texts of the era recommended weaning at a year, so it is possible that Drinker began ovulating right after she weaned, got pregnant right away, and miscarried at about two months, as in a previous miscarriage she recorded at "8 Weeks gone." [72] It is also possible that Drinker weaned Billy at the point when she discovered she was pregnant, since medical texts advised that breastfeeding during pregnancy was unhealthy. In that case, she would have miscarried at around five or six months' pregnant. Whether it was an early or a late miscarriage, it was not an event that inspired her to record the kind of anguish evident in the account of her child's death or the sadness Abigail Adams expressed after her stillbirth.

A miscarriage, unlike a stillbirth or the loss of a child, could even be seen as a blessing depending on the circumstances. Abigail Adams wrote to her sister about their mutual friend, Anna Greenleaf Cranch, who suffered a miscarriage in 1800, after giving birth to her first three children in quick succession in 1796, 1797, and 1799. "She, poor thing, has had a mishap. I rather think it good than ill luck however, for it is sad slavery to have children as fast as she has. She has recovered tho she is thin & weak." Cranch would go on to have seven more children, her last born in 1819. Her miscarriage, as physically challenging as it was, seemed less burdensome to Adams than having another tightly spaced baby to birth and nurse. For women who spent much of their adult lives in childbearing, miscarriages seemed a natural and even necessary part of a larger project of building a family.[73]

* * *

Childbearing was at the center of colonial American women's lives. Women were celebrated for their fruitfulness, and their fertility was regarded as their greatest contribution to their families and communities. But at the same time that women found their greatest rewards in childbearing and tremendous pride in their large families, they did not place too many hopes and expectations on any given pregnancy, especially in its early months. They knew from experience that not every pregnancy becomes a baby. They also knew all too personally that while losing a desired pregnancy was disappointing and sometimes scary, it was not the same thing as losing a child. Colonial life put miscarriage into a certain perspective: a miscarriage was a mishap on the way to having another child. It was part of a long and sometimes bumpy journey to a family as large and healthy as God, in his mysterious ways, might grant.

CHAPTER 2

✧

Planning the Baby

Fertility Control From Withdrawal to the Pill

"I'VE SET A DATE!" broadcast journalist Jennifer Borget announced on her personal blog in June 2009. "August or September. That's when I'm planning [on] turning my baby makin' machine 'on.'" Borget started writing her blog, babymakingmachine.com, when she began thinking seriously about having her first child, but she and her husband were not quite ready yet. For the first six months, she blogged about her growing baby fever, her husband's desire to finish his education and establish financial security, and her own mixed feelings about having to balance work and family. She wanted to feel sure and fully prepared before she got pregnant.

Borget and her husband were teenagers at Brigham Young University when they met. As is common for Latter Day Saints (Mormons), they were happy to find a mate and settle down young. Less common among Mormons was their interracial marriage—Borget is African American, and her husband is white. After their college years, they moved to Austin, Texas, where Borget would establish herself as a weekend news anchor and her husband would train to become a police officer.

When Borget made her announcement, she calculated that by August, "I'll have been off hormonal birth control and taking prenatals [vitamins] for five months." During their five years of marriage, she had taken the pill and other forms of hormonal birth control, to ensure she and her husband did not have a baby while they were still in school and launching their careers. She only set contraception aside once she had made a focused and explicit plan to become pregnant. "I've said before that I don't think I'll have the 'in-between' stage of 'not trying, not preventing.' In my eyes I either want to have a child, or I don't. And when I'm not preventing anymore I'm going to be *trying* to get pregnant." There would be nothing casual about her efforts.[1]

For Borget, as for many Americans, birth control was a crucial tool in realizing her American Dream: marriage to the love of her life, college, a fulfilling career path, and then, once everything else was in place, children. It had given her the freedom to plan her future, invest in her and her spouse's education and career, and feel confident she could nurture and support a baby. By the time she stopped using birth control, she was eager for a child, and getting pregnant was the next milestone she would strive for. She prepared her body with vitamins and yoga, readied her home by making plans for a nursery, and bought a stash of home pregnancy tests. Years of using reliable contraception gave her a strong sense of control over her life, her body, and her fertility. She would bring this sensibility into her baby-making efforts. But after years of successfully preventing pregnancy, would getting (and staying) pregnant be something she could also control?

REVOLUTIONARY STIRRINGS OF THE DESIRE
TO CONTROL FERTILITY

Evidence of the first inklings of Americans' desire to control their childbearing appeared in elite women's letters and diaries starting around the time of the American Revolution. Their private dreams echoed the revolutionary values that were transforming American political, intellectual, and social life. In public, women supported their husbands, fathers, and sons in demanding political self-determination, freedom from the yoke of a patriarchal king, and equality for all citizens. Privately, they began to wonder if they might be able to have rewarding lives as individuals, apart from constant childbearing. Esther de Berdt Reed, a prominent Philadelphian, wrote shortly after her wedding in 1772 that "a large family . . . [would] be a heavy weight."[2] She pictured an ideal family with two children, one boy and one girl, with time for travel, self-improvement, and political activity. While Reed's desired family size might have been especially small for this era, even women who looked forward to bigger families were not necessarily willing to simply accept however many children they might naturally bear. Benedict Arnold's wife Margaret Shippen Arnold wrote to her sister, Elizabeth Shippen Burd, "It gives me great pleasure to hear of your prudent resolution of not increasing your family . . . I have determined upon the same plan; and when our Sisters have had five or six, we will likewise recommend it to them."[3]

To realize the new ideal of self-determination, women adopted new ideas about personal responsibility. Much was made, during the American Revolution, of the values of prudence, forethought, and self-control. A republic could only succeed if its citizens behaved rationally and exercised good judgment on their own behalf and in their efforts for their communities. Women absorbed these values as enthusiastically as their male counterparts. To support the war effort, they gave up luxuries such as fine imported cloth and daily comforts like tea, intelligently operated large households on small budgets, and orchestrated household production of daily needs and wartime supplies. Not surprisingly, when women began to dream of their own self-determination and think of themselves as prudent, rational planners, they started to want to plan the aspect of their lives that dominated all others: their fertility. They started to reject the fatalism of their foremothers and creatively and persistently sought ways to reduce their childbearing.[4]

Women also began to challenge the authority of the family patriarch and favor more egalitarian marital relationships. In a heated argument with a judge in her community, Rachael Van Dyke, the teenage daughter of a prosperous New Jersey farmer, insisted in 1810 that she "would never promise to *fear* and *obey*—and if ever I got married I would omit that part of the ceremony or else my husband should say the same."[5] A female essayist agreed, arguing that promising to obey her husband would effectively turn her into his slave, when marriage was supposed to be a mutual and reciprocal relationship.[6] A schoolteacher published a song with joking but inflammatory lyrics: "The lords of creation men we call/ And they think they rule the whole/ But they're much mistaken after all."[7]

Privately, women harshly criticized men who they perceived to be abusing their privileges in the bedroom. Ann Warder, a prominent Philadelphia Quaker and eventual mother of ten, wrote in frustration about her "much to be pitied sister Polly Emlen." She complained of Emlen's "husband who exceed the desription of my Pen for Insinsibility—Her Children are presented Yearly which, keep her in constant Ill health."[8] Women began to expect husbands to respect their wives' need for self-determination and control over their bodies and wanted their cooperation in limiting their families.

In the long term, this budding expectation of reproductive self-determination would set modern American women such as Jennifer Borget up to expect near-perfect control over pregnancy. But the path to this was far from straightforward, and during the intervening centuries, a mix of old and new modes of fertility control interacted with a newfound determination to limit family size in sometimes surprising ways. In their zeal to create smaller, more emotionally intense, and financially prosperous families, nineteenth-century Americans devalued early pregnancies, which for most women came much more easily and frequently than was ideal. Any specific pregnancy was likely to become "wanted" only once it appeared to inevitably be leading to the birth of a child. Women who hoped for children also welcomed some early "misses," because only a mix of the two would result in the small families they wanted and believed they could care for well.

TRADITIONAL REMEDIES, NEW USES

Nineteenth-century women began their efforts to limit family size by intensifying their use of traditional remedies for spacing children. Women had long brewed their own emmenagogues—medicines designed to bring down the menses. Since regular menstruation was regarded as crucial to women's health and stopped-up menstruation was understood to cause disease, emmenagogues held an ambiguous status as both remedies for disease and fertility regulators. Pharmacopeia and women's handwritten recipe books contained emmenagogic brews to be made from plants growing in both the old world and new. After the Revolutionary War, these medicines were increasingly patented, advertised, and sold under brands such as Hooper's Female Pills and Dr. Ryan's Worm-destroying Sugar Plumbs.[9] Women bought them from druggists and by mail, responding to the advertisements that peppered the margins of newspapers and promised miraculous cures for ill health and late periods. Women were beginning to use emmenagogues not just in exceptional circumstances, such as when a woman was frail and her health would be further threatened by a suspected pregnancy, but more regularly and prophylactically, as insurance against any closely spaced pregnancies.[10] Patent medicines became ubiquitous during the nineteenth century, and "women's complaints" were one of the primary ailments they were advertised to treat.

Women also advised each other to breastfeed each child longer. Writing to her married daughter, Margaret Izard Manigault, wife of a wealthy Charleston planter, opined, "I think it is less fatiguing to the constitution to nurse this one, than to bring forth another." Elizabeth Drinker recorded in her diary that she had told her daughter that "she is now in her 39th year, and that this might possible [sic] be the last trial of this sort, if she could suckle her baby for 2 years to come, as she had several times done heretofore."[11] Groundbreaking feminist Mary Wollstonecraft, in her widely distributed *Vindication of the Rights of Woman*, proposed breastfeeding as a health-preserving practice: "There would be such an interval between the birth of each child that we would seldom see a houseful of babes."[12]

Women may have been relying on the natural suppression of menstrual cycles caused by breastfeeding, but they also may have been counting on the tradition of abstaining from intercourse until after weaning. Medical writers advised that sex was bad for breastmilk and that breastfeeding and pregnancy did not mix. While many couples ignored this advice, at least some adhered to it. Alexander Hamilton hopefully wrote home to his wife, "I shall be glad to find that my dear little Philip is weaned, if circumstances have rendered it prudent. It is of importance to me to rest quietly in your bosom."[13]

It is also likely that women increasingly employed the home remedies that have come down through the centuries as "old wives' tales" for bringing down the menses. Women and physicians alike believed that exhausting physical work, falls, and frights could affect the menstrual cycle, either dangerously halting or enhancing the flow, or causing miscarriages. Lifting heavy loads of wet laundry, and then soaking, beating, wringing, and hanging it by hand, certainly could worsen menstrual bleeding from the strain. It was plausible that this work might also bring on the menses. A fall off a horse, or a beating from a drunken husband, were known causes of premature birth. The proverbial "falling down the stairs" seemed like it might also expel an early pregnancy.[14]

Late periods and early miscarriages happened often enough that these remedies appeared to have at least partial efficacy. An example of this appears in the diary of Mary Poor, the daughter of a prominent Unitarian minister in Boston and the wife of a successful businessman. Poor, one of the few nineteenth-century diarists who recorded sexual intercourse and attempts at contraception, expressed her dismay in 1863 that she might be pregnant. She was forty-four, and the youngest of her seven children was eighteen months old. She had hoped to be finished with childbearing years earlier. She complained to her husband how ill she felt all the time, and yet she took many carriage rides and hikes. When she reluctantly admitted that her sister-in-law, who was certain Mary's symptoms indicated she was pregnant, might be right, she stopped riding for a few days and sent a letter to her physician, Elizabeth Blackwell, asking her opinion. When Mary's period came, her husband, who was more open to another child, wrote, "I see now that you ought not to have taken those long rides with me . . . Shall we never learn wisdom?" Presumably Mary herself was quite relieved.[15] In the colonial period Vice President Aaron Burr's mother Esther Ewards Burr wrote to a friend after a strenuous journey, "Found the Ride of service." She had weaned a child two months earlier and was doing what she could to ensure regular menstrual periods.[16] A doctor today would be quite skeptical that these activities could cause a miscarriage or bring on a menstrual period, but throughout the nineteenth century and well into the twentieth, even doctors regarded early pregnancies as vulnerable in the face of women's strenuous activities.

Traditional methods sometimes helped reduce fertility, but they were far from reliable. Elizabeth Drinker's daughters spaced their children much more widely than their mother had managed, averaging between four and five children each, instead of the eight their mother bore. Not everyone was so successful, though. By the time her life was cut short at age thirty-three, Esther de Berdt Reed, who had declared her intention to have two children, had already borne six, despite her husband's declared support for family limitation. Elizabeth Drinker apparently did not manage to influence her son and daughter-in-law as effectively as her daughters, as she exclaimed in her diary, "Our Son Henry at present has 6 children, and has buried two—they have been married 9 years and 8 months, nearly—O dear!"[17] Emmenagogues, breastfeeding, and heavy work surely prevented or disrupted some pregnancies, but they were unreliable as methods of birth control.

REDOUBLED EFFORTS

Americans popularized a host of additional partially reliable methods of fertility regulation during the nineteenth century. In the 1830s the first books of popular contraceptive advice particularly advocated *coitus interruptus*, or withdrawal, and postcoital douching. Indeed, these popular methods appear to have often been used together. Druggists carried a host of "female syringes," and they were advertised for mail order in widely distributed magazines.[18] A decade later, patent medicines to "regulate" menstruation and remove menstrual "suppressions" were widely advertised as well.[19]

With impressive determination, Americans managed to cobble together some effective schemes for reducing their childbearing: in 1800, women had on average seven children, but by 1900, they averaged between three and four.[20] Birth rate decline occurred first among native-born northern whites. African Americans followed suit after the Civil War, when they finally had the legal right to their own bodies; they may have also found their childbearing suppressed by especially harsh living conditions. Southern whites, too, reduced their birth rates after 1880.[21] Urban immigrants joined their native-born brethren as they acculturated in the decades around the turn of the twentieth century.[22]

It took considerable effort for women to drastically reduce their natural fertility. To conceive, bear, and breastfeed an infant occupied, conservatively, about eighteen months of a woman's reproductive life: three months' average unprotected intercourse to conceive; nine months of pregnancy; and six months' suppression of ovulation from breastfeeding (perhaps longer, with co-sleeping and breastfeeding on demand). So, for each fewer child a woman bore compared to her colonial counterpart, she had to avoid pregnancy for at least eighteen months, or an expected average of at least six conceptions. Even if she acted to bring down the menses each time, and therefore had a couple months' longer spacing between opportunities for conception, it would still take three or four pregnancy losses, whether spontaneous or induced, to substitute for one live birth. To have three or four fewer children than her colonial counterpart, a woman needed to avoid between eleven and twenty-one expected conceptions, a daunting figure given the technology available.[23]

While advice writers often advocated a single method of fertility control, many couples presumably relied on several in tandem, given the efficacy of typical nineteenth-century methods. A couple might have started by practicing withdrawal, and the woman might douche with water or an acidic solution after sexual intercourse. The wife might supplement withdrawal or douching with trying to sneeze and cough to expel semen, or dancing around the room afterward to shake it downwards and out. If she was feeling nervous, she might take some patent medicine regulating drops, advertised as medicine to "regulate" or bring on the menstrual period, each day starting a few days before her period was due. If her period was late, she might take a carriage ride over bumpy roads or wash heavy loads of laundry. If this behavior, characterized at the time as "careless," didn't have an effect, she might diagnose a pregnancy.[24]

At that point, she might accept the possibility that the pregnancy was going to stick, continue her normal daily routine (which contained many activities physicians warned could cause miscarriage), and wait to see what happened. Or if she was really determined to not be pregnant, she might take higher doses or stronger forms of medication, try and stimulate contractions by irritating her cervix, or insert a medical sound or other long, thin object through her cervix into her uterus. She might seek out an abortionist, an increasingly common and openly advertised service in American cities.[25] Even an abortionist would try these gentler, though fairly direct, methods of inducing a miscarriage before resorting to anything resembling a modern dilation and curettage (D&C).[26]

Given this range of possible means of fertility regulation, and the un-reliability of nearly all of them, it could be hard to tell what had actually worked, short of an instrumental abortion. In the nineteenth century, distinctions between contraception, abortion, and miscarriage did not seem so relevant. In practical terms, all of the methods of birth control except withdrawal were employed after intercourse and involved washing or shaking out the man's contribution. Without pregnancy tests, it was im-possible to tell whether a woman's period came because she avoided con-ception or because she disrupted a very early conception. To a populace still steeped in traditional medical beliefs that did not regard a fetus as in any real sense "alive" until quickening, there was no obvious moral distinction between intervening before or after conception.

The distinction between miscarriage and abortion was no clearer. Since most fertility interventions were not terribly specific or reliable, there was no way to know whether a late period had reappeared because of something the woman did, or whether it would have happened anyway. "Abortion" was the medical term for any kind of pregnancy loss, regard-less of whether purposeful or accidental. Women called their miscarriages "misses," "mishaps" and "accidents," but they also called them "abortions," even in circumstances where they were clearly not induced.

By the 1840s, fertility control was common enough to garner widespread controversy and popular commentary, and by the 1860s there was a ca-cophony of often-conflicting advice on the matter in publications ranging from anonymous pamphlets hawking contraceptives to weighty medical tomes by well-credentialed physicians.[27] A few health reformers promoted the concept of contraception and advertised a panoply of contraceptive services. Those who took a more conservative approach to sex chastised married couples for having sex just for fun, accusing them of using contra-ception to make marriage into the equivalent of prostitution. Even worse, they thought, middle-class women were aborting pregnancies to limit the size of their families. Plantation medical manuals warned slaveholders that the women they enslaved used herbal preparations of cotton root and other plants to prevent conception and abort pregnancies.[28]

Amidst the cacophony, anti-abortion physicians, those who appeared best equipped and most motivated to draw a bright line at conception, fur-ther muddied the waters. They drew upon new scientific knowledge about embryology to argue that quickening, or a woman's internal sensation of fetal movement, was not a meaningful marker of fetal development. Instead, they emphasized, a new human being began when sperm and egg combined.[29] And yet, because they were as morally opposed to contracep-tion as to abortion, and because they blamed miscarriages on women who they suspected welcomed them, they blurred the lines among contraception, abortion, and miscarriage. They lumped them together as the immoral thwarting of a woman's fertility.

This conservative position on contraception and abortion showed up in popular health manuals of the day, even among health reformers who were considered "sex radicals" for advocating that wives should be the ones to decide when to have sex and be exposed to the possibility of pregnancy. For example, Thomas Low Nichols, a prominent advocate of a popular nineteenth-century alternative medical system called hydropathy, or "water cure," wrote widely read home medical manuals. In 1873 he published a twentieth-anniversary edition of his 335-page tome of reproductive and sexual information and advice. In an early chapter, he described the reproductive cycle: "Every month, one or more eggs are thrown off from the ovary, pass down the fallopian tube, lodge in the uterus, and if not fecundated, perish, and are expelled as abortions."[30] He saw these "abortions" as part of the natural order, and clearly thought about them differently from induced abortions, which he would condemn later in the book, and yet he did not name them differently. To Nichols, even an unfertilized egg was a lost opportunity to have a baby, and its loss was a sort of "abortion."

Later in the book, Nichols emphatically insisted upon the biological and moral significance of conception. He based his explanation on a scientific understanding of human reproduction that was relatively new and esoteric at the time. Nichols repudiated the common notion of "quickening" as the beginning of life. He knew that fetal movement in fact began before a woman could be aware of it and that there was no obvious biological line to draw during gestation that could serve as the modern moral equivalent of quickening. To Nichols, modern embryology supported his belief that at conception "the life of the being so formed is sacred. From the moment of conception it is a human life with all its possibilities, temporal and eternal."[31]

Nichols's purpose in drawing a line at conception was to rail against women who induced abortions. But when he proceeded to describe "abortion," he blurred any distinction between spontaneous miscarriages and induced abortions. He listed causes of abortion that sound more like what would have been considered "accidents," encompassing the risks of everyday life: sexual intercourse, especially if the woman orgasmed and her uterus contracted; vigorous activity; strong emotion, "errors of diet," "exhausting labors and cares," and the mainstream medical therapies of strong drugs and bloodletting. Surely these result in what his readers would have considered "miscarriages." Then he turned to the two methods by which "abortion is willfully procured," describing dangerous dosing with drugs and two mechanical methods, the rupturing of the membranes or the introduction of a tapered, cylindrical instrument into the cervix to induce contractions. Nichols called everything "abortion," from the shedding of unfertilized ova to deliberate instrumental interference in the uterus.

Other authors lumped contraception and abortion together in moral rather than biological terms. Like Nichols, John Harvey Kellogg was a health reformer, who in 1881 advised readers on induced abortion: "The crime itself differs little, in reality, from that considered in the last section, the prevention of conception. It is, in fact, the same crime postponed till a later period."[32] To avoid the parallel crimes of contraception and abortion he advocated sexual "continence," modeled on animals, who only engaged in sex in their procreative seasons.[33]

Many authors who were trying to convince women that inducing abortion was immoral lamented the uphill battle they seemed to be fighting, since so many women seemed unconcerned by miscarriage and, like the physicians, did not differentiate it from abortion. Dr. Hannah Sorensen, a physician who wrote an advice book aimed at the Mormon community she served in the late nineteenth century, expressed a familiar sentiment. "I have found in my practice a terrible misunderstanding in regard to foetal life. Many believe it is no sin to produce abortion before there is life, but there is always life from the moment of conception." She advised: "When a woman is subject to an abortion it should be looked upon as one of the heaviest trials of her life." Sorensen noted with frustration how women failed to distinguish between miscarriage and abortion, in practical or emotional terms: "Accidents may happen, to which we are all liable, but the carelessness and indifference manifested in this important subject is perfectly alarming. By some it is considered honorable to miscarry, and oh, how many abortions are brought about through practices and applications which are called innocent!"[34]

Just because women did not generally think of early miscarriages as morally or emotionally laden events did not mean that they were trivial. All pregnancies carried the risk of a bad outcome, and a miscarriage, especially somewhat later in pregnancy, could turn into a scary and even life-threatening medical event.[35] In the spring of 1865, Mary Adams, the daughter of modest Vermont farmers, wrote an emotional letter to her sister Eliza in California. She marked it "private," indicating that Eliza should not share it with anyone. It was a jumble of joy and distress, celebrating and bemoaning childbearing in the same page (see Figure 2.1a and 2.1b).

(a)
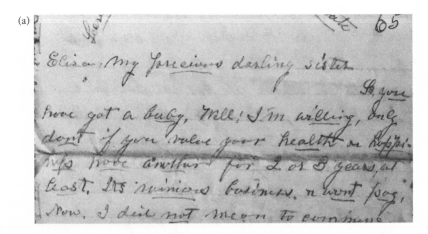

Figure 2.1a In the spring of 1865, Mary Adams wrote to her sister, Eliza, giving her advice based on her own frightening miscarriage experience. "Eliza, my <u>precious</u> darling sister[,] So, <u>you</u> have got a <u>baby</u>. Well: I'm <u>willing</u>, only <u>don't</u> if you value your <u>health</u> or <u>happiness</u> <u>have</u> <u>another</u> for 2 or 3 years at <u>least</u>. It's <u>ruinous</u> business & <u>won't pay</u>." Parker Family Letters, in the possession of Marianne Brown, Berkeley, California. Printed with permission of Marianne Brown.

(b)
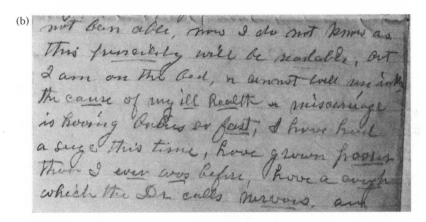

Figure 2.1b Later in the same letter, Mary Adams explained, "now I do not know as this <u>penciling</u> will be readable. But I am on the bed, & cannot well use ink. The <u>cause</u> of my <u>ill</u> <u>health</u> & miscarriage is having babies so <u>fast</u>. I have had a siege [hemorrhage] this time, have grown <u>poorer</u> than I <u>ever was</u> before, have a <u>cough</u> which the Dr calls <u>nervous</u>." Parker Family Letters, in the possession of Marianne Brown, Berkeley, California. Printed with permission of Marianne Brown.

Adams began, "Eliza, my precious darling sister, So you have got a baby, Well! I am willing, only dont if you value your health or happiness have another for 2 or 3 years at least. Its ruinious business & wont pay." After sincerely congratulating her sister, she reported on her own fragile state of health:

> I do not know as this penciling will be readable. But I am on the bed, & cannot
> well use ink. The cause of my ill health & miscarriage is having babies so fast.
> I have had a siege [hemorrhage] this time, have grown poorer than I ever was
> before . . . . I am unable to sit up more than an hour at a time, & it will be seven
> weeks day after tomorrow since I was taken sick. Its bad enough to have a baby.
> But ten times worse to have a slip [miscarriage]. I dont wonder Hattie is not
> well, if she has had one. I cannot walk without bringing on flowing [bleeding].

Because she was still so ill from her miscarriage, she had to sadly postpone visiting her sister. "I am not going to have any more [babies] for five
years. . . . Oh, how I want to see your baby." Adams was anxious over the
health of her sister's newborn, thinking of the two children she herself had
given birth to and lost in their first years. Superstitiously, she hoped her
sister's baby would not be like her own dead son, somehow too beautiful to
be allowed to stay long on earth. "I was very glad she was not as handsome
as Frankie." And then, she conveyed some worry about her own toddler,
her one living child. "Mamie was a homely little one, I hope she will be
spared to me, she is pretty looking now."

In a later letter to her parents, Mary reported that she had gotten even
sicker, bleeding so much that "I was in danger of not living for five minutes."
It turned out that the woman who had attended her during her miscarriage
had mistakenly thought the placenta had come away. In fact it had not, and
it was causing hemorrhaging. Her doctor gave her high doses of ergot and
spiced rye, which were powerful abortifacients, until she finally expelled
the placenta, fifteen weeks after the initial miscarriage. At that point, she
"began to mend at once," though she still spent several weeks as an invalid.

In the letters Mary wrote about her frightening experience with a complicated miscarriage, she worried about her own survival, her sister's health
after childbirth, and the survival of her sister's baby and her own toddler.
She had lost her first two children to early deaths, and she worried the
same might happen to her sister. And her own daughter was just over a
year old, and during the months of Mary's miscarriage-related illness, "has
been rather unwell all summer, she is teething and has had a trying time."
In an era when infant deaths were often attributed to teething, Mary was
expressing genuine anxiety about her daughter's prospects. With so much
focus on the safety and survival of living children, Mary gave no notice to
the moral and emotional status of the miscarriage.

Mary also did not resolve to avoid future miscarriages but rather to
avoid having babies for five years. She in fact had one more child, two years
after the frightening miscarriage. Like many of her nineteenth-century
counterparts, she may have welcomed any contraceptive assistance she

could get and might have regarded an early, uneventful pregnancy loss as an acceptable way to avoid more childbearing.[36]

From the American Revolution through the turn of the twentieth century, Americans were trying to seize control of their fertility in a social and technological milieu in which the practical possibilities for control were partial at best. Doctors wrote advice books listing scores of actions that might either prevent or disrupt pregnancies. Women and their partners tried many of them, but they could never be sure what would work and in retrospect were never quite sure what had actually worked. It made little sense to try and label pregnancies "wanted at conception" or "unwanted at conception," as modern fertility surveys ask. Women mostly tried not to be pregnant, at the same time that they wanted a family. They expected that their wanted children would result from pregnancies they had in fact tried to avoid.

Out of this milieu came certain central components of Americans' modern sensibility around early pregnancy and miscarriage. They gained the conviction that births could and should be planned and controlled. Women learned to be acutely aware of their fertility status and to more confidently diagnose themselves as pregnant within the first months, well before "quickening."[37]

The new sensibility was only half-developed, however. Early pregnancy loss was relied upon as an important component of fertility control. Women could not become emotionally invested in early pregnancies they rationally hoped would fail. And women did not typically express guilt or grief when pregnancies failed, even into the second trimester. In an era when it was challenging enough to keep themselves and their already-born children safe and healthy, they had not yet taken on miscarriage prevention as an aspect of maternal responsibility.[38]

* * *

In March of 2011, Jennifer Borget blogged, "I hardly ever rant . . . Or at least I try not to, but I have one topic that's been on my mind lately (like for the past six years) and I just need to let it off my chest . . . . If you abstain from sex, you won't get pregnant. If you use birth control correctly, you probably won't get pregnant. But if you do the deed during your fertile days . . . You get the idea." For a rant, it was pretty gentle.[39] "I'm not attempting to insult unplanned pregnancies, they happen every day— Heck, I'm a result of one. But I'm trying to understand. When birth control is allegedly 80-100 percent effective, why do they happen so darn often?"

While she was willing to leave a little room for technological failure, she just could not accept the fatalistic attitude she sometimes heard expressed: "If it's meant to happen it's going to happen anyway." Borget, a devout Mormon, often interpreted her childbearing experiences in terms of her faith, but this did not prevent her from taking a modern attitude toward birth control. "I don't think it's fair to blame God on the outcome of our decisions. If you don't want to prevent a pregnancy don't be shocked if it happens. If you do [use birth control to try to] prevent a pregnancy, ok, I'd be shocked too." Borget held couples responsible for minimizing the risk of an unplanned pregnancy, even though she acknowledged the value in accepting surprise pregnancies when they did happen. "Are you going to drive without wearing a seat belt because if you get in an accident and are meant to die you'll die anyway? Death is something we don't really want to take chances with. But what about new life?"

In the comments following her post, readers defensively protested that their own "surprise" pregnancies had been among the small percent of inevitable contraceptive failures. But they did not contest Borget's basic premise, that births ought to be (and generally could be) planned. And this was in the context of a discussion about married couples in which Borget felt comfortable asserting, "I'm sure the couple is going to be happy after the fact . . . but it's even better when that's what the couple wants."[40]

By 2011, it could seem reasonable to expect precision planning. Success was no longer measured only in terms of avoiding a pregnancy that would disrupt or destroy educational plans, or of having two or three kids rather than eight or ten. Even stable married couples who intended to have children together and would not consider aborting a pregnancy were expected to plan the exact number of births and their spacing. The transition from the coarse and imprecise methods of nineteenth-century family limitation to the fine-grained family planning Borget advocated took decades and significant social and technological innovations.

DISTINGUISHING BIRTH CONTROL FROM ABORTION

At the beginning of the twentieth century, the relationships among contraception, miscarriage, and abortion began to shift. Americans had long practiced birth control in the privacy of their homes, but they had been circumspect about mentioning it in public. Women might quietly share information in parlor conversations among themselves and urge their husbands to pull a brother or cousin aside to suggest some useful techniques, but it was not something to be mentioned, or even admitted, among strangers. Besides being embarrassing, in some places it was illegal to obtain birth control. Across the country, it had been against the law since 1873 to ship contraceptive and abortive information or devices through the mail, on the grounds that they were "obscene."[41]

Working to give contraception social and legal legitimacy, Progressive-era birth control advocates began a public conversation about birth control. To legitimate it, they needed to dissociate it from its sordid associations with prostitution, on the one hand, and abortion, on the other. Striving for respectability, they staked out a position on contraception that relied on its fundamental difference from abortion. As a 1917 educational pamphleteer warned fellow activists:

> In our birth control propaganda, we must be very careful to keep the question of the prevention of conception and of abortion separate and apart. The stupid law puts the two in the same paragraph, some ignorant laymen and equally ignorant physicians treat the two as if they were the same thing, but we, in our speeches and our writings, must keep the two separate, we must show the people the essential difference between prevention and abortion, between refraining from creating life and destroying life already created.[42]

Even further, one of the primary benefits of contraception was that it was supposed to prevent abortions by making them unnecessary. A woman who had access to reliable contraception would not need to have abortions, nor should she need to wish for miscarriages.

Birth control advocates ultimately succeeded in legalizing contraception and in making it "respectable" through piecemeal reforms over several decades. Margaret Sanger opened her first birth control clinic in 1916. Since her clinic was a direct challenge to the Comstock Laws—the 1873 legislation designed to disrupt the distribution of pornography and anything else having to do with sex—it proved not a simple matter to keep the clinic open or to open more of them. Sanger became a celebrity radical, enduring multiple arrests in her challenge to the law. Ultimately, it was the painful reality of the Great Depression, during which many parents could hardly feed the children they already had, that solidified public sentiment in favor of access to contraception. In 1936 the courts definitively legalized contraception for married women, at the discretion of their physicians.[43]

Margaret Sanger updated the "prudence" and self-determination of Revolutionary-era women in a twentieth-century vision of women's "self-directed guidance of the reproductive powers" involving "intelligence, forethought and responsibility."[44] She wanted to give women a female-controlled contraceptive, so that they could actually decide for themselves when they would have children. She also thought that the two most common contraceptives of the era, withdrawal and condoms, made sex terribly unsatisfying for women.[45]

The idea of valuing women's sexual pleasure was too radical for most public figures, but Sanger had a fair amount of support for the idea that women should only have children when they felt physically and financially capable of caring for them. The birth control method that Sanger offered in her clinics was a fitted diaphragm, the most effective form of birth control then available. This device was clearly a barrier to insemination rather than a way to disrupt the process after intercourse. For the women who could get one, it was a welcome improvement on the haphazard mix of pre-and post-conception methods otherwise available.

Most Americans could not get access to diaphragms, which would not gain widespread use until the 1940s and 1950s. Meanwhile, couples continued to rely upon withdrawal, douching, and condoms, with abortion as a backup. Condoms were widely available at gas stations and shoeshine stands, though they were of unpredictable quality, since they were produced and distributed in a gray market of dubious legality. Lysol was widely advertised as a douche, used in highly diluted form, and was probably at least partially effective.[46]

During the Great Depression family limitation carried particular urgency. Americans reduced their childbearing even further, averaging only two children per woman. Birth control advocates may have begun to disseminate the concept of contraception and abortion as distinct categories, but couple's practices still resembled the nineteenth-century mix of unreliable methods.[47]

Women in desperate financial straits begged for (and often received) abortions from sympathetic family doctors. Many women induced abortions on their own. Records from a Milwaukee birth control clinic in 1933 showed that 82 percent of clients had at least one self-induced abortion or had sought non-professional help before visiting the clinic.[48] Early miscarriages continued to be a welcome supplement to other modes of fertility control. Despite the legal successes of the birth control movement, couples' birth control options were hardly better than those of their great-grandparents.

With the post–World War II economic recovery women married younger than they had since colonial times, and it seemed like everyone wanted children. They hoped not for the cautious one- or two-child family of the Great Depression but for four or five kids, preferably in a nice suburban tract house with a lawn and a barbecue.[49] During this baby boom, women tended to start their families right after marriage and have their children in close succession. After they married, there was not much need for birth control, at least for a while. It took the better part of a decade to have the children, and most women started young and assumed they would spend their young adulthood focused on raising a family.[50]

In this atmosphere, an early miscarriage or two was treated casually by physicians and was likely to be accepted by a woman as well, as long as some of her pregnancies resulted in children. Pregnancy losses were not welcome in the way they had often been in previous generations: there was no reason to hope for miscarriage when parents wanted big families. But neither was there reason to dread an early pregnancy loss when they were such a common and inevitable part of having a big family, and the next pregnancy was so likely to come along soon.

Miscarriage began to receive more medical and psychological attention, though, in the context of trying to treat women with repeated miscarriages who had not been able to have children. Psychiatrists began to suggest that women who repeatedly miscarried were losing their pregnancies because they were neurotic and carried unconscious animosity toward pregnancy and motherhood. They claimed these women could be successfully treated with "talk therapy" and encouraged both psychiatrists and gynecologists to attempt this type of counseling.[51]

Physicians also attempted to develop drug remedies for miscarriage. Diethylstilbestrol, or DES, was prescribed to pregnant women in the 1940s, 1950s, and 1960s under the (mistaken) belief that it reduced the chances of miscarriage. Some doctors prescribed DES routinely, not just to women who were considered at particularly high risk of miscarriage. Not until later were the birth defects and cancer it caused in utero known.[52]

In the nineteenth and early twentieth centuries women looking to limit their childbearing had more often than not welcomed early miscarriages as a natural means of fertility reduction. And miscarriages were regarded generally as a relief, not a loss. However, during the baby boom these long-standing attitudes underwent a shift in American culture. Parents welcomed frequent pregnancies and were unlikely to regard early pregnancy losses positively. An early loss was not necessarily a tragedy, but it was an unwelcome disappointment.

* * *

When blogger Jennifer Borget announced her baby-makin' plans in 2009, her readers were warmly sympathetic and enthusiastic. Deciding to "try" was a big, meaningful decision: "Oooh I am so excited for you! Relax and enjoy the ride, you want to remember all of this. Whatever happens, this is a journey of a lifetime ☺ [.]" Borget was not alone. Another reader was on the brink of the same decision herself. "Thank you for posting this! My husband and I have been talking a lot about TTC [trying to conceive] as well, but keep putting it off. We are tentatively thinking of getting off the pill this fall. Congrats on your decision! 😊 ”

At the same time, Borget's readers also felt that they should point out that she should not assume she had control over everything. From experience, they knew that life could bring some surprises. "My advice? Roll with the punches. You may get pregnant in one year, or in one decade, just roll with the punches on this one. Remember, you have no control over anything, which by the way is a great thing to prepare you for motherhood when you relinquish most all the control over everything in life. Did I scare you? I hope not. It's all worth it." Another advised, "Relax, have fun, and wait as long as you can to take that pregnancy test. It's more accurate, you decrease the chances of getting a positive result and then being disappointed by an early miscarriage, and the first trimester definitely doesn't feel as long. Good luck and congratulations!"

Some readers' comments reflected the precision with which they, like Borget, had implicitly assumed they would be able to control the process. Having self-consciously and thoughtfully decided to "try," even a few months' delay in conceiving could be notable and significant:

> We tried for about four months before we were successful, and I have to say that in a way I'm kind of happy that we didn't conceive right away for a couple of reasons. I was a little iffy about the whole idea of starting a family. I mean, I wanted to, but I also experienced some fear that maybe I wasn't ready (kind of like everyone else who plans a pregnancy, right?). But when I got my period and found myself disappointed, I knew that we were making the right decision. Another reason is that by having to work a little bit for what we wanted, I think we appreciate it more. We've always been more of the 'work for what you want' type of people rather than the instant gratification type, and I think that always helps you appreciate what you have. Now I'm 26 weeks pregnant and we're thrilled and thankful.

This self-conciousness about "trying" to get pregnant was striking to one commentator, who reflected on how things had changed in just a generation:

> Ok, I know I'm outta the babymaking loop and all, but you gals make me TIRED just thinkin' about all the planning stuff you're doing! I have had 3 children, (the last one a major surprise). The other two? Me: 'Hey, let's make a baby!' Him: 'Ok, let's!' (Close adult activity ensued, not just for babymaking, but because we wanted to.) Then time passes (a couple of months or so), and voila!, pregnant.

There was no stress or performance anxiety. I'm too old for this stuff now, but if someone told me I had to jump on the prenatal vitamin/planning/fertility yoga bandwagon, I think it would take some of the mystery and miracle out of it. Remember, you make plans, and God laughs! You're young, you're healthy, you love your husband . . . just relax and enjoy yourselves. Let God decide the rest.

So, what happened to change the culture of pregnancy? At what point had Borget's expectation of precise control begun to arise?[53]

THE BIRTH CONTROL PILL'S PROMISE
OF PERFECT CONTROL

At the height of the baby boom came the invention that would be a tipping point: the birth control pill. Margaret Sanger had wished for an effective, woman-controlled contraceptive since her first days as a birth control activist. For decades, she orchestrated the funding and the science for this controversial project, coaxing donors and researchers into a collaboration that would result in the first hormonal birth control pill. Introduced on the American market as a remedy for menstrual disorders in 1957 and approved for contraceptive use in 1960, the pill rapidly became the most popular contraceptive. By 1965, more than a quarter of married women of childbearing age had tried the pill, and 16 percent were currently using it; by 1973 that number rose to 25 percent. By 1982, 80 percent of married women had used the pill at some point in their lives.[54]

The pill was remarkable: it worked almost perfectly and did not interfere with intercourse. Assessing its first several years on the market, the advertising trade magazine *Printers' Ink* declared it to be "the most dramatic new product of the decade . . . . We call it 'the pill.' This puts it, perhaps appropriately, on a level with 'the bomb,' worthy of an appellative of awesome simplicity."[55] Retrospectively, the pill is associated with "free love" and the sexual revolution of the 1960s, but at the time media accounts focused on what it meant for married couples. This was, finally, the device that would let women choose exactly when they would be vulnerable to getting pregnant.

The pill did not cause women to want smaller families per se. But amidst the women's liberation movement and an increasingly open job market, the pill was the tool women seized upon to create a new ideal of a satisfying life. This widely shared ideal entailed a family with two children, as well as a personally and financially rewarding career for mom and dad alike.

The pill was a crucial tool in this transformation in women's lives. Economist Martha Bailey has quantified its early influence. By comparing the birthrate in the early 1960s in states which made access to the pill legally easier to those in which it was legally impeded, Bailey found that in the states with explicit bans, the birth rate remained significantly higher until the Supreme Court struck down these laws in *Griswold v. Connecticut* in 1965. From the comparison, Bailey estimates that at least 40 percent of the reduction in the birth rate in the 1960s can be attributed to the pill.

Bailey also found that in states where unmarried eighteen- and nineteen-year-olds were able to legally get pill prescriptions in the 1960s and early 1970s, fewer women had their first births before age twenty-two, and more were in the workforce. The effect in women's lives extended far past age twenty-two; early birth control facilitated family and career planning that resulted in increased workforce participation for women through their early thirties.[56]

A second highly reliable contraceptive method, less heralded but nonetheless extremely important, was also newly popular in the 1960s. Sterilization had long been available, but it was a surgery most people had regarded with distaste, if not horror. It had been forced upon criminals and other wards of the state, not chosen by respectable people. In some hospitals doctors coerced poor black women into being sterilized immediately after childbirth, often without their knowledge or full understanding. Nevertheless, by the mid-1960s, middle-class Americans who had completed their families saw vasectomies and tubal ligations as appealing alternatives to other contraceptives. Outside the South, many of them had to fight hospital policies that imposed a "120 rule," requiring their age multiplied by their number of children to exceed 120 before they could receive surgery.[57]

During the 1970s, as restrictions on sterilization were gradually lifted, and less invasive endoscopic surgeries were developed and disseminated, Americans increasingly chose tubal ligation or vasectomy to end their childbearing. A study of married white women showed that in 1965, 14 percent of those who intended not to have more children and were using some sort of contraception were relying on sterilization; by 1975, that figure had increased to 42 percent.[58] Later studies, which included women of other races and unmarried women, found that by 1990, among women who felt finished with childbearing and were using contraception, 70 percent were relying on sterilization. This increase in sterilization was consistent across racial groups and income levels.[59]

Between the pill and sterilization, Americans had the tools they needed to home in on their ideal family size. Remarkably, more than 35 percent of women who started their families in the late 1960s and early 1970s had exactly two children, and another 35 percent had one or three children. While average childbearing was about the same as it had been during the Great Depression, it was a far cry from the cautious, anxious, hope-for-the-best family planning of the 1930s. During those hard economic times, while some women had more children than they could support, others were so cautious they ended up with fewer children than they had hoped for. Almost a quarter of women who reached their twenties at the start of the Great Depression ended up childless. In contrast, during the 1970s and after, only 16 to 18 percent of women did not have children (see Figure 2.2).[60]

The pill and sterilization also dramatically reduced unwanted births. Data from national surveys conducted between 1960 and 1965, before the new methods of birth control had really taken hold, showed that only 45 percent of births to married women had been planned pregnancies. More than 30 percent of births were "mistimed" babies who were conceived significantly before their mothers were hoping to have a child, and almost a quarter were unwanted. By the early 1970s, after the birth control pill

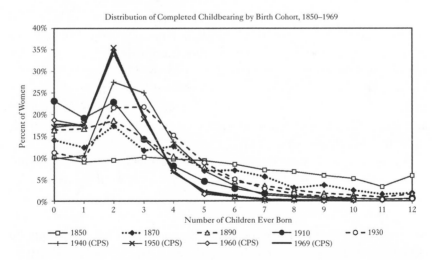

Figure 2.2 This graph shows, for selected years between 1850 and 1969, the percentage of women born that year who had each number of children when their families were complete. Women born in 1850 were as likely to have many children as few. Starting with their daughters, generation by generation, women were increasingly likely to have exactly two children. This trend reached its current peak by the time women born in the 1950s were having their children in the 1970s and 1980s. From Martha J. Bailey, Melanie Guldi, and Brad J. Hershbein, "Is There a Case for a "Second Demographic Transition?": Three Distinctive Features of the Post-1960 Fertility Decline," in *Human Capital and History: The American Record*, edited by Leah Platt Boustan, Carola Frydman, and Robert A. Margo (Chicago: University of Chicago Press, 2014).

and sterilization were entrenched but before the legalization of abortion, these statistics had shifted dramatically. In a 1975–1976 national fertility survey by the Department of Health and Human Services, women reported 63 percent of their births as wanted, about a quarter as mistimed, and only 12 percent as unwanted.[61] Married women, at least, were much less likely to be hoping for miscarriages.

When the pill first came on the market, women across a range of ages, from newly married teens to women near menopause, tried it, at least for a little while. Mothers of the boomer generation used it to end their childbearing, especially in the years before sterilization became the norm. Younger women used it to delay childbearing. It seemed useful to a wide range of women, many of whom had already struggled to keep their families as small as they wished.

Many women, though, were reluctant to stay on the pill for years on end. It could have unpleasant side effects, such as headaches, weight gain, and mood swings, especially in its earliest, high-dosage incarnations. Physicians often recommended limiting its use to a few years. No one knew if it carried long-term risks, since no one had taken it for more than a few years, even in research studies. And by the late 1960s, evidence was accumulating that it occasionally caused a fatal blood clot or stroke. Some women used it for decades anyway. When women's health activist Barbara Seaman led a fight against what she saw as the irresponsible foisting of an understudied drug on unsuspecting American women, she met substantial resistance. One annoyed woman insisted, "I don't care if you promise me cancer in five years, I'm staying on the pill. At least I'll enjoy the five years I have left. For the first time in eighteen years of married life I can put my feet up for an hour and read a magazine."[62] But many women used it only at the stage of life when they felt they most needed it.

A common pattern emerged among American women over the course of the 1970s and early 1980s. As young women, they used the pill to keep from getting pregnant before they married and to postpone children until their marriages were stable and financially secure. Then they switched to condoms and the rhythm method once they felt like they were ready for children. After two or three children, they got their tubes tied or their husbands got vasectomies.[63]

Effectively, women used the pill and sterilization to narrow the window of time in which they were susceptible to pregnancy. This way they could have the number of children they planned during the stage of life when they were ready for them. These were wanted pregnancies and planned in the sense of arriving when they could be welcomed. Since childbearing could be ended with sterilization, women no longer faced the nineteenth-century problem that children arriving too quickly meant too many children in total. A woman was much less likely to be hoping for a miscarriage, and much less likely to regard early miscarriage as a convenient form of fertility control.

Pregnancies were not typically planned down to the month, though. Many couples threw away the birth control when they felt ready to have children and left the rest to fate. Fertility monitoring was not yet a major industry. Other couples used birth control methods that were less reliable and assumed that they might fail. Many of these methods, such as condoms, sponges, and diaphragms, could be used sporadically, and often were, since they were annoying and interfered with intimacy. Couples often got careless about them when they were not specifically trying to prevent pregnancies. A resulting pregnancy might be a surprise, but that did not mean it was unwanted.

In the 1980s, refinements to the pill enabled an even more precise sense of control over pregnancy and even higher expectations of being able to plan pregnancies. From the beginning, drug companies had vied to develop lower-dose pills that would have fewer side effects without losing contraceptive efficacy. By the 1980s, many brands of birth control pills had just a tenth of the hormonal dosage of the original Enovid brand, with a sequential delivery of estrogen and progestin that, it was hoped, mimicked the natural cycle more closely.[64] Considerably fewer women reported intolerable side effects. Physicians felt that safety concerns had been narrowed to select groups of women, such as smokers over thirty-five years old, who appeared to bear most of the risk. A progestin-only pill safe for use during breastfeeding came on the market. At that point, it was possible for a woman to go on the pill as soon as she became sexually active, go off the pill when she actively wanted to become pregnant, and go back on it again after birth before she resumed sexual relations. No cycle need be left up to chance.

In 1995, the Institute of Medicine convened an expert Committee on Unintended Pregnancy comprising public health researchers, physicians, and sociologists. Their primary recommendation was that "the nation adopt a new social norm: All pregnancies should be intended—that is, they should be consciously and clearly desired at the time of conception."[65] In fact, many women had already adopted this norm. The committee wanted to see it spread more broadly across socioeconomic groups and in particular to give poor women—who often did not have access to the resources to plan their lives—the means to do so.[66]

For over two centuries, American women had sought control over their family size, and in a sense, this report was supporting this long-term shared goal. But it is striking how the committee defined "intended." This was certainly not the typical nineteenth-century pregnancy, "wanted" only once it appeared inevitable. But neither was it the "wanted" pregnancy of the baby boom, or even the 1970s, when couples accepted their pregnancies when they happened to arrive, so long as it was in the right life stage. This "intended" pregnancy was starting to look like the kind blogger Jennifer Borget was seeking.

* * *

Once Borget threw away her birth control, she got pregnant within two months. She had a mostly cheerful pregnancy that produced an adorable baby girl. Within a couple of months of the birth, she was pondering what the right spacing between children might be. She was excited to have more children, but also treasuring her time with her daughter. "I won't look back on these days and regret wondering about a number two. I'm going to spoil my daughter with light and love like no other. Because this is her time to shine, to have my full love and attention. Her time to be my one and only."[67] Still, she was soon blogging about when she ought to have her second. "I guess there's no perfect answer, or it's different for everyone, but for now, I'm thinking two and a half years would be a nice not-too-close not-too-far gap for me."[68] She debated the pros and cons of different birth spacings, wondered when her husband would feel ready, and took a First Response Fertility Test. And then scolded herself for worrying. "I should probably give #2 the same privilege of reading how seriously thought-out, loved and anticipated they were before they arrived right? Wrong? Oh, I haven't a clue!"[69]

When her daughter was almost two years old, she confessed, "All of a sudden I'm baby crazy. There's no question, I'm ready for another."[70] It took a couple of months to get her husband on board with her plan, but soon she was trying to conceive, though still trying to take a more laid-back approach. "This time is NOTHING like last time. There's no temperature taking, pill popping, sex-natzing, stressing, or tracking. I'm going to enjoy being Lil' J's mommy and focus on her, and when it happens, it happens. At least now it CAN happen. (I say all of this now, but check in again in a few months.)"[71]

Yet within a month her resolve to let it happen in its own time had broken down. After one period, she bought ovulation test kits. After the second, she almost scheduled an appointment with her gynecologist to discuss her fertility. She knew that what she was doing might seem crazy—she was only in her mid-twenties and had gotten pregnant easily with her daughter. It was certainly not the model of relaxed "letting it happen" that she had intended. She pointed out, though, that part of the reason it seemed crazy was that she was admitting it in public on a blog, not that she was the only woman to think these things. She didn't get her next period, because she was pregnant. She had a healthy pregnancy and a healthy son. And then she went back on birth control, so that she and her husband could decide exactly if and when they would have another.

* * *

At the time of the American Revolution, the very concept of deliberately controlling one's fertility and planning one's family was a barely articulated, novel idea. In the two and a half centuries since, a fine-grained family planning has developed that many women take for granted in their personal lives, and that national public health agencies articulate and institutionalize. Throughout the nineteenth and early twentieth centuries, while women might have hoped to control the overall size of their families, they could not expect to control the circumstances of each conception and pregnancy. Wanting to limit family size paradoxically meant accepting and welcoming a certain number of pregnancy losses even during the years in which couples was still building their families. Once the technology for controlling fertility caught up with our ambitions, it was realistic to prevent unwanted pregnancies rather than having to hope for miscarriages.

This can give us a greater sense of control over our family building than we really have. While conception can be prevented quite effectively, a certain proportion of pregnancy losses is unavoidable even if they are no longer welcomed. Such technologically sophisticated and effective birth control can create an illusion of control over the entire process of childbearing and family planning.

CHAPTER 3

✦

Bonding with the Baby

The Changing Meaning of Parenting

In a 2010 peer-to-peer discussion forum on whattoexpect.com, an off-shoot of the bestselling pregnancy manual *What to Expect When You're Expecting*, a pregnant woman asked for reassurance that she would be a good mother. In fact, barely three months into her pregnancy, she was worried that she was already a bad mother.

> I was just wondering if anyone out there has hard time bonding with the baby you are carrying now because you had a miscarriage before?
>
> I had a miscarriage not long before I conceived this baby. When I found out I was pregnant with the first baby, I was so excited and I daydreamed all the time about the little baby I was going to have. What a joy this baby will bring to my life! I was writing in the journals, talking to my tummy, shopping for baby stuff....Then I miscarried the baby. If you ever experienced this, you know the physical and emotional pain you had to go through. It really broke my heart. To this day, I can't talk about this miscarriage without having teary eyes.
>
> So now I am pregnant again. I am happy about this pregnancy, but I just can't seem to bond with this baby. I know motherly love should be unconditional, but I sort of have this condition of "If you survive, then I will love you." I know it sounds sad. People seem to be really excited and happy for me when they find out I am pregnant, but honestly, I am not too excited. I am almost 3 months pregnant, and I haven't written anything in my journal, I don't really talk to my tummy (other than "please stay alive..."), I don't even daydream about what the

baby will look like. Not that I am expecting to have another miscarriage, but because of what I went through last time, I guess it's hard for me to give my heart to this baby. I know it sounds so unfair and it's not this baby's fault that I had a miscarriage.

I know I will learn to love this baby as I get to know him/her. But at this point, it's hard for me to "own" this baby. I hope this baby won't have any psychological scars later because his/her mother didn't love him/her from the beginning!![1]

Women in similar situations responded by offering support: "Right now I'm feeling the same way, mostly because I'm scared if I start to bond and I lose another I will be crushed. You are not alone!!!" Others had ideas about how to cope. "My suggestion. . . just be patient. Getting over the 'loss of innocence' takes some time. The baby will be moving soon and give you reassurance it is okay. You will bond with the baby, but you may also have a fear that lasts with you until you hold the baby in your arms. Take a deep breath and just relax. Good luck and many blessed wishes for the little one!" A third reassured, "I think that probably every single one of us who have had a mc [miscarriage] worry the next pregnancy, and probably feel slightly detached at the beginning, for fear of going through all of that hurt again. Each doc's visit, I keep waiting for the other shoe to drop and find out that things didn't work out . . . again. Personally, my milestone is my next appointment this Fri (which is around the same time I lost the baby last time) and if all is well, then hopefully i can finally start to embrace this pregnancy fully. I guess it just takes time and the baby will never know!" A fourth recounted her experience with a successful pregnancy after a miscarriage. "Don't feel badly for how you're feeling. At some point, even if it's after the baby arrives, you'll feel that rush of love and it'll be like you never had these feelings at all." These women all thought that maternal "bonding" during pregnancy was a good idea, but at least did not think that a pregnant woman needed to be hard on herself if she could not fully embrace that ideal.

This online community relieved the original poster's feelings of guilt, though it could not banish her regret. "Thank you ladies for being so honest and encouraging. I feel so much better knowing I am not alone in feeling detached from the baby I am carrying. I felt so bad for feeling this way and I thought I am such a bad mother-to-be! I know I will probably worry throughout the whole pregnancy and I can only relax and really love after the baby is born and healthy. I really envy those pregnant women who can enjoy the whole pregnancy and love their babies with all their heart from the beginning." The series of posts triggered a comment recognizing how difficult it is for women to lose pregnancies. "I have not experienced a miscarriage but I just wanted to say that I think all of you are so AMAZING! I can't imagine what you have gone through and how you find the strength to keep going and keep trying after emotional and physical setbacks. You all are so brave and so strong, it's truly inspiring." Several of those who commented had miscarried more than once, making their experiences particularly challenging. But this comment also highlighted just how devastating miscarriages can be in a culture in which maternal bonding is expected from the first moment of pregnancy.

And still, not everyone was ready to let the original poster off the hook. The final comment on the thread made it clear that failing to bond in the first trimester is truly, in some people's eyes, a genuine maternal failure, no matter how understandable it may be. "I feel sad for all you ladies that cannot love their babies right now due to fear. Life is too short to not live in the moment. I hope it all gets better for you . . . Fear for our children lasts our entire lives. Wanting them safe, wanting a good life for them . . . no need to not love due to fear . . . Good luck. I hope you're able to love soon and live in the moment because it's so wonderful when you let go and enjoy life. I can't wait to see all our babies!! What a moment that will be." When women and their partners are expected to begin relating to a "child" based on a positive home pregnancy test, unconditional parental affection is supposed to begin even before a baby can be felt kicking or makes itself noticeable in a recognizable "baby bump," never mind before it makes its appearance in the outside world.

MOTHERING IN THE NINETEENTH CENTURY

Ideas about maternal bonding originated at the turn of the nineteenth century when some American women began to write about their delight in their babies from the moment of birth. This was a new phenomenon. Earlier, colonial women and their husbands had written diary entries to praise God for the deliverance of "a living mother of a living child."[2] Physical survival and God's grace by no means disappeared as priorities in the nineteenth century, but they were extolled alongside the emotional connection between mother and child.

Victorian women continued to be grateful for surviving birth, but they often directed their sentimental feelings directly to their babies, rather than to Heaven. Elizabeth Sedgwick, proprietor of Mrs. Sedgwick's School for Young Ladies in Lenox, Massachusetts, described the birth of her first child: "At 6 o'clock on the 7th of January 1824 I was a *mother* and experienced that delightful transition from suffering, danger and anxiety to happiness and that intense delight, that unspeakable sentiment which pervade the heart at its first maternal throb."[3] Elizabeth Child wrote to her daughter, "I remember that while I looked you opened your eyes . . . and as they met mine I thought they mutely recognized the new tie."[4] This expectation of immediate affection between mother and child was so new that the experience took some mothers by surprise. Caroline White, a prosperous New England matron, reflected, "The dear little fellow, I did not think I should love him so well so soon."[5]

Birth was the emotional milestone for nineteenth-century women; pregnancy was regarded differently. Anti-abortion activist and physician Hugh Hodge complained that "women whose moral character is, in other respects, without reproach; mothers who are devoted, with an ardent and self-denying affection, to the children who already constitute their family [are] perfectly indifferent respecting the fetus in the utero."[6] Hodge, who condemned both contraception and abortion, was partially referring to women who employed mechanical or medical means to limit their births. But he was also thinking about the ambivalence and fatalism with which women often regarded the process of childbearing. When they thought about their pregnancies, women worried primarily about surviving the birth. Having personally known women who had died from miscarriages and difficult births, they understood well that even women who survived might be permanently disabled. Pregnancy led most immediately to the suffering of childbirth. Once that hurdle was overcome, they could focus on the baby.[7]

As they cared for their beloved babies, these well-off Victorians were creating a new culture of the American family, one that would eventually have a profound impact on how Americans of all social classes thought about mothering and pregnancy. They were the first American women to "stay home" while their husbands "went to work." Colonial American women had typically contributed to the household economy alongside their husbands, planting gardens, milking cows, and making cloth. They raised babies while they worked. But in the nineteenth century, men's and women's daily lives began to diverge. Well-off men developed businesses and professions that took them outside the home to work. They became solely responsible for the family income. Their wives, on the other hand, supervised the household and raised the children. Instead of contributing tradeable goods, useful objects, and a passel of hard-working children to the household, affluent Victorian women established themselves as the emotional center of the family. They were idealized as "angels of the house," creating a warm and loving haven in a heartless world.[8]

Women who could hire servants to perform the strenuous and tedious household labor could focus a great deal more emotional energy and sentiment on their children. While some wealthy women left their children in the hands of hired nannies much of the time, others clearly spent a great deal of time in their nurseries with their children. They recorded their children's first steps and first words. They wrote to relatives about adorable things the children did and described cherubic faces and sweet smiles.[9]

Unlike their forbears, these Victorian women spent a substantial amount of time with only their children for company, forming intense bonds with them. Victorian culture idealized and reinforced these tight mother-child bonds. In the nineteenth century, it was a source of pride rather than embarrassment for a son to be "tied to his mother's apron strings."[10]

These family relationships were also more emotionally intense because there were fewer children needing attention. Well-off families were the first to limit their childbearing. While nineteenth-century farm families still might easily have ten or twelve children, and enslaved women continued to have many children and little control over their sexual or reproductive lives, the urban middle class was beginning to see three or four offspring as a new norm. This meant mothers had more time and energy to spend on each child and could regard each as a distinct individual.[11]

When children got sick, mothers still prayed for their health, but they took much more responsibility for their children's survival onto themselves. They read medical advice books that promised they could save their children if they used the right treatments. They tried new medical systems, like homeopathy, searching for the safest treatments for children.[12]

Despite mothers' best efforts, children sometimes died. In fact, children died just as often as they had a century earlier, from the infectious diseases and summer diarrhea that no one yet understood how to prevent.[13] And mothers, distraught at their losses and no longer so willing to see children's deaths as God's will, developed an elaborate culture of mourning. Americans began to see children's deaths, compared with the passing of adults, as especially tragic.[14] The death of a young innocent seemed particularly poignant. Life was supposed to have a certain trajectory, and a child's death repudiated that expectation. Puritan parents had emphasized to their children that death could come at any moment and had stressed the importance of being spiritually ready.[15] In contrast, Victorian parents knew that children were vulnerable, but strove to protect them, and perhaps themselves, from the reality of the threat of mortal illness.[16]

When a child died, her parents mourned deeply. Victorian parents commissioned portraits of their deceased children, and many of the earliest photographs were of children laid out for burial or resting in their cribs for the last time. Mothers recorded intense grief. And unlike many of their colonial-era forbears, they did not look for solace in the assumption that another child would come to take the place of the child they had lost.[17]

And yet, nineteenth-century motherhood was not completely transformed, even among the urban middle class. It was not yet entirely focused on forming affectionate bonds and nurturing children as individuals. While economic pressure to have children was attenuated, it was not erased. A mother was likely to rely on them for some degree of economic support, particularly later in her life. A woman would assume she could count on her sons to take care of her in her old age.[18]

Women also continued to feel traditional cultural pressures to procreate in service to God as well as her family. Women were clearly expected to have children on behalf of fathers and husbands. Her children carried on her husband's family line. Women commonly described their children as their "tender pledges" of affection and devotion to their husbands.

Affluent Victorian women made America's first foray into "intensive parenting," albeit with older parenting values and methods mixed in.[19] They intensively invested tremendous attention and affection in each child as an individual, in contrast to the earlier tradition of extensive childbearing. They set parenting standards for the wider society in many ways, even though it would be a long time before the majority of Americans could possibly follow their lead.

TWENTIETH-CENTURY PARENTING

Gradually the affluent Victorian model of parenting began to make sense for a larger portion of Americans living in more modest circumstances. At the turn of the twentieth- century economic reasons for having children no longer applied as widely. The American economy was shifting, and fewer families were able to take advantage of children's labor. Americans were moving away from farms, where even young children had traditionally helped the family make a living, to cities. In the late nineteenth century, many working-class and immigrant families sent their children to work in mills and factories, but Progressive-era child labor laws restricted that practice. It no longer made sense to have a big family to boost one's immediate economic prospects. Working-class families shrank, just as wealthier families had a few decades earlier.[20]

Working-class women also began to stay home with their children if they could afford it. More men supported their families by taking jobs for wages, and if their wives worked outside the home, it was often only after children were in school. A wider swath of American mothers could spend time and energy cultivating their children as individuals.[21]

Concomitantly, as sociologist Vivian Zelizer has described, the early decades of the twentieth century saw a wider embrace of the belief that children were precious primarily for the emotional satisfaction they brought to their parents. Children might be expected to help their parents financially in the long term, supporting parents in their old age, but in the short term, they were actually a financial expense. Parents justified the expense not by speaking of long-term investment, but rather of the joys of parenting.[22]

As an example of this shift, Americans changed the ways they adopted children, in line with these new values. In the nineteenth century, children were most likely to be adopted if they were older boys, already capable of pitching hay and hauling feed. Small children ended up at orphanages, or worse. Babies were almost impossible to place, and many died in "baby farms," where mothers who couldn't keep their children paid a fee for their care. In the 1920s, the situation reversed. The idealized adoptee was a blonde, blue-eyed baby girl. Adopted children were not supposed to be useful anymore; they were supposed to be cute and lovable. Their adoptive parents were more likely to be older professionals who primarily wanted the emotional reward of childbearing and did not need any financial benefit.[23]

During this same time, child mortality dropped dramatically. In New York City in the mid-1880s, a quarter of babies died before their first birthdays. By 1915, that figure stood at less than 15 percent. Many cities improved their sewage management and water quality and ran clean milk campaigns, preventing annual epidemics of deadly summer diarrheal disease. Parents increasingly had the luxury of focusing on their children's emotional well-being, rather than simply working to keep them alive.[24]

By the mid-1940s, many fewer women died in childbirth, as well.[25] The Lamaze movement could depict childbirth as an exhilarating experience, and women could regard it with more excitement and less dread.[26] As childbirth became safer, it was possible to imagine pregnancy as a time of happy and relatively carefree anticipation. It would be several decades before the months of pregnancy would be widely regarded as pleasurable in themselves, but the stage was set.

EMOTIONAL DEMANDS

At the same time that American parenting was becoming more emotionally intense and pleasurable, it was becoming more demanding as well. While Victorian mothers could consult a few advisors in widely distributed health manuals, parenting advice came into its own in the twentieth century. Self-appointed experts, from doctors to psychologists to society ladies, publicized their opinions about the right and wrong ways to parent. Victorians had believed that good mothering was God-given, but modern experts insisted that the only good mother was the well-informed mother.[27]

In the early twentieth century, advice on babies differed from advice about older children. Baby advice focused on health: teaching some basic hygiene and nutrition could save babies' lives. Older children, though, could benefit from well-informed intellectual and social grooming. Ellen Key, an influential feminist writer, acknowledged that a college-educated woman might legitimately feel "the drudgery of baby-tending to be incompatible with her attainments," but urged her to find inspiration and challenge in making a study of child development, observing and responding to her children as they grew.[28] At least when it came to older children, in early twentieth-century books, magazines, and newspapers, experts urged mothers to be informed about child-rearing and thoughtfully involved in all aspects of their children's development.

By mid-century, parents were under substantial pressure to have the "right" kind of intense emotional relationship with their children, and a variety of psychologists, psychotherapists and behavioral biologists were ready to act as judges. Freudians accused women of causing their children's autism and schizophrenia: "refrigerator mothers" supposedly instigated mental illness by withholding affection. On the other hand, journalist Philip Wylie's best-selling *Generation of Vipers*, published in 1942 and reprinted through the 1950s, blamed a host of social ills on overbearing and overinvolved mothers. Wylie coined the term "mom-ism" to describe the social and personal adulation of mothers he believed he saw around him, and the immaturity and over-dependence he thought it caused. A good 1950s mom was all-giving, yet not emotionally needy herself. She found her main personal fulfillment in staying at home with her young children, but she knew when to cut the apron strings.[29]

THE SCIENCE OF ATTACHMENT

In this cultural milieu, a cluster of particularly influential psychiatrists and biologists developed the concept of "attachment" to describe the emotional relationship they believed ought to exist between mothers and their young children. It was a description of what they believed came naturally, biologically and psychologically, when a woman bore a child. At the same time, it was a prescription for how mothers ought to behave and how they ought to feel about their children. Developed in the 1950s, the concept would have great cultural staying power, despite eventual skepticism from within the scientific disciplines that had birthed it. And it expanded the focus of cultural discussion about child-rearing from older children to babies and toddlers.[30]

Psychoanalyst John Bowlby first proposed his theory of attachment in the early 1950s. Around the world many children who were orphaned or who spent much of World War II sheltered in group homes away from their families showed signs of psychological damage. The World Health Organization commissioned a study to ask how to rehabilitate these children and produce healthy, functional citizens. Bowlby, the leader of the study, drew on a combination of psychoanalytic theory, psychological studies of children, and biologists' observations of maternal behavior in animals. He concluded that to become psychologically healthy adults, children needed to develop an intense and loving "attachment" to a primary caretaker. He, like just about everyone around him, assumed that this caretaker would almost always be the child's biological mother, except in unusual circumstances such as adoption.[31]

Bowlby turned to biologist Konrad Lorenz's work on imprinting in Greylag geese to bolster his ideas about attachment. Many Americans in the 1950s had seen magazine photographs of Lorenz traipsing through a meadow with a gaggle of geese behind him.[32] In his popular book *King Solomon's Ring*, Lorenz described how Greylag geese "imprinted" on the first moving object they saw during a critical period in the second day after hatching. Usually, this would be the hatchling's mother, but Lorenz induced goslings to imprint on him instead. The geese that imprinted on Lorenz followed him faithfully. As adults, they directed mating rituals at people rather than other geese. Even a brief encounter very early in life appeared to shape the broad outlines of their psycho-sexual development.

The process of imprinting had an effect on the mother, too, according to Lorenz. In the birds he studied, seeing a newborn chick triggered caregiving behaviors such as feeding the baby and chasing away predators. Extrapolating to humans, Lorenz asserted that women and girls found baby humans and animals particularly cute and appealing because they triggered maternal instincts.[33]

Bowlby, with Lorenz's enthusiastic endorsement, speculated that animal-type imprinting was a crucial component of human attachment. He saw it as the natural, instinctive beginning of the kind of caring parental relationship he thought was necessary to healthy human development. He believed it was important for a small child to have a single, primary person continuously fulfilling his emotional and bodily needs. Studies had shown that institutionalized children suffered emotional damage; Bowlby attributed the problem to the absence of the mother specifically, rather than a more general lack of loving care and social stability.

Importantly, in Bowlby's conception of attachment, the mother's conscious and unconscious feelings toward her child were as important as her actions. The child would not be happy and securely attached unless he felt, consciously and unconsciously, that his mother loved him and was 100 percent devoted to him. The mother would not truly be able to fully devote herself, as Bowlby believed was necessary, unless she derived her primary satisfaction in life from her relationship with the child. Her biological instincts were supposed to lead her to dedicate herself to childrearing. In Bowlby's model, there was no room for the good mother who needed some time to herself. If a mother didn't always enjoy her children, Bowlby seemed to suggest, there was something wrong with her, and she would likely damage her children.[34]

Bowlby's ideas took flight at a time when middle-class Americans were retreating from the frightening Cold War world into suburban tract homes and fantasies of family togetherness. Many women had entered the workforce during the war, and there was a strong cultural push urging them back home. Some went willingly; others resisted. Everyone debated what would keep families safe and strong. Bowlby's ideas fed Cold War concerns but also offered an apparently achievable solution: families would be happy, healthy, and produce strong citizens if mothers wholeheartedly embraced their role. Bowlby publicized his views in popular magazines such as *Ladies' Home Journal*, and his concept of attachment was enthusiastically received in American popular culture.[35]

By the peak of the baby boom in the late 1950s and early 1960s, American parenting culture had evolved into something resembling the contemporary version of intensive parenthood. Baby-boom families were large, parents typically started their families in their late teens and early twenties, and the culture lionized full-time mother-homemakers. Mothers were still seen as the primary parents, particularly of young children, but the import of their role was interpreted by scientific experts rather than sentimental writers.[36] Good mothers were to dedicate themselves fully to their babies and young children in order to foster healthy attachment. But then they were to encourage healthy separation as their children grew.

Mother love was regarded not just as a God-given blessing but also a biological necessity for a child's development. Mothers were not simply assumed to love their young children but were mandated to feel constant (appropriate) affection, consciously and unconsciously, or risk undermining their children's long-term well-being and ability to function as citizens.

Victorian mothers had aimed to set a moral example and inculcate a sense of shame and personal responsibility through their demonstrations of love; baby-boom mothers were supposed to provide love as the necessary and natural environment for the growing child.[37]

Baby-boom parenting ideals coalesced around the concepts of attachment and family "togetherness." Women strove to provide unremitting maternal love and affection to their young children as their primary role and central responsibility. The psychological experts' message to mothers was: love your children fully and correctly, or risk irreversibly damaging them. The broader culture reinforced the message. Whether or not individual mothers actually managed to stay home to raise families behind suburban white-picket fences, they took the message seriously.

ALL YOU NEED IS LOVE

With the arrival of the seismic cultural shifts of the 1960s and 1970s, *Leave it to Beaver* family togetherness seemed under attack from all quarters. Almost nothing about the American family was left unquestioned. Feminists asked whether it was inevitably women's destiny to bear and raise children. Beatniks advocated sex for pleasure, not baby making. Hippies shrugged off the authority of family patriarchs. Environmentalists wondered if so many people should have children on an overburdened planet.

Ironically, while traditional family values appeared to be under siege, each of these trends in its own way made children all the more precious to their parents. The countercultural movements dramatically reduced the scope of legitimate reasons to have children. By the time they receded, it would seem that the only remaining good reason to have a baby was an overwhelming desire to love and nurture and relate to a new being.[38]

In 1968, activist-scientist Paul Ehrlich published *The Population Bomb*, which urged Americans to take personal responsibility for the dangers of overpopulation by having fewer children. Ehrlich contended that overpopulation was an even bigger threat to human survival than the possibility of thermonuclear warfare. He was by no means the first to sound the alarm about population growth; scientists and policymakers in the 1940s and 1950s observed with growing concern the population explosion around the world. Before Ehrlich, though, the most prominent population control advocates blamed overpopulation on developing countries. They worried about political instability and the possibility of being "overrun" by people from formerly colonized nations or impoverished Americans from the nation's inner cities. Ehrlich's vision was somewhat more egalitarian: he was unwilling to absolve middle-class Americans' personal responsibility for population reduction.[39]

Following on *The Population Bomb*, Ehrlich founded Zero Population Growth (ZPG), an activist organization whose mostly youthful members pledged to have no more than two children. ZPG never had that many adherents, but it held a significant place in the public imagination. *Life* magazine's coverage, while ZPG was rapidly growing in the early 1970s, was bemused. "America has always been a growth society. But today an organized challenge is being mounted against the heart of that concept. . . . The movement [to stop population growth] is serious, thoughtful, responsible—and certainly debatable." Accompanying photos showed high school and college students cheerfully handing out environmentalist leaflets and participating in an educational demonstration of exponential growth.[40]

A couple of months before its article on ZPG, *Life* had featured a professor who had a vasectomy as, the headline announced, "One Man's Answer to Overpopulation."[41] Walter and Betty Brainerd, of Tenafly, New Jersey, shared the details of their decision. Surprisingly little was left to the imagination. The article included a discreetly shot photo of Walter on the operating table, with his white-draped surgeon standing over him explaining last-minute details of the surgery while Walter gestures his acknowledgment (see Figure 3.1). And there's another photo of Walter walking cheerfully out of his doctor's office after the surgery. Like Ehrlich, who spoke widely about having a vasectomy after fathering one child, the Brainerds felt "deeply worried by this country's wildly expanding population and the grim fact that people just like them—young, successful, educated—are producing more children than any other group." They acknowledged their disappointment that, having two girls, Walter would not be passing on the family name. Betty thought she might have enjoyed having another baby. Still, they were committed. They regarded childbearing as something they did solely for their personal satisfaction, despite its negative impact on the world around them. Having babies was something one did in spite of the common good, not in its service.

Some environmentalists loudly supported Ehrlich's and ZPG's calls for all Americans to limit their childbearing as a matter of personal responsibility. The Sierra Club, in fact, published *The Population Bomb*.[42] Stewart Brand, who would go on to found the Whole Earth Catalog, organized a rally to support Ehrlich's cause.[43] Ehrlich put his arguments in environmentalist terms, berating middle-class Americans for monopolizing natural resources and contributing disproportionately to environmental degradation.[44] Like

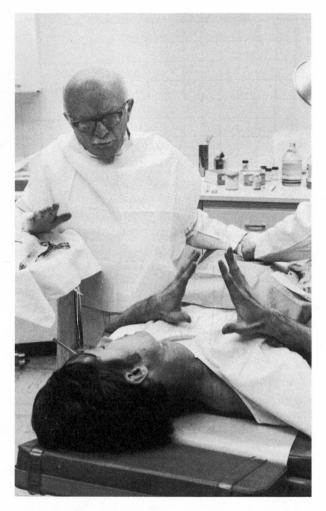

Figure 3.1 In the 1960s and 1970s population control advocates argued that it was ethically responsible to limit one's childbearing. This 1970 *Life* magazine story showed a couple choosing vasectomy as a way to prevent future pregnancies. Here, the surgeon explains the procedure. *Life*, March 6, 1970, page 45. Leonard McCombe/The LIFE Picture Collection/ Getty Images.

Betty and Walter, environmentally concerned Americans felt responsible for weighing the public interest in protecting the planet against the personal fulfillment of childbearing.

Feminists raised a different set of challenges to traditional ideas about childbearing. At the beginning of feminism's second wave, in the early 1960s, those challenges were relatively modest. In *The Feminine Mystique*, Betty Friedan spoke forcefully about "the problem that has no name"— the disaffection and alienation of middle-class homemakers—but she assumed that most women wanted children. Primarily addressing women who were already raising children, she observed that they loved and cared for their families, but for many women this wasn't enough to sustain them throughout a lifetime. They were beginning to ask, "Is this all?" Friedan asserted that women could be fully realized, fully feminine wives and mothers and simultaneously enjoy meaningful careers. She believed that childbearing was insufficient as the only source of meaning in a woman's life, though she regarded it as important and fulfilling. She protested the false choice women were told they had to make between family and career, insisting that they could have both if only the wider culture would support them.[45]

As the women's movement grew, radical feminists pushed Friedan's critique much further. They questioned everything that had been taken for granted about women's lives: that they should defer to men; that they should live and sleep with men at all; that women were inherently or necessarily "feminine"; and that childbearing was necessary or even desirable for many women. Shulamith Firestone famously predicted that artificial reproduction would someday enable women to eliminate patriarchy, as women would no longer be biologically tied to the project of bearing children.[46] Firestone and other radicals were committed to demolishing the feminine mystique altogether.[47]

Radical feminists' male peers were no more committed to raising families. They infuriated their feminist sisters by assuming that women would continue to take care of traditional tasks of cleaning, cooking, and sexual availability. But this did not mean they were looking forward to lives of traditional domesticity. They assumed that women would take responsibility for birth control and turn themselves into sexually adventurous playmates. Sex was for entertainment, and pregnancy did not inevitably lead to a shotgun marriage. As far as they were concerned, sex had been liberated, even if women had not. Liberated sex was supposed to be about seizing pleasure and living in the moment, not about making babies.[48]

Even once a couple decided to have children, the counterculture influenced the advice they received about childrearing. Experts adopted a new tone in parenting manuals, suitable for parents bewildered by their hippie children, and equally for the new kind of parents those hippie children would strive to be. Guides such as *Parent Effectiveness Training* called upon poet Kahlil Gibran, a beloved counterculture figure, rather than the Bible. *Parent Effectiveness Training* author Thomas Gordon offered a new way for parents of this rebellious generation to think about their relationships with their children. A parent could share her values by her example, explained Gordon, but she could not force them on her children without risking profound alienation. Treat your children as fully fledged people, respect them as separate human beings who will live their own lives, he instructed, and you will enjoy them more and earn their respect. Parenting was about the personal satisfaction of mutual enjoyment. Sustaining a loving connection to a child was ultimately more important and more attainable than inculcating specific religious or cultural values, insisting on deference, or shaping the family line.[49]

By the mid-1970s, a thoughtful couple could be so torn between the expected fulfillment of parenting and its anticipated personal and social costs as to be paralyzed by the decision about whether or not to have children. Social scientist Elizabeth Whelan's *A Baby? Maybe. . . A Guide to Making the Most Fateful Decision of Your Life* (1975), was emblematic of the new self-consciousness about childbearing. Young couples who considered their options in the 1960s and 1970s made their family-building decisions amidst clamorous challenges to patriarchy, tradition, and the nuclear family. In a world where nothing could be taken for granted, couples who earlier would have embarked on a family without a second thought were asking new questions.

When Whelan began researching her book, she found no shortage of opinions on, as one Planned Parenthood campaign put it, "Dumb Reasons for Having a Baby." Whelan listed the "dumb" reasons on billboards plastering the New York City subway: Because it would make the grandparents happy. To patch up a rocky marriage. To give a wife something to occupy her time. To solicit help from relatives. To prove one's virility. To have a boy this time (or a girl). Because it is a woman's destiny. All of these reasons would have seemed more or less reasonable to most Americans only a few years earlier, before the counterculture, the women's movement, and the population control movement.

If those were the wrong reasons, what were the right ones? Whelan spoke with psychologists and counterculture activists as well as young married couples who struggled to articulate why they planned to have children. Without traditional justifications, it was not so easy for them to explain why they planned to sacrifice relaxed marital contentment, career ambitions, and free time in favor of bringing children into their lives. Whelan concluded the only good reasons to have a baby were, as she put it, "selfish." Whelan was graciously willing to defend couples who thoughtfully explained their desire for emotional security in old age, their intention to deepen a strong marriage bond, or a woman's desire to make child-rearing her primary vocation. Still, the very best reason to have children, perhaps the only truly legitimate reason, was because a couple treasured the experience of parenting in itself.[50]

Not everyone was as accepting as Whelan of 1970s culture and its new-fangled way of thinking about babies. Prominent members of the religious Right publicly and vigorously defended traditional ways of thinking about childbearing. "Family Values" entered the Republican Party platform in 1976.[51] A year later, evangelical leader James Dobson founded Focus on the Family, a nonprofit organization that produced and disseminated conservative media and advocated for conservative views on family life. On his popular daily radio show, Dobson urged women and men to commit to traditional marriages, with breadwinner husbands and homemaker wives and mothers. Along with many televangelists and evangelical leaders, Dobson condemned homosexuality, abortion, and sex outside of marriage. Dobson's Family Research Council translated these messages into political advocacy, strongly influencing the Republican Party.[52]

In an important sense, however, there was no going back, no matter how much conservatives might have wished to recapture the past. Traditional childbearing could no longer be taken for granted. Even those who did their best to maintain tradition could no longer do so unselfconsciously and in easy harmony with their neighbors. Ordinary Americans were suddenly much more self-conscious about their gender roles and their parenting. The political and social implications of intimate decisions were obvious to countercultural feminists, who declared "the personal is political." A lesbian couple's public avowal of a committed, sexualized relationship was clearly a political statement. In a culture in which traditional family life could no longer be taken for granted, patriarchal marriage and childrearing became political statements as well. The wife-and-mother role was a choice, not a requirement. Having a large family was not only an explicit choice but went against the grain of contemporary trends. Keeping an inconvenient pregnancy was a choice rooted in faith, not an acquiescence to fate.

Defending conservative patterns forced Americans to justify the old ways, consciously choose them, and articulate them to critics. Explicit commitment to childrearing traditions intensified and sentimentalized the meaning of those traditions for those who defended them and adhered to them. For conservatives as much as for liberals, the emotional import of childbearing intensified and crystallized in the cauldron of the sexual revolution and culture wars of the late twentieth century.[53]

BONDING AT BIRTH AND BEFORE

For those in the 1970s who made the momentous decision to become parents, the moment of birth took on new importance. The generation that vowed to "make love, not war" and rebelled against bureaucratic authority of all kinds, thirsted for a more natural and more affectionate mode of giving birth. If they were going to choose to have babies, they were going to make their children's entrance into the world meaningful and rewarding. Becoming a parent was emotionally significant and deserved to be treated as such. They found the official backing they needed to challenge dehumanizing hospital rules in the theory of maternal-infant bonding developed by neonatologist Marshall Klaus and pediatrician John Kennell.

Bonding theory was an extension and update of baby-boom parents' attachment theory. Klaus and Kennell observed that parents of very sick newborns kept in the neonatal intensive care unit (NICU) often had trouble relating to their infants once they went home. They speculated that even healthy infants were not bonding optimally with their parents due to hospital rules that newborns be thoroughly inspected by nurses, put through a regimen of preventive health care, and kept in germ-free centralized nurseries. Based on formal observational studies of mother-newborn interactions, they theorized that the relationship formed through constant, intimate contact between mother and baby during the hours immediately after birth was crucial to setting the stage for secure attachment.[54]

Klaus and Kennell's theory had an enormous cultural impact. Hospitals moved quickly toward policies of keeping mothers and babies together after birth and prioritized familial visits and skin-to-skin contact between parents and newborns in NICUs. Couples read about bonding theory in pregnancy manuals and popular magazines. They wrote "birth plans" that instructed their doctors and nurses to prioritize early, close contact with their newborns. Nurses learned to facilitate the connection between new parents and new babies.[55]

When hospital procedures such as cesarean section disrupted birth plans, as they often did, new parents worried. What if they had missed the window for bonding, and their relationship with their child was permanently damaged? For every magazine article hyping the benefits of bonding after birth, another assured frantic parents that if they were separated from their babies after birth, all was not lost.[56] Close contact immediately after birth was ideal, but its absence could be overcome. Given the frequent disjuncture between the ideal birth and birth as it unfolded in its full unpredictability, parents needed constant reassurance that a disrupted bonding ritual would not doom their relationship with their child.

Bonding theory was compelling because it held both promise and threat. An amazing kind of parenting magic could happen, if circumstances allowed. A moment already regarded as special was imbued with even more meaning in American culture. An already important parent-child relationship could be enhanced and deepened, with the right rituals performed at the right moment. But it was a moment that could so easily be missed, and perhaps never quite recaptured. Americans were already learning that they should "treasure every moment" of parenting, in an ever more sentimental culture organized around children.[57] The moment of birth was doubly precious: it was a key moment in and of itself, and it might irrevocably establish the groundwork for the relationship that would develop between parent and child. Done right, it could make parenting even more rewarding. Done wrong, and the parent-child relationship might be forever emotionally stunted. Birthing couples were not willing to take chances. They earnestly attempted to supplement safe births with bonding rituals they hoped would be emotionally meaningful for themselves and healthy for their children.

Researchers studying bonding quickly posited that mother-infant bonding actually began before birth. The nurses and social workers who spearheaded research on prenatal bonding could see quite clearly that women who suffered stillbirths grieved their losses, even if they were never given a chance to see the child. Some kind of connection was developing during pregnancy, a connection they described as "bonding." Those researching prenatal bonding in the early 1980s seemed to imagine that if they could only get at-risk women to bond with their fetuses, those women would find a way to overcome poverty and addiction out of love for their babies.[58] While in retrospect it seems naïve to believe that mother-love alone could overcome embattled circumstances, the proposals testified to the power many Americans attributed to bonding.

William Sears, a popular pediatrician who would go on to make his name and fortune with the concept of "attachment parenting," was a notable booster of the concept of bonding during pregnancy and at birth. His 1982 book *Creative Parenting* assumed that "you have formed a bond probably from the first moment you found out you were pregnant, or certainly from when you first felt life." He described prenatal care as "parenting your unborn child" and thought of bonding as something that peaked at birth, rather than being initiated at birth. "The intensity of this bond reaches its climax at birth and should not be interrupted unless overwhelming medical complications prevail."[59] Sears's ideas were initially on the parenting-advice fringe but would not remain marginal.

The impulse behind the prenatal bonding research was already apparent in the broader culture by the late 1960s. Personal narratives from popular articles about artificial insemination hint at an important shift away from baby-boomer attitudes toward pregnancy. Medically supervised artificial insemination became more common and acknowledged in the 1950s and 1960s than in earlier decades, but it continued to carry the taint of quasi-adultery. In those decades, artificial insemination was justified with reference to prominent psychoanalysts' assertions that pregnancy and birth are necessary to women's "psychobiological drive," while fostering men's "fatherliness" toward children that are not biologically related to them.[60]

By the late 1960s, the meaningfulness of the parenting experience was made central in discussions of pregnancy via assisted reproduction. In 1969 a woman published the story of her artificial inseminations in *Redbook*. She initially worried about how her husband would feel about using another man's sperm. "Listen, Sandy," he assured her, "sharing the joys of pregnancy and birth would be more rewarding for me—for both of us, really—than adoption." He was right. After having two children through artificial insemination, Sandy concluded that the procedure was well worth it, because "we have had a greater share in the joys of life than those couples who adopt."[61] Pregnancy was no longer an inconvenient and potentially dangerous hurdle to be overcome to realize the ultimate goal of having children: it was an integral, rewarding part of the parenting experience.

Paradoxically, as women reaped the benefits of the women's movement and increasingly pursued full-fledged careers in the 1980s and 1990s, they also subscribed to intensive parenting standards even more tightly focused on children's happiness and parents' emotional fulfillment. By the late 1980s, the pattern was unmistakable. In her landmark 1992 study of American parenting norms, sociologist Sharon Hays described what she called "intensive mothering." She saw middle- and working-class American women avidly striving to develop close relationships with their children and cultivate happy children. Working mothers were as intent as stay-at-home mothers. Hays described a widely shared ideology in which mothers were the primary emotional caretakers of their children, whether or not they worked, and showered their children with attention, deliberate stimulation, and expensive educational toys and lessons. They centered their own emotional lives around their children and believed that this was necessary to their children's well-being and their own fulfillment. Hays observed that mothers were especially invested in intensive parenting, but fathers were also expected to be emotionally involved and available to a much greater degree than in previous generations.[62]

This cultural pattern was not nearly at its peak in 1992. In 1993 William Sears coined the term "attachment parenting," and a parenting movement coalesced around him.[63] Sears advocated a set of particularly intensive practices around caring for infants and toddlers that he insisted was the only way to make children happy and parents fulfilled. An attachment parent, almost inevitably a mother, spent every moment with her baby. She slept with her baby, breastfed whenever he wished day and night, carried him on her body in a sling all day, and never left him crying. She let him decide when he was ready to wean and sleep in his own bed. Attachment parenting advocates acknowledged that mothers occasionally needed to use the bathroom or take a shower, though they were vague about the practical logistics of having a private moment when a baby might feel that he urgently needed to nurse at any moment.

It might seem like an exhausting regimen, but Sears was encouraging (or perhaps disingenuous). Sleep when your baby sleeps, he told new mothers, and you'll get enough rest. Put the baby in the bed next to you, and he can nurse without really waking you. Carry him around all the time, and he won't cry, so he'll be an easy baby. People think it sounds hard, but actually, it's easier once you embrace it!

Attachment parenting was a replay of the attachment theory of the 1950s, taken up a notch. It reiterated the same basic idea: a mother who fully gives herself over to mothering will find true, deep emotional fulfillment. Her baby will feel her unconditional love and sense of complete satisfaction, and he will be happy and secure. Only this time around, what it actually meant to promote attachment in practical terms was much more demanding. Nineteen-fifties babies generally slept in cribs, ate from bottles, rode in strollers, and played in playpens. Mothers needed to change diapers, but they didn't need to think it was fun. In the 1990s mothers were made to feel guilty for every moment they weren't physically attached to their babies. This vision of attachment was much more physically intimate and strenuous, with an inflated sense of the importance of every fleeting, irretrievable second in the first years of a child's life.[64]

PARENTING BEFORE BIRTH

What did this all mean for how women experienced pregnancies since 2000? Expectations about the emotional investments and rewards of parenting continued to grow. Between 1995 and the mid-2000s, working and at-home parents alike substantially increased the amount of time they spent helping kids with homework, taking them to sports games and medical appointments, and otherwise caring directly for them, largely at the expense of their own free time.[65] Attachment-style parents of babies added a new level of parenting ambition with "elimination communication," or diaper-free parenting, requiring continual attunement to baby's subtle signals indicating he was about to pee or poop and needed a toilet.[66] The home birth movement gained momentum and attention. Even a highly medicalized hospital birth might involve a cesarean section with epidural rather than general anesthesia, immediate contact between mother and baby, and a lactation consultant to offer breastfeeding support. Parenting was supposed to be the best thing in life, and the hardest.[67] From the moment they conceived, many parents seemed amped up, stressed out, and intent on having a rewarding and fulfilling parenting experience and emotionally healthy and happy children if it killed them.

Shortly after the turn of the twenty-first century, the concept of "bonding" during pregnancy, even very early in pregnancy, entered public consciousness, and soon peppered advice columns on pregnancy and parenting websites. Nursing and social work researchers had already begun talking about it in their professional journals in the early 1980s, and William Sears mentioned it in his early book *Creative Parenting*, but the Internet made "bonding" a regular way to refer to the maternal-fetal relationship.[68] Pregnancy manuals had been careful to describe bonding as something that happened at birth and reassured parents that it might be more gradual than they imagined, even if it was important. But as baby and parenting websites became primary sources of pregnancy advice, in the early 2000s authors online began to casually suggest that "bonding" was a pleasant and important activity during pregnancy. They didn't need to define it; "bonding" had already entered colloquial American pregnancy talk.

For readers already comfortable thinking in those terms, it seemed only natural to extend the emotional intensity of parenting earlier and earlier into pregnancy. They responded to exuberant articles advocating all sorts of prenatal bonding practices: talking to one's belly, having one's husband read children's books aloud or sing a special baby song each night, writing letters or journal entries to the baby, taking highly aestheticized semi-nude photos of the "baby bump" each week. Many enjoyed the suggestions. Some felt guilty for not feeling like bonding quite yet. No wonder it could be difficult—by 2015, BabyCenter was telling women to begin a twice-daily bonding ritual, hands cradling their not-yet-a-bump, at nine weeks' pregnant (seven weeks after conception), still six or eight weeks away from quickening.[69] Morning sickness and fatigue might signal pregnancy, but they were significantly less charming than feeling the baby kick. And yet, there was that impulse—a pressure but also an urge—to feel like a parent from the first moment, and to feel that it was wonderful to be a parent.

* * *

In colonial America, childbearing had partially been about creating loving bonds, but it was equally about fulfilling God's commandment to be fruitful and multiply, producing descendants in a traditional patriarchy, and ensuring financial security in old age. Most of these reasons for parenting have since faded away, save one: the pleasure of creating a loving relationship with a child. Simultaneously, the responsibilities and pleasures of parenthood have moved earlier and earlier, first to the moment of birth in the early nineteenth century, then into pregnancy in the twentieth century, and finally into the first weeks of pregnancy in the twenty-first century. Given this twenty-first-century understanding of pregnancy and parenting, early pregnancy losses can take a tremendous emotional toll.

CHAPTER 4

⚭

Taking Care of the Baby

Prenatal Care at the Doctor's Office and Beyond

"I seriously love this app . . . . It gives you a picture of what the baby looks like each day and has tons of fun facts each day. Here is what my baby is looking like at 5+2. Not much like a baby, but it is growing a spine! I love it!" This enthusiastic participant in one of Babycenter's "birth clubs" happily shared the picture she had received on her phone that day, showing an embryo at five weeks and two days. One of hundreds of thousands of women who have downloaded a pregnancy app, she, like many other women, gave Glow Nurture a rave review.[1]

Other users loved its many logs and prompts for keeping on track with daily vitamins, water intake, exercise, pregnancy symptoms, weight, and doctor appointments. One laughed ruefully, "It may be turning my first pregnancy into a video game where I try to always get 100 percent health each day!" Some particularly liked being able to log symptoms so they could remember to share them with their doctors at appointments.

The logs served multiple purposes. In addition to maintaining a health record, they allowed women to record their thoughts and feelings. One woman was excited that the app could compile the logs for download afterward, noting, "This is an incredible memory for your baby book." For women who use Glow Nurture and other apps and websites like it, pregnancy is intensely monitored, often from its very first moments; users often roll over to Glow Nurture from Glow, a fertility tracker.[2] A pregnancy managed by a prenatal care app entails daily and even hourly requirements to eat, drink, do, and think the right things to keep the pregnancy healthy. The associated reward is equally frequent opportunities to learn and dream about the growing baby.[3]

For twenty-first-century expectant mothers it can feel like a requirement to use one of the many available pregnancy apps. As the Huffington Post editorialized,

> For most first-time expectant moms, there's nothing more thrilling than tracking baby's development (that's why your Facebook news feed has at least one fetus-compared-to-fruit status a week). But pregnancy apps are about more than just pregnancy trivia and measuring babies against kiwis and cantaloupes. They can be important tools for maintaining a healthy pregnancy, too.[4]

The Huffington Post highlighted ten apps that it approved for their detailed medical advice, cute interfaces, and logging possibilities that ran the gamut from integrating self-monitoring with physicians' records to baby-bump photo timelines.

Contemporary pregnancy is full of health dos and don'ts, doctor appointments, and science lessons on embryonic development. Most people assume that pregnancy is a medical condition, or at least a unique bodily experience requiring professional medical care. Women are supposed to be constantly self-conscious about their pregnancies so that they take care of themselves, and especially their developing babies, to the standards of modern scientific medicine. How did pregnancy come to be regarded as an exceptional health challenge, requiring constant self-monitoring and regular medical attention?[5]

EMPHASIZING MOTHERING OVER MAKING BABIES IN THE NEW REPUBLIC

Attitudes toward the physical demands of pregnancy began to alter noticeably around the time of the American Revolution, as beliefs about the role of mothers began to change. In the colonial period, pregnancy had been seen as a natural and routine, if uncomfortable, part of a woman's fertility cycle through much of her adult life. In the new republic producing babies was to be only part of women's role in society and not, perhaps, the part held in the highest esteem. The revolutionary generation emphasized women's minds, morals, and rationality over their bodily accomplishments. Women would do their part to build the country by educating its children into a citizenry capable of exercising self-determination.[6]

As patriarchal family norms softened, mothers took on much of the moral and practical authority that had previously been reserved for fathers and focused their attention more on the intellectual than on the physical aspects of parenting. In 1815, eighteen-year-old Mehitable May Dawes wrote enthusiastically in her diary about new proposals for women's education. "What an important sphere a woman fills! . . . [H]ow thoroughly she ought to be qualified for it." Dawes, who would go on to have six children, believed that mothers shaped the world by virtue of the education they gave their children, especially their sons. "All men feel so grand and boast so much . . . If their mothers had not taken such good care of them when they were babies, and instilled good principles into them as they grew up, what think you would have become of the mighty animals—oh every man of sense must humbly bow before woman."[7] Mehitable and her peers still focused their energy on family life, but they glorified the intellectual endeavor of childrearing more than the physical efforts of pregnancy, birth, and breastfeeding.

The religious renewal of the Second Great Awakening also helped push Americans to redefine mothers as educators rather than as baby makers. Pastors who led the religious revival of the late eighteenth and early nineteenth century realized that the devoted women who dominated their congregations were their primary audience. The archetypal woman in their sermons was no longer Eve, the sexual temptress consigned to bring forth children in pain as a permanent reminder of mankind's proclivity to sin and fall away from God, redeemed only through the repeated suffering and mortal risk of labor.[8] Instead, pastors emphasized the role of Christianity in raising people out of the natural condition of bestiality and regarded women as especially capable of reaching new heights of moral purity and serving as models for male kin. Many women embraced this new view of women's nature, satisfied to accept the novel idea that women could be "passionless," able to escape sensuality in favor of an elevated moral and spiritual sensibility.[9] In this new theology, sex, pregnancy, and childbirth no longer defined the essential nature of women.

As the physical act of childbearing was made less central to women's identity, women were less willing to take its burdens for granted. One response was to try and exercise some control over the number of births a woman would endure in her lifetime. Extended breastfeeding, male "continence" or withdrawal, and various folk remedies for preventing pregnancies came to seem more appealing and more reasonable.

A second response was to complain about the outsized physical toll pregnancies and births took on a woman's health, and potentially her life. Pregnant women and their husbands began to use the terms "unwell," "sick," and "indisposed" as euphemisms for pregnancy, rather than the earlier terminology of "teeming," "breeding," "lusty," and "thriving."[10] Some explicitly regarded non-pregnancy as a state of good health.[11] In letters and diaries, eighteenth-century stoicism gave way to dramatic expressions of fear and anguish. One New Year's Eve in the 1820s, a pregnant Sidney Carr wrote to her sister, "Oh my dear Jane how can I ever get through[!] I feel as the time approaches that I would rather die than bear so much pain. What a fool a girl is ever to get married, if I should be so fortunate as to have a daughter my first lesson to her shall be to despise everything that wears breeches." In 1812, Ann Barraud, the wife of a Virginia physician, wrote to her friend Ann Cocke about her worry for a mutual friend. She was "in a very gloomy state of Mind. . . she expects the birth of her child will put a period to her existence as her constitution is far too exhausted to bear the distresst state to which she is exposed in childbirth."[12] Even at a time when women could still expect to have many pregnancies, they were beginning to regard pregnancy as a time of exceptional danger and distress, and to see non-pregnancy as a baseline healthy state rather than a state of unaccustomed infertility.[13]

DOCTORS IN THE BIRTH ROOM

As the physical demands of childbearing came to be seen as an exceptional challenge to a woman's health, women began looking to physicians for care. It happened first with regard to birth. During the nineteenth century, middle-class women increasingly sent their husbands to fetch the doctor rather than the midwife when they went into labor. In earlier centuries, physicians were only called to births when they had gone disastrously awry. They had been charged with the gruesome task of dismembering an irremediably stuck (and usually stillborn) baby to extract it or desperately attempting to halt a life-threatening hemorrhage. As women increasingly saw pregnancy as an illness and birth as a health crisis, those who could afford doctors began to see them as the best attendants at normal births.

If a woman and her family called the doctor, he would be immediately available in case of emergency, and he would bring with him a host of tools meant to speed and ease labor. Doctors brought ergot to stimulate contractions, opium to mask the pain, and forceps to pull the baby through the birth canal. In hindsight, it is clear that physicians did at least as much harm as good with their interventions and brought far more of the bacteria that caused deadly puerperal fever into birth rooms. In most times and places, wealthier women have safer births, but in the nineteenth century, women who could afford to hire doctors died at a higher rate than their poorer sisters. Nonetheless, women inclined to see childbirth as a health crisis turned with hope to physicians as a source of authority and assistance.[14]

By the 1850s, physicians also brought with them a groundbreaking innovation: anesthesia to dramatically reduce the pain of labor. It was not without controversy. Many physicians felt pressured by their patients to provide chloroform or ether but were nervous that it might not be safe. After all, in large doses it could suppress respiration to the point of death. Arguing against anesthesia, a few physicians made the religious claim that God had decreed that women were to suffer in childbirth, but that view was mostly seen as old fashioned and misguided. A few others made a novel argument about the benefit of pain, claiming that a child brought forth with much suffering and sacrifice would be all the more precious to its mother. On the other side, arguing in favor of anesthesia, some doctors claimed that middle-class women had become so high strung and delicate that their nerves would be wrecked by the pain of birth. Others who were dismayed at the falling birth rates of middle-class women hoped that pain-free birth would encourage them to have plenty of children. Those commentators had misread the situation: in fact, women were beginning to regard childbearing as an exceptional burden even aside from the pain of labor, and the use of anesthesia during labor contributed to the common view that birth was a health crisis one wouldn't want to repeat more times than absolutely necessary.[15]

Physicians were pleased to attend normal births as a way to build up their practices. Women were generally in charge of medical care for their entire family, and if a woman liked the doctor who attended her birth, she was likely to hire him the next time a family member was ill enough to need a physician. Doctors were happy to encourage the idea that they were more qualified than midwives and by the later decades of the nineteenth century were actively campaigning to remove midwives from the birth room. Bringing physicians into the birth room raised concerns about modesty and propriety at a time remembered for an exaggerated sense of decorum and prudery. Obstetric textbooks showed doctors how to manually examine a patient while reaching under her skirts, with the idea that touching was less voyeuristic than looking. Women and their husbands were willing to deal with male doctors despite their reservations because of the medical benefit they expected from a doctor's presence.[16] A new definition of modesty would have to be based on the formalized expectations of the doctor-patient relationship.

While birthing women still often asked female relatives or friends to assist them at their births, the communal aspects of the birth room had gradually been dwindling since around the time of the American Revolution. A smaller group gathered, and instead of celebrating the baby's emergence with a "groaning party" hosted by the birthing woman and her family, female friends and relatives made quiet visits to greet the baby once the mother was ready to "sit up," a week or two after the birth.[17] As Americans became more likely to move away from their extended families, they were less likely to have female friends and relatives to call to a birth.[18] The communal female birth ritual of old was being displaced by a medical ritual. Middle-class families developed an expectation of privacy and propriety based on the physician-patient relationship rather than the traditional community of women.[19]

In the last decades of the nineteenth century, not just birth but pregnancy too was increasingly sheltered within the private space of home and family. Victorian prudery had become so exaggerated that some medical writers asserted that "good" women were free of sexual desire and only wanted sex in order to have children. Anything to do with the body was a source of shame, especially if it was connected to sex. Women began to feel that they should not be visibly pregnant in public. Since at that point many middle-class women had only a few children, it was not entirely impractical to hide for the last few months of each pregnancy. It was a far cry from the colonial era's matter-of-fact acknowledgment of pregnancy. Children could be told that the stork brought babies, and as far as anyone outside a woman's immediate family could tell, it might as well have been true. As a result, pregnancy came to seem like an even more exceptional state of being.[20]

NINETEENTH-CENTURY PREGNANCY ADVICE MANUALS

In the late nineteenth century, too, some medical writers began to encourage women to see pregnancy as a stage of life that required special medical and scientific knowledge to handle correctly. A blossoming genre of advice literature, intended for mothers to give to their daughters to educate them as they embarked on married life, was authored mostly by physicians, many of them women. It was premised on the assumption that middle-class women, increasingly protected from vulgarity by Victorian mores, might know none of the "facts of life" before marriage. So the books combined sex education, moral admonishment, pregnancy and birth preparation, and baby-care advice.

It can be both surprising and discomfiting to read these manuals from a twenty-first-century perspective. These books had none of the warm and reassuring tones of the late-twentieth-century bestseller *What to Expect When You're Expecting*.[21] Some of them began with a diatribe against abortion and a strict warning to the reader that abortions were dangerous, unnatural, immoral, and illegal. Just at the turn of the century, Mrs. Emma Drake, MD, in *What a Young Wife Ought to Know*, scolded mothers for teaching their married daughters how to abort and pleaded, "Shall we teach our daughters that the institution of marriage is for home and children, and that unless they are prepared to make the home and desire children, they are committing a grievous sin by entering its sacred portals?"[22] Elizabeth Scovil, associate editor of the *Ladies' Home Journal*, told her reader (incorrectly) that from conception, abortion was considered murder and punishable by death in some states.[23]

In those decades, physicians were feeling the stress of being caught between new laws criminalizing abortion and their patients' frequent requests for help. Women physicians could be especially harsh and indignant, as they were tired of being mistaken for the euphemized "women doctors" who advertised in the backs of newspapers their services in "restoring menstrual cycles."[24] Advice book authors told women in no uncertain terms that it was their responsibility to care for the developing babies in their wombs, not destroy them.[25]

These authors assumed, probably correctly, that many women of the late nineteenth century had inherited an attitude of carelessness and fatalism toward their pregnancies, especially in their early months. Despite a century of advice literature encouraging women to take precautions to protect their pregnancies, a proactive approach had yet to become mainstream. Historian Shannon Withycombe has shown, based on a close examination of women's letters and diaries and cases that physicians reported in medical journals, that nineteenth-century women who miscarried did not express guilt or responsibility, even if they might be able to pinpoint a likely trigger that they believed precipitated the miscarriage. Neither did they describe making any special efforts to try to care for their pregnancies as the books instructed. Rather, early miscarriages were often welcomed as a crucial piece of the contraceptive puzzle, a natural and accepted way to keep overall childbearing low.[26]

The tone of the nineteenth-century advice literature set certain precedents for the genre as it evolved. Most crucially, it told middle-class women that they could produce healthy babies if they did the right things during pregnancy. In its most basic form, this meant not trying to have a miscarriage or procure an abortion, but it was elaborated to include a broad array of positive steps to take. Some authors named this "prenatal culture." A pregnant woman should take care to adjust her activities to avoid all potential causes of harm and create opportunities for positive exposures to elevate the physical and moral constitution of her unborn child.[27] Women were held responsible for the health of their pregnancies, and in a time of high abortion rates, when a pregnancy failed, the pregnant woman was suspected of sabotaging it.

In addition, pregnancy advice authors began to describe embryonic and fetal development in detail and expected pregnant women to take an interest in it. Physician-authors believed that exciting developments in embryology deserved rapt attention from a middle class increasingly fascinated by all things scientific and eager to embrace a scientific modernity. The new science of human embryology had gained great momentum during the nineteenth century. Physicians had begun to collect miscarried human specimens from women's bedsides to display at medical meetings and write about in medical journals. They no longer regarded miscarried bits of flesh and gushes of blood as evidence of "moles" and uterine mistakes but searched them for evidence of tiny expelled embryos and enthusiastically shared their findings. Sketches of embryos were published in biological and medical textbooks and journals and also made their way into educational books for laypeople.[28]

Authors compared human embryos to insects and gave dry, scientific descriptions. Illustrations often depicted tadpoles and chicken embryos, because they were more readily available for study than human embryos. For example, in his 1873 treatise for laypeople, *Esoteric Anthropology*, Dr. Thomas Nichols illustrated fish and chicken embryos and described them at length, before turning to the human embryo. "On the thirteenth day the embryo is as large as a horse-fly, and resembles a worm bent together. There are as yet no limbs, and the head is larger than the rest of the body. When stretched out, the embryo is nearly half an inch long." Dr. Alice Stockham, in her 1887 *Tokology*, reiterated these insect and worm metaphors. Dr. Seth Pancoast's 1865 *Ladies' Medical Guide* contained more illustrations of fully formed fetuses, yet they were alien looking and skinny, far from anything we would be inclined to call "cute" (see Figure 4.1). Still, women were supposed to take from these scientific developmental narratives the lesson that this was a baby inside from the beginning, not simply a blob of congealing fluids or, as earlier medical theory metaphorically described it, the curdling of menstrual blood by the addition of semen.[29]

These two characteristics of nineteenth-century pregnancy advice—the idea that women could proactively prevent problems and ensure healthy babies through their behavior, and the fetal development timeline as an anchor for understanding pregnancy—would be preserved even as the tone of the pregnancy advice literature changed dramatically.

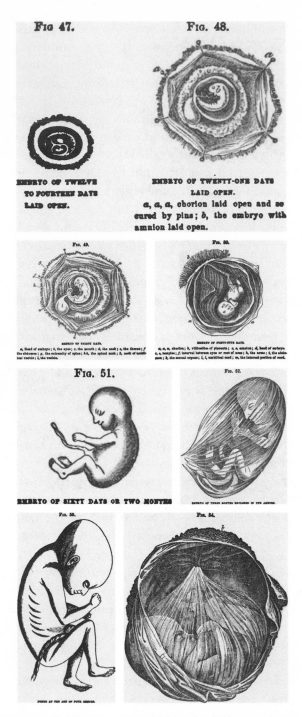

Figure. 4.1 Sketches of embryonic development from Dr. Seth Pancoast's 1865 *Ladies' Medical Guide*.

PREGNANCY GOES MODERN (EVENTUALLY)

Late Victorian mores around pregnancy were remarkably persistent in the first decades of the twentieth century. Women felt ashamed to be seen pregnant and hid at home if they could. They fretted about the pain and danger of birth and justifiably so: while infant and child mortality dropped substantially in the decades surrounding the turn of the century, mothers continued to die during and after birth at alarming rates, and newborn mortality rates remained high. The risks of childbearing seemed more pronounced at a time when Americans were generally becoming healthier and living longer. The World War I generation compared mothers to soldiers, ready to lay down their lives for a noble cause.[30]

When women did talk with each other in private about pregnancy, they often told "war stories" to match the men's. While surely some advice was practical and reassuring, "childbirth gone wrong" was a popular genre. Experienced mothers spoke of blood, pain, and death as well as heroism, miracles, suffering, and, above all, personal sacrifice. Women commiserated with each other and brought young women pregnant for the first time into the private society of women's talk, filled with gossip, one-upsmanship, and camaraderie. Young women learned about pregnancy from the personal stories and traditions passed down by female relatives, friends, and neighbors. It would have been hard not to be fully (and frighteningly) aware of all that could potentially go awry.[31]

Through the 1910s, women were assumed to be caring for themselves and their pregnancies without direct medical supervision up until the birth, and the advice literature rarely recommended earlier doctor's care. Obstetrical textbooks listed many reasons why a woman might consult a doctor, but preventive care was not one of them. The Children's Bureau's first *Prenatal Care* pamphlet, published in 1913, did recommend that women engage a doctor and send urine samples to the doctor to be tested for albumin throughout the pregnancy. But it conceded that the doctor "may have very little to do beyond giving advice and making the routine examinations of the urine."[32] A 1920 Lydia Pinkham pamphlet, distributed in conjunction with her eponymous patent medicine, perhaps gives a more realistic sense of what women might do: the extent of prenatal care Pinkham recommended was sending a urine sample to the doctor in the last months of pregnancy should symptoms of toxemia (now called preeclampsia) arise.[33] This would soon change, between medical advances that made some prenatal care more effective, and ebullient, overcharged optimism that prenatal care could prevent most maternal and infant mortality if women were supervised closely enough.

THE MODEL OF A MODERN PREGNANCY

A new crop of advice books imbued pregnancy with the can-do spirit of the 1920s. Women were told to be optimistic, proactive, and modern. They were to embrace science and medicine and to regard the doctor as their guide, rejecting tradition and superstition. They were also supposed to be matter-of-fact and frank about pregnancy, dispensing with Victorian prudery and embracing dressing in cute maternity clothes rather than hiding at home. Pregnancy was back in the public eye.

In 1922, Carolyn Conant Van Blarcom, a respected expert in obstet-rical nursing, simultaneously published a popular pregnancy guide, *Getting Ready to be a Mother* and a textbook, *Obstetric Nursing*.[34] She was determined to set a new tone and a new standard for prenatal care. Her guide gained a popular readership and was reprinted in ten editions through the 1940s. Van Blarcom, alongside her medical and public health colleagues who made similar efforts, launched a new way of conceptualizing pregnancy.

Van Blarcom's work was part of a larger movement for maternity care reform, which began as a Progressive cause in the 1910s and blossomed in the 1920s. Progressive reformers began to imagine a more proactive, op-timistic, and modern way for all women to handle pregnancy. Unlike their nineteenth-century middle-class predecessors, they did not regard their middle-class habits as valued markers of distinction, but instead wanted to spread middle-class habits and values to everyone.[35] When it came to maternity care, they were convinced that women would have safer and healthier pregnancies and births if they rejected tradition and supersti-tion, had their medical issues addressed by a doctor during pregnancy, and better educated themselves about self-care.

In the first pages of *Getting Ready to be a Mother*, Van Blarcom asked her reader to choose sides. "How does it seem to you—the coming of a baby? Does it seem the most amazing of miracles, so stirring in its beauty and mystery that you are eager to make ready and prepare for it fitly? Or have you, perhaps, come to share the general feeling that motherhood is a nat-ural state which one accepts when it comes, but need not prepare for?"[36] Since her reader had purchased a pregnancy manual, the right answer was obvious. Van Blarcom nevertheless elaborated. She acknowledged that she was arguing against "a very old and deeply rooted conviction that, as women always have had babies and have had them through the working of one of Nature's laws that has been operating over and over throughout the ages, they doubtless will continue to have them in the same old way, and the entire matter may well be left to take care of itself." Van Blarcom blamed too-frequent dire outcomes on this traditional fatalism and on the custom of waiting until labor to call the doctor. "All too often the mother has died, because of this tardy care, been injured or become an invalid, while equally sad things have happened to the baby—and needlessly so." Van Blarcom promised that medicine was poised to save the day. "[N]ow, happily, a great change is taking place in the realm of mothers and babies . . . [W]omen are more and more generally seeking and being given 'prenatal care,' which is care before the baby is born, together with advice and instructions which fit them to assume motherhood safely and successfully."[37]

Van Blarcom carefully described the pregnant role models she wanted her reader to emulate:

> Many women, nowadays . . . begin by consulting a doctor as soon as they know that they are pregnant, because they appreciate the importance of doing so. They study eagerly the questions relating to motherhood; the structure and workings of those parts of their own bodies which are concerned with the baby's creation; how he evolves within them; what he needs during those nine months of development; what practices, what conditions are bad for the baby and themselves; what they can do to avoid or correct these and how they can help to make things go smoothly.

She concluded that "the women who face the facts of motherhood in this way generally go through the entire adventure normally and successfully, as Nature intended they should." Van Blarcom's book was arranged to support each of these aspects of a conscientious pregnancy.[38]

Van Blarcom gave her reader strict instructions on who she must and must not consult for pregnancy advice. The doctor was to guide the process from start to finish, aided, perhaps, by the wisdom of a medically sanctioned advice book. Mothers and mothers-in-law were worse than useless, with their war stories and their traditions; they sabotaged the doctor's best efforts. "One factor which keeps some expectant mothers from seeking medical care is the well meaning but dangerous counsel so freely offered by older women who claim fitness to advise by virtue of having had several children of their own. Their lack of success, as evidenced by miscarriages, stillbirths, children dying in early infancy, as well as injuries and disabilities of their own, is usually overlooked as they press their superstitions and remedies upon the inexperienced and bewildered younger woman. When disaster follows, as it so often does, it is very likely to be ascribed to the will of God, and the mother's needless sacrifice does not even serve as a warning to others who are in line for the same kind of advice."[39] Van Blarcom was so sure that scientific medicine could remedy all ills that she blamed the older generation for their own reproductive tragedies, suppressed realistic warnings about what could go wrong, and disavowed any attitude of fatalism or acceptance.[40]

Surprisingly, given her grand rhetoric, Van Blarcom could offer only a few modern medical innovations. The most important and effective innovation was a treatment for syphilis. Syphilis caused many stillbirths and grave illness in children born with it. The arsenic-based compound Salvarsan, introduced in 1909, could cure syphilis in a pregnant woman and prevent congenital syphilis in her baby.[41] This was indeed the kind of miracle medicine Van Blarcom promised, but the stigma of sexually transmitted diseases meant that she could not directly discuss it.[42] But a blood test at the kind of early prenatal care check-up Van Blarcom advocated would have been checked for syphilis, and treatment could be started right away.

Most of Van Blarcom's advice was aimed at preventing convulsions, the term then used for eclampsia. Often fatal for mother and baby alike, convulsions were one of the most common and feared of the serious complications of pregnancy. Then called "toxemia" in the medical literature, it was believed to be caused by the buildup of toxins in the body at a time when the body's systems of elimination were working overtime. Accordingly, Van Blarcom gave a great deal of dietary advice focused on preventing and relieving constipation and indigestion, and she urged women to drink plenty of water, allow their skin to breathe, and take baths to wash away perspiration. If toxemia was caused by a gradual buildup of toxins, then a woman should make sure that all her small daily habits were promoting their release. Van Blarcom also wanted women to go to the doctor for regular check-ups because modern medicine had shown that protein in a woman's urine was a signal of the beginning of preeclampsia. She assured her reader that "after looking over the records of many thousands of mothers who have had prenatal care, it seems almost safe to say that the expectant mother who follows such a course [of studiously following Van Blarcom's regimen and consulting a doctor] will not have convulsions."[43]

In this case, Van Blarcom's faith in modern medicine far outstripped the reality, as the only effective way to treat preeclampsia is to deliver the baby.[44] Van Blarcom believed that her and her physician-colleagues' treatment of preeclampsia was successful. She must have explained away cases that resulted in full-blown eclampsia, discounting evidence that would have thrown doubt on her prescribed regimen. Perhaps, too, Van Blarcom presented what she knew was an overly optimistic picture because she truly believed that if only women scrupulously followed medical advice, they would all be saved from the sometimes deadly convulsions of pregnancy. Perhaps she thought that medical advances in detecting preeclampsia meant that doctors had control of the situation. And perhaps she was willing to provide a bit more reassurance than the situation justified because she believed that pregnant women fared best when they anticipated a good outcome.

Like today's pregnancy apps, the regimen Van Blarcom prescribed laid out schedules for meals, sleep, and exercise, and insisted that these must be carried out precisely to give baby and mother the best chance at good health. Yet, unlike the alerts pinging from pregnancy apps, those details were supposed to become quickly absorbed and ingrained as unconscious habits. She advised her reader to "try to forget that you are pregnant, so far as you can do this and still remember to take proper care of yourself." Thinking about it too much led to dwelling on the potential complications, which then carried its own risks. "Above all, don't worry. Worry will interfere with your sleep and it will also upset your digestion quite as seriously as will wrong food." It was a tricky balancing act she expected from pregnant women. "Try not to be too self-centered or too watchful of your symptoms, but at the same time avoid the dangerous habit of thinking that any unusual condition which develops is due to your being pregnant, for a sick pregnancy is not normal." Van Blarcom's long and minute list of dos and don'ts laid the initial groundwork for intensive monitoring of pregnancy.[45]

When it came to miscarriage, as with eclampsia, Van Blarcom promised far more than she could deliver. She explained, correctly, to her reader that "at least one out of every five pregnancies ends in abortion [i.e. miscarriage]." But then she claimed that "the tragedy of this [is] that it is very largely a preventable disaster . . . . The prevention of [miscarriages] is of such obvious importance and there is so much that you can do to this end, that we shall take up the question at some length."[46] She gave women a long list of suggestions, all variations on the traditional strictures, including no jolting, no heavy lifting, no sex, no sweeping, no running a foot-pedaled sewing machine, no jumping, no dancing, and no traveling. Her message in her handbook was that a responsible woman would not have a miscarriage.

Yet, in her textbook *Obstetrical Nursing*, Van Blarcom admitted that a large portion of miscarriages were inevitable: "Dr. Mall, of Johns Hopkins University, showed after years of investigation that at least one-third of the embryos obtained from [miscarriages] were malformed and would have developed into monstrosities had they lived to term." She admitted, too, that women might want to know about this finding. "It is often a great comfort to the expectant mother who loses her baby early in pregnancy to realize that had she carried her baby to term it might have been a monster, and that, therefore, she has not lost a beautiful, normal child. Just why these abnormalities occur is not known, nor is there any known method of preventing or correcting them."[47]

Why did Van Blarcom encourage women to blame themselves for their miscarriages when she knew that a substantial portion were due to genetic anomalies? Partly, she seemed to have believed in all the traditional explanations for miscarriage, despite evidence that challenged medical tradition. Long-standing explanations were too deeply ingrained to abandon in one generation, and Van Blarcom and her medical peers would continue to suspect that heavy lifting and sex caused miscarriages. As late as 1970, the fifth edition of Dr. Nicholson Eastman's *Expectant Motherhood* estimated that 80 percent of early miscarriages were due to chromosomal anomalies and yet still suggested that "it would seem prudent for every expectant mother to follow the dictates of common sense and avoid long automobile trips, lifting heavy weights and any form of activity which involves jolting."[48] It would take several more decades for scientists and physicians to fully debunk traditional ideas about why miscarriages happen. These traditional explanations make such intuitive sense that many women still wonder about them when they miscarry. Nonetheless the up-to-date science Van Blarcom cited challenged these traditional views, and she was deeply invested in modern science. Presumably, she did not want to share Dr. Mall's statistic with pregnant women because she believed it would reinforce the sense of fatalism she was trying so hard to change. She was willing to induce undeserved feelings of guilt over miscarriages in order to get women to take their prenatal care seriously.

MODERN PREGNANCIES FOR ALL

Initially, maternity care reformers aimed to bring prenatal care to isolated, struggling farm wives and poor immigrant women living in squalid tenements, because those women and their children were more obviously suffering. Since the 1890s, Progressive organizations such as Hull House in Chicago had provided education and social support in an effort to assimilate the tremendous influx of newcomers into American life. Maternity care reformers shared this goal and likewise tended to assume that scientific rationality and middle-class habits naturally went together. Some studies showed that clinics offering comprehensive prenatal and maternity care had lower maternal and infant mortality rates than their surrounding communities.[49] In the 1920s and 1930s, the Kentucky Frontier Nursing Service provided trained nurse-midwives to poor, isolated farm wives for their prenatal care and home births. Ten times fewer women died under their care than the average rate for the country, a remarkable testament to the value of nursing care.[50] Being delivered by one's local doctor was still a risky prospect, but comprehensive, nursing-based prenatal and maternity care brought improved results.[51]

Even if many of the specific protocols Van Blarcom and her colleagues prescribed were not effective, the overall impact of high-quality prenatal and maternity care was, and continues to be, real. Van Blarcom and her colleagues were also observing a general trend toward better health and longer lives for adults and children alike, beginning in the late nineteenth century and accelerating in the 1920s.[52] From their perspective on the ground in the 1920s, maternity care reformers believed their efforts would quickly bear fruit and were happy to take credit for the improvements they witnessed.

Not everyone was as persuaded as Van Blarcom and her colleagues. Some women felt that the reformers were nosy busybodies who had no business intruding upon something as private as pregnancy. The Maternity Center Association, founded by a group of doctors and New York society women activists in 1918, sent nurses to poor New York neighborhoods to knock on doors and invite pregnant women to attend free prenatal care clinics and classes. Early on, many women simply slammed the door in the nurse's face.[53] From New York to Boston to San Francisco, clinic directors and physicians complained that women refused prenatal care. The Boston Lying In Hospital reported, "We are constantly urging upon our patients the importance of putting themselves under our care early in their pregnancy, but find it difficult to get hold of them much before the fifth and sixth months."[54]

Working-class men were also skeptical. As Van Blarcom complained, they were frequently reluctant to pay for monthly visits to the doctor for their pregnant wives, since they knew their own mothers had delivered their babies without them. Van Blarcom told a story of a farmer whose hogs won a prize at the county fair, but whose baby was a dismal failure in the Better Baby contest. She scolded him for his unwillingness to treat his wife with as much care and respect as the hogs he carefully raised with scientific methods and substantial financial investment. At the end of Van Blarcom's (likely apocryphal) tale, the husband was persuaded to apply modern, scientific methods to human pregnancy as well as to his hogs, and the couple's second baby won the next county fair prize.

Even general practitioners were much less supportive of prenatal care than their obstetrician colleagues. At the 1927 Detroit meeting of the National Medical Association, the dominant medical organization for African American physicians, Dr. Leon Wilson observed that wealthy women received excellent care and destitute women sometimes had access to good care at free prenatal clinics; but woe to the woman who turned to her general doctor to help her through pregnancy and birth. "As a general thing urine analyses are seldom if ever run, blood pressure likewise, and often a simple physical examination not to speak of an obstetrical examination is never made. He is called at labor, rushes there, haphazardly examines the patient, may or may not use gloves, nature helps him and away home he goes. If things do not run smoothly he is very soon at sea, and in an effort to do something, does the wrong thing and the mischief is done."[55] Writing from his experience as a physician in Salt Lake City, Dr. William Hunter complained that even when women received a prompt from their insurance company to seek prenatal care, not much good came of it. "One line italicized in this pamphlet reads: 'The first and most important thing to do, consult a doctor as soon as you know or think that you are pregnant.' When these patients consult some doctors he too often takes the name and address, estimates the date of confinement, and rests on his oars until the time of delivery."[56] Prenatal care was still the province of obstetric specialists and public health clinics in many places, and general practitioners often hewed to tradition.

Still, not every tenement dweller and farm wife resigned herself to bearing whatever came with pregnancy. One Tennessee woman wrote to the Children's Bureau, a federal agency that distributed pamphlets on baby care and pregnancy, to ask for support pushing against the traditional attitudes of her spouse. "My husband does not see any necessity of any extra care of my health now, and says it is only foolishness. So I am quite at a loss to know what to do." Like Van Blarcom, the assistant director of the Children's Bureau, Florence McKay, urged the supplicant to shame her husband by pointing out that he treated the animals better than he treated her. "It is quite important for a mother during pregnancy to have especial care for her health. Farmers realize this in regard to their livestock and it is even more important to the mothers of children."[57] Many women wrote letters to the Children's Bureau begging for advice about how to have a healthy pregnancy and birth and asking for familial and medical assistance.

The most eager adopters of prenatal care were middle-class women who could comfortably afford medical care and were adopting modern styles in everything from bobbed hairdos to Kotex.[58] They filled classes at the Maternity Center Association, bought books like Van Blarcom's, had their babies in hospitals, and saw doctors for regular prenatal check-ups.[59] They buoyed reformers' efforts to remake maternity care into its optimistic modern model and embraced the reformers' message: that pregnancy could be safe, even rewarding and happy, if they trusted the doctor, sought up-to-date science-based care, and listened to the reassuring messages of Van

Blarcom and her colleagues rather than the war stories of their mothers and grandmothers.

Maternity care reformers were pleased to reach middle-class women as much as poor women at a time when many political and intellectual leaders were fretting about demographic shifts that threatened the dominance of white Anglo-Saxon Protestants in America. Leaders nationwide held prejudices against new immigrants from southern Europe and African Americans and wished that middle-class white women would have larger families, not smaller ones. If middle-class women could be convinced that pregnancy and birth could be made safe, they thought, perhaps they would be willing to return to raising larger families. Whether rich or poor, women would be well-served, reformers believed, by a rational, modern, scientific approach to pregnancy and birth.[60] By the beginning of the postwar baby boom, the modern, middle-class style of pregnancy favored by maternity care reformers would become the aspirational norm.

SENTIMENTAL SCIENCE

A key feature of modern pregnancy manuals was an illustrated chapter about *in utero* development, from conception through birth. While not as elaborate or sentimental as the timelines of today's e-newsletters from WhatToExpect.com or notifications from the Glow Nurture app, they were a far cry from their nineteenth-century predecessors. Typical earlier manuals had included a few dry paragraphs and a picture or two, but the modern manuals beginning in the 1920s were more expansive. Often written in a tone of breathless scientific wonder, development was described in detail as the story of a perfect pregnancy from gametes to baby.[61]

This narrative combining sentiment and science served maternity educators' dual purpose. First, educators believed that scientific knowledge was the key to improving health generally and that the more science education people had, the better they would know how to take care of themselves. Second, as Van Blarcom explained it, "I have given some space to a description of the course of the baby's development in order that his mother might have an abiding sense of his reality and his need of her protecting care from the very moment of his origin."[62] It was not logically obvious that these scientific descriptions would improve medical outcomes or tug at a parent's heartstrings, though. Pregnancy manual authors and modern readers alike had to agree to invest technical descriptions with emotional meaning and regard them as an impetus for care.

Scientific descriptions of development were not directly applicable to prenatal care. A woman would not know any better what to eat, for example, by knowing how the baby grows. Public health pamphlets aimed at the least literate Americans implicitly acknowledged this fact. They left out the science in favor of practical advice, assuming that their readers would be unable or unwilling to follow the technical language.[63] Rather than science having some direct application, authors felt that it made people feel modern, engaged, and in control of their destinies when they shared a scientific understanding of their bodies with their physicians. This engagement was presumed to inspire women and their husbands to trust doctors' advice and adhere to prenatal care guidelines.

Before the 1960s, many women would have encountered pictures and descriptions of embryos for the first time in relation to their own pregnancies. Someone with the right connections might have gained more knowledge as a young person; in her cutesy 1944 pregnancy guide *ABCs for Mothers-to-Be*, Jean Aaberg guessed that

> all of you during some shadowy period of your life have probably been introduced to the wonders of medical books and the full page color plates therein. You had an uncle who was a doctor, or a friend who had such an uncle; and one idle afternoon, sure as anything, you found yourself in possession of the treasure. There were the pictures, month by amazing month, all graphic and lurid; and in them the unborn babies always stood placidly on their heads, and in the face they looked alarmingly like one of the Dead-End Kids.

Medical books were not the only possible source for upper-crust girls: "Even if you had no such furtive experience, you probably had lots of long discussions after the lights were out at boarding school. Or you may have taken an enlightening course in elementary biology."[64]

But those who were not related to doctors or attending boarding school were unlikely to learn the scientific details until they had children, and then only if they took the initiative to buy books about it or ask the doctor for a reproductive anatomy lesson.[65] Even Aaberg was unwilling to completely presume, because "on certain issues there is still a startling amount of misinformation, and the girls still ask their eager questions . . . . It's nice to have at least a sketchy chart of the course you propose to travel."[66]

Modern timelines in pregnancy manuals described development in much more sentimental and human terms than their nineteenth-century predecessors, as part of their effort to teach women that motherly care for a baby ought to begin at conception rather than birth. This required both a new descriptive language and a new attitude toward human development.

Before this shift, embryos, in the view of many authors, appeared almost repulsive and hard to recognize as human. In a description of first trimester development, the 1835 *Home Book of Health and Medicine* had explained that the fertilized

> ovum, as soon as it becomes visible, appears like a small vesicle, attached to some part of the uterus, generally to its upper part; and all the organs of which it consists, seem to be confusedly blended. . . . A foetus of four weeks is nearly the size of a common fly; soft, mucilaginous, and, in appearance, suspended by the belly; its bowels covered by a transparent membrane. At six weeks, it is of a somewhat firmer consistence, nearly the size of a small bee; the extremities then begin to shoot out. At three months, its shape is tolerably distinct, and it is about three inches long.[67]

Later in the century, some health guides drew upon German biologist Ernst Haeckel's idea that embryos had to "recapitulate" the stages of evolution of their species as they developed, rendering early embryos as humans' non-human evolutionary predecessors.[68] Through the nineteenth and early twentieth centuries, medical and scientific authors conveyed a sense of wonder at how something so alien and animal-like could develop into a human being.

In contrast, Van Blarcom, writing in 1922, saw the first-trimester fetus as most certainly a baby, not a fly or a pre-human evolutionary ancestor.

> These different kinds of cells rearrange themselves and grow in such a manner that some of them begin to form the different parts of the baby's body and others develop into two thin membranes that finally enclose the baby in a double sac. He is attached to the inner surface of the sac; the space which he does not occupy is filled with fluid and the sac itself is attached to the uterine lining at the point where the cell mass happened to stop and bury itself. . . . At the end of the second month, or eighth week, his head is fairly well shaped: bones are beginning to develop, webbed hands and feet are formed and the little body is about 1 inch long. At the end of the third month, or twelfth week, his entire body shows marked development and is about 3 1/2 inches long. His fingers and toes are separated and bear soft nails; the teeth are forming, the eyes have lids and the umbilical cord has taken definite form.[69]

A pregnant woman could almost imagine cuddling the tiny baby of Van Blarcom's description. While looking at the same embryonic images as her nineteenth-century predecessors, Van Blarcom focused her description on the ways in which embryos were like babies, instead of the ways they were different.

The Maternity Center Association (MCA) likewise carefully shaped its developmental descriptions to inspire parental care. Describing the first seven weeks of embryonic development, the organization's 1932 *Maternity Handbook* explained, "When the two tiny cells began to grow they did not look much like a baby. There is nothing more wonderful than the way the cells arrange themselves to make the baby's body as they grow from two to four to eight to sixteen and on up into the millions. Each day some new part of the baby's body is being made—and it can't be done over the next day. So every day matters." Pointing to a series of line drawings from twelve days after conception to six and a half weeks' gestation, the author explained, "This is a picture of the baby as he grows for the first few weeks and begins to look like a baby"[70] (see Figure 4.2). The MCA wanted to make sure its clients saw continuity in the developing embryo as a baby, even when the developmental images it provided seemed to belie that description.

For the 1939 World's Fair, the MCA collaborated with respected obstetrician-gynecologist-cum-sculptor Robert Latou Dickinson to create a beautiful display known as the Birth Series. Twenty-four models depicted pregnancy from conception through birth. As historian Rose Holz has observed, Dickinson and his sculptor-collaborator Abram Belskie intended to emotionally move their audience as much as educate them. They created

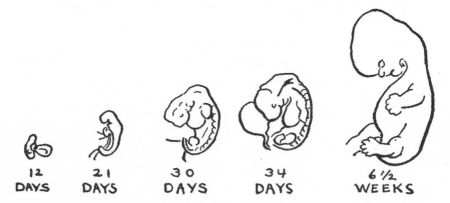

Figure. 4.2 Sketches of embryonic development in the Maternity Center Association's 1932 *Maternity Handbook*: "This is a picture of the baby as he grows for the first few weeks and begins to look like a baby."

aesthetically compelling models out of white plaster, evoking the white marble of Michelangelo's *David*. Their reverence for the creation and development of human life was palpable. (This did not, however, imply a political message about abortion: Dickinson was an activist for birth control and a vocal supporter of abortion rights.) Through his sculptures, Dickinson told a story of human development that combined his Christian religious reverence for humanity, his obsession with accurate and detailed scientific observation, and his appreciation for the aesthetic beauty of human bodies. In Dickinson and Belskie's rendering, the earliest embryos might not be self-evidently babylike, but they were part of a through-told story of the awe-inspiring beauty of human development (see Figure 4.3a and b).[71]

The MCA display, and particularly the Birth Series, was deluged with eager visitors. Critics praised its reverential and informative display at a time when sex education was controversial and often tarred as smut. Hundreds of thousands of visitors filed past the sculptures. Teachers brought their students, and parents brought their children. In the fair's winter months, the sculptures were displayed for many more visitors at the New York Museum of Natural History.[72]

When the fair closed, the MCA reproduced the sculptures for medical centers and museums around the country to be used as teaching tools for physicians and nurses, as well as schoolchildren. The sculptures were also photographed and published in the MCA's *Birth Atlas*, which was distributed even more widely to classes for expectant parents as well as to medical professionals. Versions of the *Birth Atlas* continued to be printed into the 1960s. Select images from it were featured in popular magazines such as *Life* and *Look*, used in advertising, and appeared in pregnancy advice books. The MCA published its own guide for laypeople, *A Baby Is Born: The Picture Story of a Baby from Conception Through Birth*. Dickinson's sculptures appeared in the interior, while an unattributed marble sculpture of a family, with husband, wife, and several babies and toddlers, was featured on the cover and on the final page under the label "A Family Is Born." Dickinson's beautiful, reverent sculptures were the first aestheticized representations of embryonic and fetal development to be widely distributed in the United States, and they shaped Americans' understandings of pregnancy. They told a story of a pregnancy that unfolds perfectly from conception through birth, a continuity of serene images culminating in the birth of a perfect baby.[73]

A few decades later, in 1965, *Life* magazine published Lennart Nilsson's spectacular photographs of embryos and fetuses, floating in gorgeously backlit amniotic sacs. Delicately evocative in a different but equally compelling register, Nilsson's photographs showed the reader the

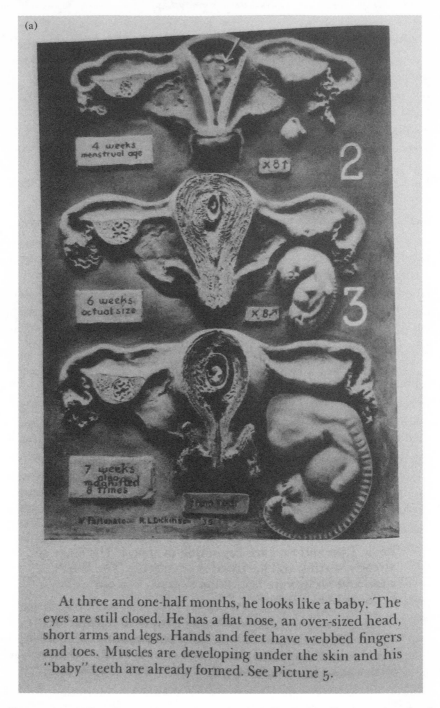

At three and one-half months, he looks like a baby. The eyes are still closed. He has a flat nose, an over-sized head, short arms and legs. Hands and feet have webbed fingers and toes. Muscles are developing under the skin and his "baby" teeth are already formed. See Picture 5.

Figures 4.3a and 4.3b Dr. Robert Latou Dickinson's "birth series" sculptures rendered the developing embryo in three-dimensional elegance. Created for the 1939 World's Fair, they were reproduced and photographed for wide distribution in educational displays and pamphlets, including this one from the Maternity Center Association. *How Does Your Baby Grow?* (New York: Maternity Center Association, 1940). In "Report of The First Year of Life. An Exhibit at the New York World's Fair. 1940," folder 7, box 39, Maternity Center Association Records, Archives & Special Collections, Columbia University Health Sciences Library. Used with permission of the National Partnership for Women & Families.

(b)

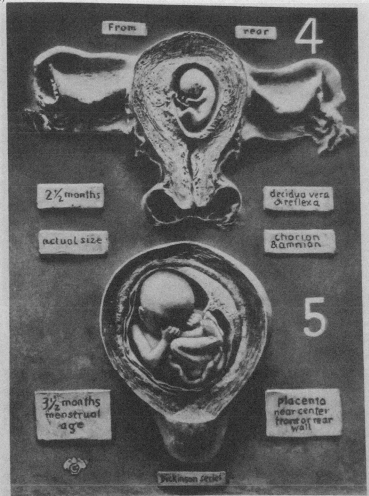

Between 3½ months and 7 months the baby becomes more like the baby you see when born. The mother feels his movements and the doctor hears his heart beat.

By the time the baby is seven months old, he is about 14 inches long and weighs about 2 pounds. He looks like a

Figures 4.3a and 4.3b Continued

semi-transparent tiny hands and feet of specific fetuses. The cover photo was labeled a "living 18-week-old fetus inside its amniotic sac," inviting the reader to imagine this peaceful child, with its eyes closed and hands tucked up under its chin, residing in its mother's womb (see Figure 4.4).[74] The description was disingenuous; while Nilsson took some photos in conjunction with amniocentesis procedures, others were from a clinic where

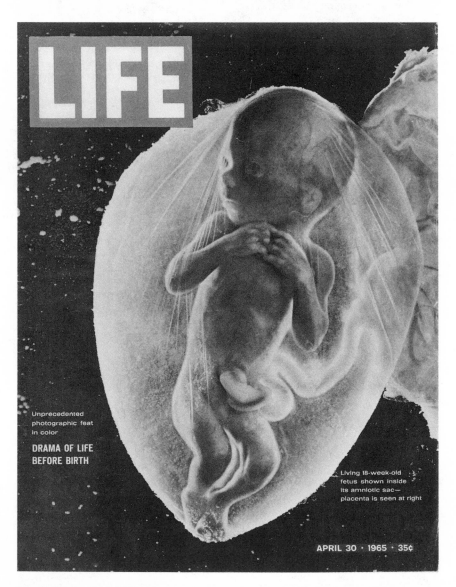

Figure 4.4 April 30, 1965 *Life* magazine cover photographed by Dr. Lennart Nilsson.

women received medically indicated abortions. Most of the embryos and fetuses he photographed would actually have resembled the pickled, jarred specimens that had been featured in educational science displays since the nineteenth century. But for the photographs he rendered the surroundings as black backdrops that could easily be imagined as the dark inside of a woman's body.[75]

Nilsson's photographs were widely re-published and distributed around the world to a fascinated public. *Life* magazine's entire print run of eight million copies was sold out within days.[76] That same year, Nilsson published an educational and advice book called *A Child Is Born*. The book followed a young couple week by week through their pregnancy, with parallel pictures of the developing embryo. Nilsson's Swedish press sold over fifty million copies internationally in multiple languages. These photographs became the iconic images of prenatal development for decades to come. Ironically, many of the embryos and fetuses that would become famous as representation of normal human development were only available to be photographed because they were from pregnancies that would not continue to become full-term babies. Like Dickinson, Nilsson and his publishers scrubbed their developmental timeline free of the complications of real pregnancies and real women's lives, depicting a single, ideal path directly from conception to baby.

In their descriptions of conception and development, advice writers told their readers how to feel about pregnancy through their analogies as much as through their illustrations.[77] In one prominent mid-century guide, Dr. Nicholson Eastman's *Expectant Motherhood*, sperm were described as if they were an aggressive horde of princes in a biologic fairy tale, competing in a dangerous quest that only one would complete with triumphal ravishment. "Although many million spermatozoa die in the vagina as the result of the acid secretion there, myriads survive, penetrate the neck of the uterus and swarm upward through the uterine cavity and into the Fallopian tube. There they lie in wait for the ovum." In the end, all but one of these "suitors" would die.[78] Only one could penetrate the ovum. After that came the happily-ever-after honeymoon voyage. It was a "leisurely sojourn" for the fertilized egg, whose "timing has been precisely correct; the bed is prepared and the ovum has so developed that it is now ready to dig into that bed."[79] Eastman's description was romantically appealing, but misleading. Given the large proportion of fertilized eggs that never implant, it would have been more accurate for Eastman to have extended his analogy of a perilous quest until quite a bit later in development.[80]

OPTIMISM AND VIGILANCE

During the baby boom of the 1940s and 1950s, Americans enjoyed a couple of decades of sanguine optimism about their prospects for happy and healthy pregnancies and births. The maternal mortality rate finally began to drop noticeably in the late 1930s, and the 1940s saw the diffusion of major medical breakthroughs critical to maternity care. Blood transfusion could save a woman who hemorrhaged during birth, and the drug ergometrine could contract the uterus to prevent hemorrhage. Antibiotics were crucial in combating deadly postpartum infections. At long last, women had a much better chance of surviving childbearing than had their grandmothers.[81]

Cultural expectations around pregnancy shifted noticeably. Women no longer compared themselves to soldiers but adopted a cheerful modern outlook on pregnancy. Women wanted childbearing to be fulfilling right from conception. Abandoning the traditional sensibility of cautious foreboding associated with pregnancy, women and their families and friends set a new standard for pregnancy as a happy time, leading to the joyful welcoming of a healthy baby.[82] While surely some pregnant women worried and wondered, it was no longer acceptable to express too much ambivalence. During the 1950s baby boomers' parents set a new expectation for happy pregnancy, a standard that has persisted.

That baby boom happiness was not to continue unmarred, however.

At the same time that Nilsson published his spectacular and intimate full-color pictures of embryos and fetuses in *Life* magazine in 1965, American women were coping with a devastating and well-publicized epidemic of rubella, also known as German measles. Rubella caused miscarriages, infant deaths, blindness, deafness, heart malformations, and mental retardation.[83] If a woman contracted rubella in her first weeks of pregnancy, her child had a 50 percent chance of being affected.[84] The only "remedy" was an abortion.

Americans reacted with alarm to the news of rubella because they had been primed by news of the damage done by thalidomide, a drug prescribed in Europe as a supposedly innocuous sleep aide. Thalidomide caused babies to be born with short, flipper-like limbs for arms and legs, and Americans had seen widely circulated pictures of babies born with these visible birth defects. The drug had not been approved in the United States, so Americans were largely protected from the direct impact of its unexpected side effects. But they learned that babies could be harmed by seemingly innocuous exposures at a critical stage of early pregnancy.[85] Women were still expected to be happy during pregnancy, but with the recognition of the dangers of rubella and thalidomide, they were also supposed to be vigilant against threats they could not easily predict or control.

Recognition of prenatal dangers continued to increase. In 1971, news broke that diethylstilbestrol (DES), a drug prescribed since the 1950s to prevent miscarriage, was not just ineffective but dangerous. It caused unusual cancers and reproductive tract damage in young women who had been exposed in the womb. Research on alcohol exposure during pregnancy led to a 1973 consensus on the diagnosis of fetal alcohol syndrome. Evidence of the dangers of cigarette smoking in pregnancy, accumulating since the late 1950s, finally led to the 1985 Surgeon General's Warnings that smoking "May Complicate Pregnancy" and that "Smoking by Pregnant Women May Result in Fetal Injury, Premature Birth and Low Birth Weight."[86] Women needed to worry about prescription drugs, alcohol, cigarettes, and infectious diseases. The placental barrier was clearly more porous than earlier researchers had realized. What other dangers might be lurking?

In the 1980s, concern about prenatal exposures and the uterine environment soared. Pregnant women came to be seen increasingly in terms of the threat they posed to their expected children's well-being. Physicians and the public became alarmed about the crack cocaine epidemic and what was widely assumed to be the damaging impact of the drug on so-called crack babies. In some locales, law enforcement began to charge pregnant women with prenatal child abuse. The punishment of cocaine-addicted mothers soon extended to alcoholic mothers. Women were seen as possible or likely adversaries of their expected children and often punished rather than treated for their addiction.[87] In 1980 the Food and Drug Administration issued a warning that caffeine might cause birth defects and recommended that pregnant women avoid coffee and soda.[88] While the science behind the recommendation quickly came under question, pregnant women found themselves publicly censured for drinking coffee.[89]

Public health efforts in the 1980s and 1990s increasingly sought to leverage individuals' choices to improve health on a population scale, emphasizing personal responsibility rather than communal solutions such as political action to clean up health hazards in the environment.[90] Messages aimed at reforming the behavior of pregnant women often tried to persuade women by implying that those who failed to comply with mainstream prenatal care were unloving mothers. For example, the March of Dimes, a nonprofit organization committed to preventing birth defects and promoting good birth outcomes, ran "Healthy Baby Week" campaigns to encourage women to take better care of their unborn children. One March of Dimes public service announcement that played on the radio in 1983 instructed, "If you're pregnant, show you care with early and regular prenatal care. It's the kind of love your baby needs right now. Please, don't take chances with that little life that depends upon you. See a doctor now and follow medical advice." The message implied that a woman who did not seek early prenatal care was demonstrating that she didn't love her baby. Another March of Dimes radio message urged, "Babies don't thrive in smoke-filled wombs. . . . If you're pregnant—picture a tiny baby puffing away the next time you reach for a cigarette. Your unborn baby will thank you."[91] Mother love and guilt harnessed to individual responsibility and initiative were supposed to produce better birth outcomes across the nation.

One of the caring actions pregnant women learned to take during pregnancy was swallowing a daily folic acid supplement. Folic acid had long been recognized as a treatment for macrocytic anemia during pregnancy, which was sometimes deadly to women who were malnourished. In the 1980s, researchers hunting for magic-bullet solutions to birth defects discovered that folic acid also helped to prevent neural tube defects such as spina bifida in babies. Public health organizations ran publicity campaigns to urge doctors to prescribe folic acid to their pregnant patients and recommended that women of childbearing age take a daily folic acid supplement just in case. Folic acid is effective only if taken very early: a month before conception, to build the woman's bodily store of the substance, and during the first weeks of pregnancy, a stage when many women do not yet know they are pregnant. In 1994 the United States added folic acid to the grain supply to try and ensure that women would not be folate-deficient when they got pregnant. The generalized supplementation reduced neural tube defects by 19 percent, but the March of Dimes estimated that if every woman of childbearing age took a supplement, defects could be reduced by 70 percent. In 1999–2001, the organization ran a comprehensive publicity campaign to teach women and their doctors that every woman of childbearing age, regardless of whether she was planning a pregnancy, should take a daily folic acid supplement. This magic bullet cure was cheap and easy to distribute, but it only worked if a woman incorporated it into her pregnancy plans from the very beginning, ideally before conception.[92]

The concern about the uterine environment extended far beyond avoiding specific dangerous substances and taking a prenatal vitamin. Women were increasingly urged to do their best to perfect the uterine environment, not just to avoid a few specific dangers and follow their doctors' advice. Fetal alcohol syndrome was not well understood, but the consensus was that it was better to be safe than sorry: the public health message was that no amount of alcohol was known to be safe during pregnancy and therefore not a single drop should be swallowed.[93] Women worried themselves sick over a few drinks imbibed before they got positive pregnancy test results.

The list of specific hazards grew longer, and the bad outcomes they might cause were increasingly rare. Don't change the kitty litter, don't eat unpasteurized cheese, avoid sushi, heat your lunchmeat until it is steaming. In 1984 *What to Expect When You're Expecting* introduced the "Best Odds Diet," with the principle that "you've got only nine months of meals and snacks with which to give your baby the best possible start in life. Make every one of them count. Before you close your mouth on a forkful of food, consider, 'Is this the best I can give my baby?' "[94] The standard of good prenatal mothering was perfection.

The idea that every choice a pregnant woman made affected her baby, combined with a punitive and adversarial attitude toward pregnant women, resulted in a widespread attitude that pregnant women were appropriate targets of demeaning free advice and shaming. The pressure on pregnant women was already oppressive by the mid-1980s, well before the deluge of public health campaigns and advice literature of the 1990s. Writing in *Glamour* in 1984, commentator Sue Mittenthal described her experience of "the propaganda expectant mothers are battered with today. They're warned to refuse so much as a sip of wine during pregnancy and urged to resist even the mildest dose of painkiller during labor out of panic that the drug will leave mother and baby too groggy to begin bonding instants after birth." As critical as Mittenthal was of absolutist and unrealistic rules for pregnant women, it could be hard to resist. "I find this fanaticism appalling, yet somehow infectious; it's hard to live with the thought that you might not be doing all you possibly can for your baby."[95] Plenty of advice-givers were happy to promote pregnant women's fanaticism, at considerable expense to the pregnant woman's mental state, if they thought it would be in the best interest of the expected child.

A substantial portion of the public still sometimes reacted to public health messages with skepticism or fatalism, to the dismay of public health organizations, which continued to press people to take all threats to pregnancies seriously. In 1997, the March of Dimes commissioned a "Brand Identity Development" study to try and understand why its messages did not seem to energize more people, perhaps especially donors, to take action to improve pregnancy outcomes. The study concluded that too many women were complacent because they did not expect rare bad outcomes to actually happen to them; they were distracted by more immediately pressing concerns such as housing and job security; they were fatalistic, believing there was not much they could do to prevent them; or they were so frightened by the possibility of a child with a birth defect that they were in denial altogether. The report concluded that the March of Dimes needed more messages that conveyed both urgency and reassurance: urgency in addressing all possible causes of poor birth outcomes, and reassurance that with earnest effort, poor birth outcomes truly could be prevented. The problem with this approach was that while the interventions recommended by the March of Dimes prevented some percentage of poor outcomes, the public was right that in many cases the pregnant woman did not have control over her and her child's fate, no matter how urgently she acted to protect her pregnancy.[96]

PREGNANCY ADVICE IN REAL TIME

Over the last couple of decades, websites and smartphone apps have increasingly taken over as the main source of information and education for pregnant women. This new format has made generic pregnancy advice feel more personalized, more urgent, and more overwhelming to women who look to it for support.

BabyCenter.com, Whattoexpect.com, and other online pregnancy websites and apps began delivering developmental timelines and prenatal advice in real time in the late 1990s and early 2000s. They urged women to register their due dates and sign up for newsletters, like BabyCenter's "MY PREGNANCY THIS WEEK®," so that they could receive pregnancy information timed to their exact stage of pregnancy.[97] Pregnancy advice books had occasionally labeled their developmental descriptions of embryos and fetuses as "your" baby since the 1950s, but the real-time delivery of e-mail and text newsletters made the connection between the ideal pregnancy, as described in the educational materials, and the reader's own pregnancy much more direct.[98] A newsletter subscriber would be constantly reminded of how far along she was in her pregnancy. The newsletters also implicitly offered misleading reassurance that the subscriber's pregnancy was unfolding just like in the developmental timeline.

Websites offer readers as much information about pregnancy as they are willing to digest, far more than could fit in a paper pregnancy manual. The content of the major websites is so voluminous, from articles by medical experts, to "promoted content," to peer-to-peer forums, to interesting opinions and perspectives from bloggers, that it would be possible to spend one's entire pregnancy reading it. Since websites measure their success by "reader engagement" and "click-throughs," they are organized to keep a pregnant woman engaged and returning frequently.

The website format encourages online advice-givers to break their proffered information down into discrete chunks linked together in unending combinations, which readers experience alternately as an overwhelming cascade or a tempting rabbit hole. Without the guiding hand of a single author, a woman might never encounter an article discussing the possibility of miscarriage. Or, she might click through on every article about pregnancy complications and get the impression that anything can happen with equal likelihood: from miscarriage to stillbirth to a deadly amniotic fluid embolism.

Websites became such a dominant advice format that they influenced the organization of paper pregnancy manuals. Early editions of *What to Expect When You're Expecting* embedded developmental descriptions in sections called "What You May Be Feeling" and featured diagrams of a pregnant woman at each month of gestation, with inset descriptions of the embryo. The edition published in 2008, several years after the website was launched, featured a new section called "Your Baby This Month." It featured sentimental week-by-week descriptions and illustrations of embryonic development, like those on the website. Illustrations of the pregnant woman became an afterthought, on a separate page. The website organized its newsletter around bite-sized, weekly developmental updates, as the most enticing material for attracting and maintaining a sustained readership. Once materials were developed for the website, they became the organizing principle for the book. The through-line was the standard pregnancy, unfolding along an idealized embryonic development timeline, and the reader was encouraged to engage with it in real time.

Smartphone pregnancy apps, introduced in the twenty-first century, are pregnancy websites on steroids. By pinging their users frequently, they aim to keep women engaged and thinking about their pregnancies all day every day. Many are finer-grained adaptations from the websites that spawned them, but some have pioneered new ways to drive users' engagement. Exploding in popularity in recent years, many free and others by subscription, they appear poised to become a standard feature of American pregnancies.[99]

One popular innovator, Glow Nurture, promises its users personalized insights into their pregnancy health, derived from data that users are asked to supply daily.[100] For example, "Laura F." signed up with Nurture on May 14, 2017.[101] She told the app her last period was three weeks and two days earlier, on April 21. It was five days before her expected period, the earliest possible day she could detect hCG using a home pregnancy test.

Nurture asked Laura twenty questions, ranging from her weight to her alcohol intake to her sleep duration, as the basis for a daily log. Some questions required further clarification, such as check boxes about her mood and the condition of her cervical mucous, a slide bar to show how much water she drank, and a place to fill out the names of ovulation and

pregnancy tests she might have taken. Nurture displayed three dials, labeled "Prenatal," "Physical," and "Emotional," allowing Laura to see if she
had tracked enough elements of her pregnancy to push the dials to full.

The app does not require perfect behavior to fill a dial, just perfect
tracking. Laura could get 100 percent even when she slacked. On days when
she admitted to skipping her exercise, or drinking only seven glasses of
water, though, Nurture delivered lectures on why pregnant women needed
to exercise regularly or drink eight to ten glasses of water every day. When
she appeared too reserved in reporting her emotional state and did not con-
fess to emotional upset, Nurture wondered whether she might be hiding
something. "You did not have any emotional discomfort. It's fantastic that
you are feeling great. Women often experience a range of emotions during
pregnancy and it is important to track them to observe patterns. Please be
sure to log any emotions into Glow." The next day, it rearranged the checklist of emotions so that all the negative ones showed up first. Perhaps the
Nurture programmers were simply trying to encourage honesty. But perhaps it is bad for business when users feel complacent and contented.

Nurture is based around daily logging, and this daily interaction
structures its other features as well. Where BabyCenter and WhatToExpect
websites and apps give weekly developmental updates, Nurture delivers
them daily. Laura was given the chance to click on pictures and information about "your baby" for each day separately, enhancing the impression
that it was delivering real-time updates on her womb.

Whenever Laura failed to fill out a daily log, Nurture texted her a reminder. "The more you log. . . the more helpful we can be. So keep letting
us know what's happening," it urged. "Complete your log! We get a little
more effective at personalizing your experience every time you log." Laura
only remembered to fill out her log three or four times a week, so she got a
lot of these reminders. "Don't forget to log! Nurture can help you stay on
top of your pregnancy symptoms and help you see important patterns."
Nurture wasn't content with only sending the reminders to her; it wanted
to get her husband involved. "Pregnancy is a shared journey. . . .Did you
know that Glow Nurture comes with a partner app? Let us tell your partner
what's happening so they can be as supportive as possible." If Laura wasn't
motivated enough to log for her own sake, perhaps she would engage more
with the app if she included her spouse.[102]

Nurture insists that it is collecting logs for its users' benefit. Its checklists
enforce habits that physicians and advice book writers generally recommend to pregnant women. In its "insights," Nurture directs women to brief
articles relevant to what they have logged, sharing standard pregnancy advice targeted to the behaviors or concerns a woman has recorded. It gives

women the opportunity to record information from doctors' appointments and organize data to share with their doctors. The database its engineers are building from women's data may eventually give new insights into prenatal health. The Nurture creators are probably genuine in their declared intentions to help women have healthier pregnancies.

Nurture, however, is a business at heart, and its public health efforts must at the very least align with its money-making interests. To make money, it must attract women to the platform and convince them to engage with it frequently. Currently, it collects money from premium subscriptions; in the future, it is likely to begin to show ads among the advice, as the BabyCenter and WhatToExpect apps do.[103] Nurture has every incentive to maximize women's attention to and investment in their pregnancies, whether or not that is a good approach for every woman and every pregnancy.

Just because a particular self-care recommendation is sensible and generally sanctioned by obstetricians doesn't mean hewing to it perfectly will produce an even better result. Regular exercise is helpful during pregnancy. Feeling pressure to exercise every single day per Nurture's guidelines might be counterproductive. Like *What To Expect*'s "Best Odds Diet," too-perfectionist standards and too-microscopic monitoring can make pregnant women feel like they are failing their future children. For many women the checklist is unrealistic and may induce feelings of guilt and inadequacy over "failures" that health-care providers would agree really don't matter.

At eight and a half weeks gestation, Laura told Nurture that she was spotting and that she felt anxious. Nurture delivered two separate "insights": first, that "anywhere from 20-30 percent of women experience some degree of bleeding during the first trimester. If you are bleeding, you should always wear a pad or panty liner so you can monitor how much and the type of bleeding that is occurring. If worried, please check with your doctor." Second, "5 to 16 percent of women struggle with an anxiety disorder during pregnancy or postpartum. This is perfectly normal." Nurture's algorithm apparently is not yet sophisticated enough to register the connection between bleeding and anxiety. In the same day's updates, Nurture explained, "You won't be aware of your developing baby's activities inside the uterus for some months yet, but the fact that his elbows are forming allows him to make some small movements; the wrists do not yet move. Your baby is looking more human by the day. His vertebrae and ribs are now in place, and his fingers are gradually lengthening. His body is less curled up than it was a few weeks ago" (see Figure 4.5). Delivered to someone who had begun to bleed, this was a rather optimistic and insensitive account of what was supposedly happening inside.

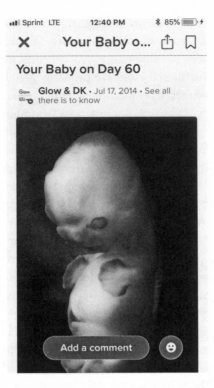

Figure 4.5 Screen shot of a Glow Nurture article delivered at eight and a half weeks' gestation, showing "Your Baby on Day 60."

When Laura told Nurture a couple of days later that she had red bleeding, she was given a list of "warning" signs that would indicate that she should see her doctor. It was coy about naming the reasons for concern. "Vaginal bleeding during early pregnancy could be due to many causes, some serious and some not. Watch for vaginal bleeding, cramping pains (worse than menstrual cramps), and tissue passing through the vagina. If you experience any of these symptoms, please consult your doctor right away."

Soon after, Laura needed to tell Nurture she had a miscarriage. It was not obvious how to do it; she had to ask Google and found that she needed to change her "status" to "healing from loss." Nurture asked for some details, invited her to come back when she was ready to log another pregnancy and suggested she check out their other great apps about fertility and parenting.

Laura searched the app for guidance about miscarriages and found an article about it among a continued stream of pregnancy health tips. It shared the common wisdom about miscarriage from pregnancy manuals and online experts. "It really doesn't matter how far along the pregnancy was when the miscarriage occurred, you and your partner are still going to feel upset, and the woman, especially, will have to go through the stages of grief before feeling more balanced again."

Laura had even more trouble updating her status in the BabyCenter app, and for a while she gave up trying. For several weeks she found text updates on the opening screen of her phone. "You're 13 weeks pregnant. Your baby's tiny fingertips have fingerprints, her veins and organs are clearly visible through her still-thin skin, and her body is starting to catch up." She opened the app to find the headline, "Your baby is about the size of a peapod." She tried again to tell Baby Center that she had miscarried. She opened "My Profile" in order to "Edit my family." In "My Children" she found the blank labeled "Baby's name," which she had not yet filled out, and her due date, "Jan 26, 2018." It turned out she could not fix this in the app; she needed to go to babycenter.com and log in again to edit "my family." In her profile, she had to scroll past questions such as "Has your baby arrived?" to get to the options to "report a loss" or "remove child from profile." She chose to "report a loss." It told her, "We're deeply sorry for your loss. We'll stop sending you emails and notifications related to this child, and won't customize our site or apps for this child any longer." In order to continue she had to choose again to "Remove child from profile." It warned, "This will erase all photos, milestones, and announcements associated with this child on our website and mobile apps."

She hesitated. Then she clicked the button to update.

* * *

In colonial America, pregnancy had been a regular part of life for women in their twenties and thirties. Women treated pregnancy as a normal, if often uncomfortable, state of being, and its physical demands as an inherent part of womanhood. During the nineteenth and early twentieth centuries, as women exercised more control over their fertility and spent more of their parenting energy nurturing each child, they came to see pregnancy as an exceptional physical demand on their bodies, requiring specialized medical care to keep themselves and their children safe and healthy. During the twentieth century, nurses and doctors offered elaborated care regimens, supplemented with education about embryology designed to encourage pregnant women and their husbands to be highly engaged and invested in pregnancies, rather than taking a "wait and see" attitude until the birth. The twenty-first century has seen the rise of websites, pregnancy apps, and regimens of self-care and education that mandate heightened attention, early emotional investment, and round-the-clock concern. Although more medical attention to pregnancy has no doubt saved the lives of many women and children, and enhanced the health of many more, the current mode of intensive monitoring has also encouraged women and their partners to become highly invested in early pregnancies destined to miscarry. Too often it has given women a false sense of control over the outcomes of pregnancies that cannot come to fruition no matter how conscientiously a woman cares for her expected child.

CHAPTER 5

✿

Buying for the Baby

Marketing to Expectant Parents

On November 16, 2012, lararesearch@gmail told babycenter.com she was four weeks pregnant.[1] It did not feel as public as, say, posting a positive home pregnancy test to Facebook, but she was essentially giving that information to strangers. It had seemed so easy, even unavoidable. She was browsing the website and a popup immediately offered a chance to figure out her due date with BabyCenter's handy due date calculator. She told BabyCenter that her last period was exactly four weeks earlier, and BabyCenter replied, "Congratulations! Your baby is due on or around: Friday, August 23, 2013. Right now you're about 4 weeks pregnant and your baby is the size of a poppy seed. See your personalized calendar below for a list of exciting pregnancy milestones." And then, "What's next? Personalize your BabyCenter experience and receive free weekly newsletters about your baby's development. Join now." The e-mail signup took just a few more clicks, and she was in the system: BabyCenter and its sponsors were privy to her most exciting and intimate news (see Figure 5.1).

BabyCenter, the behemoth of online pregnancy and parenting websites, was peddling more than developmental updates. Lararesearch@gmail was offered a chance to sign up for ads from BabyCenter affiliates and sponsors, offering coupons, deals, and information. Even the weekly developmental updates came with sponsors' ads and offers, as well as links to interesting and relevant articles surrounded by yet more advertisements. The e-mails started immediately, with a welcome message:

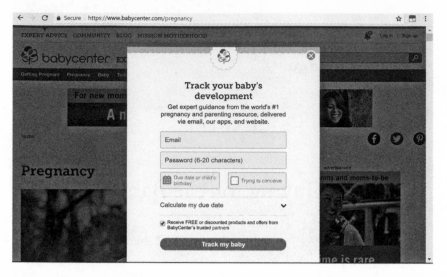

Figure 5.1 Popup at Babycenter.com, encouraging a visitor to the website to sign up for developmental updates by revealing her baby's birth date or due date.

> Congratulations on your pregnancy! Having a baby may be the most challenging thing you ever do—and the most amazing. And BabyCenter will be at your side every step of the way. We'll help you get answers to all your questions about your pregnancy and baby, with thousands of expert articles, helpful tools, and a warm, supportive community of parents like you.[2]

BabyCenter promises sound and supportive advice, and for the most part, it delivers. Its medical advice is up to date. It solicits and produces essays and videos from respected experts across a range of fields, from obstetricians and midwives to lactation consultants and doulas. It is progressive in its presentation of natural childbirth and breastfeeding. With occasional exceptions, it does not give the impression of having "sold out" to its advertisers.[3] A pregnant woman's health-care provider could feel as comfortable referring her to babycenter.com as to popular mainstream advice books such as *What to Expect When You're Expecting*.[4] Women who participate in the online forums BabyCenter organizes by due date find them fun, reassuring, and community building.

At the same time, babycenter.com delivers on promises it makes to its advertisers. A premium advertiser can choose to be included in BabyCenter's popular e-mail updates. "Timed to Mom's exact life stage and with industry leading open and pass along rates, our email is the gateway to her BabyCenter experience—and the start of her emotional connection with your brand." High-quality educational content is not only geared to learning. "Our award winning video library combines advertising with orig-inal content on pregnancy, baby, parenting, and beyond to engage moms, build awareness, and drive sales." Health recommendations could become product recommendations: "From seasonal specials and nutrition guides to baby naming trends and health alerts, align your brand with original content, written by BabyCenter editors, supported by industry experts."

Advertisers are also offered the opportunity to shape certain edito-rial content: "Tell us your objective. We'll hand-pick influential voices on the BabyCenter Blog and across our extensive network of Mom Bloggers to craft a campaign that resonates." The information about due dates collected from women like lararesearch@gmail means that "We deliver your marketing message so it's perfectly timed to Mom's exact stage and mindset, across both web and mobile platforms. No wonder our audience says we're psychic." Women's active participation in online forums and surveys is monetized as market research. "Get Mom insights that will in-form how you think about, market to, and connect with the most pow-erful consumer in today's marketplace. It's a real-time focus group, without the traditional research setting." And all of this content and advertising are served to BabyCenter visitors on home computers and smartphones linked to Facebook, Pinterest, Twitter, and Instagram. An expanse of top-notch, appealing content is designed to draw as many pregnant visitors as possible, keep them on the site, and show them the maximum number of relevant advertisements, while collecting their opinions and behavior to compile into saleable market research.[5]

So has BabyCenter.com found the perfect synergy between its audience's needs and its advertisers' desires? Has it avoided seemingly inevitable conflicts of interest? When it comes to early pregnancy, the answer is no.

BabyCenter's advertisers want to reach women as early in their pregnancies as possible to beat out their competitors. So BabyCenter has an incentive to attract newly pregnant visitors and hold their maximum possible attention and interest. Visitors are likely to come to the site al-ready excited to think about and plan for their babies, and BabyCenter has every incentive to amplify this excitement, even when many visitors' pregnancies are destined to miscarry.

Between four-week and five-week developmental updates, in addition to e-mails about "what you should know about ultrasounds" and "10 icky preg-nancy side effects," BabyCenter sent an invitation to lararesearch@gmail to "join the BabyCenter Moms Panel," because "it's our members who are the real parenting experts." Barely pregnant enough to trigger a positive home pregnancy test, lararesearch@gmail had already been declared a "mom" by eager market researchers. Shortly after came "the nine pregnancy products you can't live without," linked to "the baby gear you'll really need." And then, even before the six-week update, came the first of many ads from the stem cell bank that is a major babycenter.com sponsor. "You've already won! We don't need to tell you that your wonderful baby bump is your 'grand prize.'. . . REGISTER TO WIN our 2nd Grand Prize: FREE Cord Blood Banking from StemCyte." The ads continued, fast and furious. Before the eight-week developmental update, lararesearch@gmail received additional ads for Huggies diapers, Britax carseats, diapers.com, and Town & Country, miscellaneous "free stuff and great deals," as well as two more e-mails urging her to join the Moms Panel. Interleafed were developmental updates and two features on choosing baby names.

Why does BabyCenter feature baby-naming articles often and early? "100 most popular baby names" is the top-featured article in the five-week developmental update.[6] Choosing names is on the first-trimester portion of the "ultimate pregnancy to-do list."[7] Baby-name articles are promoted because they are appealing. Women who visit the site find them enticing and spend a lot of time looking through lists of baby names, perhaps also glancing at the advertising banners and sidebars. In featuring baby name articles so early, BabyCenter is trading on women's excitement, encouraging them to be highly involved and emotionally attached to their pregnancies, and bringing them into contact with a panoply of advertisers at an early stage of pregnancy.

More directly, BabyCenter encourages site visitors, particularly those who sign up as members, to shop early and often. Like browsing baby names, shopping is one of the enjoyable aspects of pregnancy for many women. BabyCenter functions as a sought-out source of information and leads on baby-related products as much as a source of health advice. Visitors can find articles and blog entries about product categories such as carseats, diapers, and strollers, reviews of specific products from BabyCenter members, and plenty of coupons and special offers. And as BabyCenter points out in its marketing materials, women change many buying habits as they prepare for a baby, so BabyCenter and its sponsors provide advice about everything from family-friendly cars to financial services to organic clothes and food. Since visitors come to the site looking for shopping tips and links, visitors' and advertisers' interests are often aligned. But as with the developmental updates and baby-naming articles, BabyCenter's business model tends to encourage shopping for baby gear at an earlier stage of pregnancy than might be prudent. If lararesearch@gmail took advantage of the coupons BabyCenter sent before they expired, she would have owned a carseat, a stroller, and a large box of diapers before the end of her first trimester.

BabyCenter and its ilk did not spring whole cloth from the minds of Internet entrepreneurs of the twenty-first century. Lararesearch@gmail's interactions with babycenter.com reflect the culmination of two centuries of developments in how pregnant women and their families and friends prepare their homes for a new baby. Before babycenter.com could exist, families would need to routinely purchase (rather than make) their baby gear. A lucrative and attractive market for baby things would need to develop. Marketers and advertisers would need to become sophisticated enough to perceive the value of pregnant customers and figure out how to reach them. They would need to become clever and competitive enough to find women at the very beginning of their pregnancies, the time when miscarriages are most likely.[8]

FROM MAKING TO BUYING

Following a long tradition, women in colonial America prepared what they called "child-bed linen," which included a variety of baby garments, from basic clothing to special wrappings and hats intended to strengthen the infant's floppy spine and close the soft spot on the skull. Women made these baby items, as well as a few postpartum and nursing garments for themselves, either while they were pregnant with a first child or as part of preparing for marriage.[9] This was understood as material and emotional preparation for motherhood. In English legal tradition, women who gave birth to stillborn children in suspicious circumstances were often acquitted of infanticide if they could demonstrate that they had prepared child-bed linen.[10] Hand preparation of baby clothes continued to signify maternal love well past the colonial era. In 1964, humorist Betty Rollin poked fun at the sentimentally coy euphemisms for pregnancy in her era. She described a fictitious woman who was too reserved to announce her pregnancy directly to her husband: "He came home and found me knitting . . . tiny garments . . . for the precious cargo . . . And I had a glow."[11] Rollin considered that approach old-fashioned, but it was not yet long out of date.

Beyond bed linens, a colonial American infant claimed few material goods. A family might own a small cradle and a walker. Even an older child had few possessions aside from the clothes on her back, perhaps a rag doll or a whip top. Children were expected to participate in the household economy and learn productive roles early. "Play dough" did not come in plastic tubs; it was a handful of dough from the main loaf, given to a young girl so that she could keep herself occupied and begin to learn housekeeping skills while her mother baked. Adults had few leisure-related possessions, and neither did children. Neither infants nor children inspired parents to shop.

Gradually these long-standing cultural patterns changed, as Americans' wealth increased and industrialization led to the production of cheaper commercial goods. Americans in 1800 had many more material possessions than Americans in 1700. Even those with fairly modest incomes had a table and chairs for mealtimes, rather than a moveable plank and roughhewn benches of earlier times. There were enough chairs that children were not required to stand to eat, and each person might have his or her own plate and utensils. Tea sets and mirrors were no longer privileges of the wealthy. Adults were likely to own more than one set of clothes and make them out of purchased fabric rather than homespun. As the nineteenth century progressed, more and more Americans owned some personal goods beyond their basic needs. Wealthier families set up nurseries for children, for the first time formally separating children's sleeping quarters from adults', and gradually added the accoutrements associated with babies' special needs: elaborate cribs, high chairs, bathing basins, child-sized utensils. As Americans spent more on themselves, they spent more on their children as well.[12]

At the same time, communal practices around childbirth also changed. Middle-class women began to feel that old-fashioned "groaning parties," where the groans of the laboring woman were accompanied by the feasting of her friends and supporters, were unseemly. Births became quieter occasions. During the early twentieth century they would move to the hospital, where the traditional female helpers would be banished entirely. Women still wanted to support and encourage each other, but they would need a new occasion for gathering together to celebrate birth and bolster new mothers.

TWENTIETH-CENTURY PARENTS-TO-BE ENTER THE CONSUMER AGE

At the turn of the twentieth century, an American culture of consumption bloomed rapidly and, with it, the market for babies' and children's goods flourished. It was in the twentieth century that children became an excuse to shop. Continuing industrialization and improved transport brought a panoply of consumer goods to Americans everywhere. City dwellers shopped in new department stores, while the Sears catalog and the Wells Fargo wagon served the countryside. Retailers targeted a range of new customers, from the established middle class to working parents who scrimped and saved to buy a special outfit or two and a modern, hygienic bottle and nipple for a new baby.[13]

Advertising and selling grew more sophisticated. Advertising developed from simple lists of available products and prices to its own genre of persuasive literature. Marketing and sales developed into full-blown professions with an array of specialized trade journals.

As historian Gary Cross has documented, advertisers and marketers cannily observed that Americans had come to treasure the perceived innocence of their children and helped create a vision of "wondrous innocence." Parents could re-live an idyllic childhood through their children's eyes by sharing with them new and wonderful toys and other material goods. And they could justify it as morally acceptable because it was pleasurable consumption on behalf of their beloved children, rather than money spent on themselves.[14]

A new baby increasingly seemed to require a mountain of purchases, and retailers gradually learned how to make the buying process easy, even fun, for expecting parents. In the 1920s, department stores began experimenting with "infant" departments, innovatively organizing goods based on the customer's identity, rather than on product categories such as shoes or toiletries. The idea was novel enough in 1921 for the *New York Times'* business pages to feature an extended interview with Mrs. E. Gilman, a manager of wholesale infants' and children's wear with the Bush Company in New York City. She told the reporter, "If there is anything that appeals to the prospective mother when she goes to shop . . . it is being able to find nearly everything she wants and needs assembled in a single part of the store. She does not want to have to go to the fabric section to buy some baby muslins and then have to go to the drug sundries department in some other part of the store to get a bath thermometer. I am a mother, and I know from experience."

Mrs. Gilman coached hundreds of department stores in this type of reorganization. She advocated putting the baby linens with the cribs and assembling "maternity baskets" and "obstetrical baskets" to prepare for home births, with products recommended by prominent local physicians. She included toys and cute dresses, along with clothes, furniture, and toiletries. The reporter seemed especially struck by Gilman's suggestion that maternity corsets and gowns be stocked in the infants department as well.[15]

Hundreds of product lines from all around the store were to be gathered in the infants department to give "prospective mothers the very best kind of service that can be given them, in that it helps them conserve their strength at a time when they need it most." Not coincidentally, it would give a shopper more ideas of what purchases might be necessary or desirable.

Ideally, the department would be staffed by a saleswoman who was also a mother, perhaps a widow who would be earning her family's keep, as well as a friendly trained nurse.[16] A pregnant woman shopping in an infants department could relax and enjoy herself, supported by a knowledgeable and friendly staff and an inventory arrayed to promote comfortable browsing and thorough purchasing.

These retailing innovations were not limited to sophisticated city women. The Sears catalog, a staple of rural shopping, initially scattered baby goods across almost every category in the "big book." A woman browsing the 1897 catalog would have had to flip through nearly seven hundred pages to find what she needed. An "elastic abdominal supporter," illustrated with a picture of it wrapped around a clearly pregnant belly, was tucked in underneath jock straps and above "soft rubber catheters" and a "ladies' elastic doily belt" meant to be "worn by ladies during their menstrual period, for the convenience of attaching the napkin and is indespensable [sic] for comfort." Infant dresses were mixed in with women's dresses, and infant underwear was in the general underwear section. Cotton diapers were pictured with towels and tablecloths. Baby swings and jumpers came after extension ladders and corn baskets, and before dairy supplies. A shopper certainly could find everything she needed, but she would either need to start from a list and make good use of the index, or be willing to spend hours browsing the enormous catalog for ideas.[17]

Beginning in 1907, more than a decade ahead of the department stores, Sears experimented with a new way of marketing to pregnant women and new mothers. It hired Mrs. Eliza Emerson Goff to organize all its maternity and baby goods, from maternity corsets to nursing blouses to layettes, rattles, and doctors' kits for home births, into a single catalog.[18] The *Baby Book* was intended for "every mother, present or prospective."[19] A woman could start shopping while she was pregnant and order additional items from the catalog as her baby grew (see Figure 5.2a and b).

Sears advertised its catalog in *Woman's Home Companion* and other women's magazines, with a personal note from Mrs. Goff: "Let me send you a free copy of THE BABY BOOK. It will tell you many things that will interest you and will introduce you to the most exclusive and most beautiful baby clothes to be obtained anywhere. *Address me personally*. I want to handle your correspondence myself."[20] *Printers' Ink*, the major advertising trade journal, praised the approach as "introducing the human element in a way that seems sure to prove effective."[21] Mrs. Goff, perhaps with help from silent assistants, was the equivalent of a retail store's baby department matron, giving reassurance, making suggestions, and ensuring that the new mother's preparations would be complete.

(a)

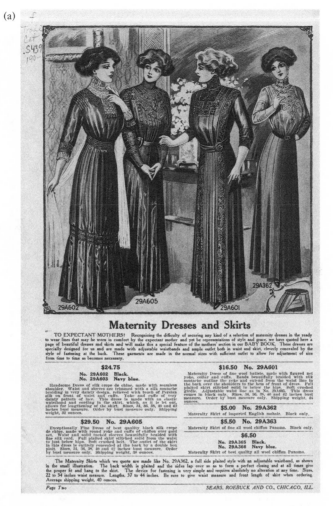

Figures 5.2a and 5.2b Sears' innovative *Baby Book*, published in 1907, was a comprehensive catalog for pregnancy and infant needs. Sears, Roebuck and Company, *The Baby Book* (Chicago, IL, 1907), ID #08078751, Hagley Museum & Library, Wilmington, DE 19807, pages 2 and 15.

Mrs. Goff not only brought the whole panoply of baby items into one catalog, she also created sets of infant clothing and toiletries that would become known in future catalogs as "layettes." They came in several price points, from $5.99 for twenty-eight pieces to $18.98 for sixty pieces.[22] Cascades of little dresses, diapers, bedding, and talcum powder boxes illustrated the many items included. Text box inserts explained the purpose of the sets. "For the benefit of the young mother who is inexperienced in the requirements of the babe's first wardrobe we have greatly simplified the task of selecting the necessary articles by assembling in complete outfits

(b)

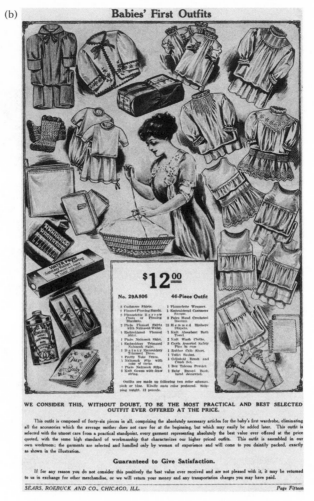

Figures 5.2a and 5.2b Continued

the various articles of wearing apparel and toilet accessories essential to baby's arrival."[23] What could be an overwhelming number of choices became a matter of simply choosing between fancy and plain. Women could feel reassured that they had not missed anything crucial. At the same time, Sears could take the opportunity to help define what was "essential" in baby care, perhaps expanding the scope of what would come to be considered necessary expenditures.

Many of the catalog's baby items could easily be purchased after the birth. But Sears intended for women to buy the layettes ahead of time. They were the first major item intended for purchase during pregnancy, not for the mother's health and comfort, but for the expected baby. Many women presumably did buy them during the later stages of pregnancy, rather than scrambling to obtain bedding and diapers once the baby was born. But plenty of women must have waited, because in the 1940s Sears added an innovative, if gimmicky, incentive to purchase ahead: "If it's Twins or Quints! Let us do the worrying! Order your Layette at Sears and if there's more than one arrival, send us the certificate which you will find enclosed with your first Layette, together with a signed statement from your physician or minister, and we will send you the extra Layette (or extra Layettes) postpaid—absolutely free!"[24]

While Sears was an early innovator with its *Baby Book*, Mrs. Goff's marketing strategy did not inform the organization of the Sears *Big Book* right away. The 1908 edition of the main Sears catalog looked just like its counterpart from a decade earlier. By 1925, a shopper could find layettes complete with a baby-care advice book, followed by several pages of baby items. Still, children's furniture and toys were listed with their adult counterparts, while maternity corsets and dresses were with women's clothes. And someone using the index to find baby stuff would still have to know exactly what she needed, since the listing unhelpfully read, "Babies'—see name of article wanted."[25]

In 1931, the Sears catalog experimented with putting maternity clothes in the section of baby clothes and gear, just as department store expert Mrs. Gilman had done a decade earlier. This might seem like savvy marketing: perhaps a woman who only meant to buy herself a maternity dress at that moment would be drawn in and start browsing for baby things earlier than she had intended. But Sears may have had reservations about the new organization, since by 1935 maternity wear was back with women's clothing, scattered among corsets, dresses and "supports." By the 1940s, baby items and maternity gear had coalesced into two distinct departments, though they were well organized and listed in bold in the index. Sears, like many retailers, groped its way toward targeted marketing techniques, unevenly applying the insight that informed its 1907 *Baby Book*.

In addition to prospective parents, friends and relatives shopped the infants departments and catalogs for gifts for the expected little one. "Stork showers," the precursor of baby showers, began among well-off women in the late nineteenth century. Socially, these parties were a replacement for the birth-room gatherings of previous generations. A few weeks after a birth that had been attended only by a doctor and couple of close confidants or professional nurses, a new mother would be feted by her circle of female friends and relatives. At this new social ritual, gift-giving was reversed. Instead of the new mother providing a party to thank her friends for helping with the birth, her friends brought gifts to celebrate her new baby. In 1914 the *Los Angeles Times*' social pages recorded the elaborate surprise party Miss Minnie Burchhardt threw at her home for Mrs. Elmer Hickman. "The decorating scheme was unique, pink being the general plan, with small electric lights trimmed in pink strung from chandeliers to walls and baby dolls hung from the ceiling." Guests were treated to baby-themed party favors, sweet treats, and games.[26]

The announcement did not say whether the party took place `before or after the birth. The pink decorating scheme might indicate that the baby had been born, but colors associated with a baby's sex were a recent innovation. The following year Marion Harland, a prolific author famous for her domestic advice books, answered an inquiry from a reader in her *Chicago Tribune* etiquette column: "Please publish in your Corner the colors worn by an infant boy and by a girl. I am going to attend a 'stork shower,' and I wish to be posted upon this point." Harland explained, "Blue is the conventional color for the boy—presumably because he is to be a warrior in the 'world's great field of battle.' Blue is the soldier's and sailor's color. 'Celestial rosy red, Love's proper hue,' is gallantly awarded to the baby girl. Her conquests in the olden times were supposed to be under Cupid's banner." The stork shower host may or may not have felt obliged to hew to modern color expectations.[27]

By the mid-1920s, stork showers appear to have been more generally expected. They were not only a luxury of the wealthy, like so many of the other parties recorded in the society pages. In 1925 the *Atlanta Constitution* reported that the pre-school age circle of the Kirkwood PTA, besides having a successful candy-pulling fundraiser, was enthusiastically preparing a stork shower for a needy mother. If well-off women gathered many of their new baby goods through a shower, the PTA must have reasoned, a woman who could not afford to purchase them would surely appreciate the gifts, and a party was a friendly way to bestow them.[28]

As the twentieth century progressed, consumer marketing, inaugurated as a discipline in the 1920s, grew increasingly sophisticated. Marketers figured out more reasons and more ways to target pregnant women. Although marketing research was almost always proprietary, the scattered marketing reports that have been made public indicate that, by the 1960s, marketers were well aware that pregnant women could be valuable targets.[29]

In 1962 renowned market researcher Ernest Dichter conducted an in-depth study for Playtex, which had just launched its innovative Playtex Nurser baby bottle. Dichter, who had shaped the field of market research and invented the concept of "focus groups," listened carefully to what women told him about bottles, babies, and motherhood. His research team visited women in their homes and brought Nurser kits for them to assemble.

They also ran focus groups where women talked about the Nurser's widely circulated television commercial, explained what they liked about the product and what exasperated them, and critiqued Playtex's claims. And they conducted a large survey to evaluate the reach of the commercial and the distribution of women's current brand preferences. Dichter and his team interviewed women with babies, many of whom had older children, too, but they also interviewed pregnant women expecting a first child. Dichter had the sense that first-time pregnant women might be a somewhat different audience susceptible to different marketing techniques. Indeed, he found good reason to recommend that Playtex especially target expecting women.[30]

Dichter had developed his sophisticated approach to market research on pregnant women and new mothers in a previous study for Clapp Baby Foods. For Clapp, Dichter proposed to investigate experienced and prospective mothers' awareness of baby food brands; the factors that influenced a new mother's choice of brand; and importantly, "What is the fertile moment for brand selection among new expectant mothers?" He also proposed to find out whether reaching them early mattered. "How tentative or how permanent is the initial brand decision made by the new mother? As the new mother gains experience does she tend to switch to other brands? To what extent?"[31]

When it came to baby food, Dichter found that women did not profess much brand loyalty; it was important for Clapp to reach them with coupons and offers to put itself in consideration, but this was not especially urgent. Dichter also learned from this research, as well as a previous study on the relationships between pediatricians and mothers, that pregnant women were highly invested in learning about infant feeding and child care and development in general. As he summarized in the introduction to his Playtex report, "Mothers' attitudes . . . appear to be continually growing and developing as educational levels increase and as scientific materials become more generally available through women's service magazines, special prenatal courses for pregnant women, and a more 'scientific' relationship between doctor and patient in which the prospective mother becomes more adequately informed and more deeply interested in the physiological and psychological aspects of child feeding and child handling."[32]

Playtex's new product was designed to appeal to these highly educated and invested new mothers. The Playtex Nurser's big innovation was a disposable, sterile bottle liner designed to simplify the cleaning process and prevent the baby from drinking air bubbles and getting gas. Playtex made some big claims about what the Nurser could do. It was supposed to prevent colic by preventing gassiness; be more "natural" than other bottle systems; and keep the baby safer and the preparation easier with its sterile linings. It was relatively more complicated to assemble but claimed to be more convenient because the linings were disposable. In an era when few houses had dishwashers, a mother could avoid having to regularly boil all the bottle components to sterilize them.

Dichter found that while experienced mothers were skeptical about these sweeping claims, women who were pregnant for the first time were inclined to believe them. Experienced mothers found the bottle harder to assemble than traditional bottles and doubted it could be more convenient. They wondered how a babysitter could handle it and how it would actually work in practice. They also had a more realistic sense of the intractability of colic.

In contrast, women who were pregnant for the first time had no basis for comparison, so they were more inclined to be impressed at how modern and scientific the bottle appeared and to take its complexity for granted. One exclaimed upon opening the box, "Oh, look at all these things—my husband will go crazy putting all of this together—he will have a good time with this!" Another mused after putting it together, "The whole thing was not really that bad and I'm not mechanically minded. As a matter of fact it was kind of fun. I can just see my husband with it—I bet he will find it fun too." Dichter concluded, "The attitude throughout, as indicated by test results, show inexperienced prospective mothers as a much more positive and accessible market for the Nurser than experienced mothers."[33]

Given that the task was to reach women who had not yet had their babies, Dichter considered how Playtex might best market the Nurser. He noted that pregnant women did not think of bottles as one of the more fraught baby purchases. First-time mothers naively assumed that bottles were more or less all the same. The women he interviewed bought whatever they could find at the drugstore just before or after the birth, or added a set as an afterthought at the department store infant section after shopping for furniture and clothes. To capture these purchases, Dichter recommended that Playtex hire demonstrators who could make the bottle's assembly look easy and tout its benefits, and arrange for them to staff department store and drugstore infants' sections. He also strongly advocated direct-mail appeals, with coupons and educational literature, since prior research for Clapp's baby foods had demonstrated that women were highly receptive to them.

Dichter and his team spent a lot of effort interviewing women about their attitudes toward breastfeeding versus bottle feeding, as well as their personal history or intentions. He concluded that women had strong convictions about what would work best for them and implicitly recommended against Playtex trying to convert breastfeeders to the bottle. But he thought that the Nurser was appealing to women who wanted to breastfeed but for physical or psychological reasons could not, because of its claims of being a more "natural" sucking experience for the infant than other bottles. Besides reaching prospective mothers at the drugstore, department store, and through the mail, he advised Playtex to get its product into hospital obstetric wards, pre-natal clinics, and pre-natal classes. Anywhere a pregnant woman was learning about how to feed her child, Playtex should be there.

Dichter advised many direct, targeted appeals to pregnant women, but he was particularly impressed with the impact of Playtex's 1962 TV commercial. The large majority of his interviewees had seen it, and many could describe it in detail:

> The very special psychological climate which envelopes a household expecting or raising a baby, together with the profound psychological changes and developments which occur among both men and women who are expecting or rearing a baby, create an almost unobstructed access for baby product advertising. Within this sensitive and differentiated atmosphere, the Playtex Nurser ad has created intense impact and product-interest.

He found that prospective mothers were particularly influenced by the commercial, more so than by word of mouth, much to his surprise: "It would seem that the Playtex commercial has a strong appeal for prospective mothers, who are looking for 'the best' for their babies, and who are interested in what appears to be a new and advanced concept in feeding."[34] Of his sample, 62 percent of the pregnant women planned to use the Playtex Nurser, as opposed to 19 percent of experienced mothers. If Playtex could convince these women to start with the Nurser and learn to take its tricky assembly for granted, it could do very well indeed.

The Playtex Nurser proved an enduring success and today is touted as "used by moms for generations."[35] Ultimately, women adopted a new and more complicated bottle technology because they were convinced it was better for their babies. And bottle technology became one more thing women felt they should evaluate before their babies' births. It is hard to gauge how important marketing to first-time pregnant women was to the Nurser's success, but Dichter's research demonstrates that shrewd marketers were aware that this could be a crucial and unique constituency. Dichter and his marketing colleagues were convinced that the quickest way to introduce a new idea or product into the mainstream of parenting culture was to reach women when they were looking forward to imminent parenthood but had not yet actually entered the culture and absorbed its traditions. Given the results, Playtex was likely convinced too. The race to be the first to reach newly pregnant women had begun.

BABY MAGAZINES DRIVE MARKETING

Since the 1920s, baby magazines have been a critical nexus between marketers and pregnant women. To reach pregnant women with effective advertising, market researchers needed to identify who was pregnant. This was a specialized and non-trivial task. Baby magazines were among the biggest consolidators of marketing lists of expecting women and also a major conduit between advertisers of baby goods and pregnant potential customers. The biggest magazines, such as *American Baby* and *Baby Talk*, have been published continuously since the 1930s, and in recent years, they could brag of reaching hundreds of thousands of new readers each month, along with several million ongoing readers.[36] Distributed free in thousands of doctors' offices and maternity clothing departments, they relied entirely on advertising revenue. They capitalized on their valuable mailing lists, sometimes conducting their own marketing research to persuade potential advertisers of the value of their ad pages, and sometimes renting out the lists directly.

In 1973 *American Baby* magazine commissioned a survey of baby toy purchasing and brand recognition using its mailing list. Greenwich Research conducted the study for *American Baby*, and its researchers sent questionnaires to women in their third trimester of pregnancy as well as women with babies under six months old. The company appeared to have quite a bit of information about the women before it mailed out the survey; it received responses from approximately equal numbers of women expecting first babies, expecting subsequent babies, caring for first infants, and caring for subsequent infants. Far fewer respondents were in their seventh month of pregnancy than in their eighth or ninth, suggesting that in 1973, it was still hard to reach women earlier in pregnancy, even if that might have been desirable. They mailed out the surveys "under a Greenwich masthead of The Institute for Baby Research," presumably a made-up organization for the purposes of this study.[37]

Remarkably, almost half of the women approached filled out the surveys and sent them back. Given the claim that this was research by an "Institute," they may have assumed the results would serve some nobler purpose than creating proprietary market research to help toy manufacturers and *American Baby* sell them more stuff. But perhaps not. Sharing opinions with manufacturers, after all, might result in them making more appealing toys or selling them at the right price point. In any case, it is clear that women, whether still pregnant or caring for an infant, had opinions about their purchasing and child care practices that they felt were well-considered and worthy.

The surviving report is focused on toys, but the appended question-naire asks additional baby-related questions. Women were asked if they intended to breastfeed or bottle feed, and, if they were going to use a bottle, which formula they intended to use. The Playtex Nurser had clearly made an impact: the bottle choices were "glass," "plastic" or "disposable liner in plastic holder." Respondents were asked which of a long list of bath and grooming items they had purchased, whether they had a crib and car seat, and whether or not they had bought more life insurance as part of preparing for the baby. These questions, along with inquiries about family income and the make and model of the family's car, might have been in-tended to help place the respondents demographically, but they may have also been useful to *American Baby* outside of the toy research.

The bulk of the questions were focused on infant toys, in the specific categories of rattles, squeak toys, cuddle dolls, mobiles, and play gyms. Women were asked which toys they purchased, which brands, and at what stores. Did they buy them for themselves or to give to others? Did they receive them as gifts? They were asked to evaluate the toys on a range of qualities, from safety to durability to imaginativeness. And they were asked how much they were willing to spend for their own children and for baby gifts.

The results must have been eye-opening for toy manufacturers. They probably helped *American Baby* sell more than a few ads, too. It turned out that women did not just buy the necessities before the birth; they bought toys as well. They received even more toys as gifts. By the ninth month of pregnancy, substantially more than half of respondents had rattles and mobiles, about half had squeak toys, a third had cuddle dolls, and a quarter had play gyms. Pregnant women were a major market for baby toys. Indeed, they bought enough baby toys that they often became sated, and the window of opportunity to reach them nearly closed within a few months after the birth. At the same time, brand recognition was very low. Women did buy toys, but they bought them generically. There was a serious brand-development opportunity here, and as with the Nurser, the results seemed to indicate that the most valuable audience would be women who were earlier in their pregnancies. Marketers would continue to work on the problem of how to find women at an earlier stage.

* * *

In 1992, journalist Erik Larson interviewed *American Baby* marketing director Patricia Calderon about how the magazine developed its marketing lists. Larson, concerned about Americans' loss of privacy at the hands of marketers, wondered how they learned of something so personal as a woman's pregnancy status. Simple, Calderon explained. *American Baby* got women to tell them. But not directly. The magazine made arrangements with doctors to display subscription cards with offers of free magazines in their offices, and if a woman submitted the card and signed up to receive the magazine, *American Baby* added her to the marketing lists they sold. In exchange for detailed information about her due date or the birth date of her baby, a woman would receive a version of the magazine tailored to her baby's age. In the early 1990s, *American Baby* had this arrangement with ten thousand doctors' offices. The magazine also supplied sign-up sheets to hospital pre-natal classes and arranged for maternity clothing stores to offer subscriptions.[38]

By this time, marketers had realized that it was not only baby clothes that women bought when they were expecting. A couple might buy a new house or car, purchase life insurance or open a savings account, switch to an organic grocery store, or investigate which gyms offered family memberships and children's classes. A pregnant woman was open to new products and brands across the entire swath of her existence, and she would soon be making choices and perhaps initiating new brand loyalties. "Life stage marketing" was designed to take advantage of this frame of mind. It wasn't the first time anyone had noticed that having a baby could spark some big purchases; a 1945 special publication from *Parents' Magazine* called "Your New Home" featured a couple who had decided to quit renting and build a home because they were expecting.[39] But the new designation formalized the common wisdom that had developed over the twentieth century and encouraged marketers for a wide range of products to start considering the value of pregnant women as targets.[40]

While *American Baby* was intent on reaching women before the birth, it did not find doing so too early advantageous. Calderon told Larson that the first trimester was not a good time to reach women. "That baby isn't real yet. You're sick. You don't feel good." But then excitement started to build, crescendoing to a third-trimester buying spree. The sweet spot for acquiring a woman's address was in the second trimester. "An advertiser wants to be there from the sixth month of pregnancy to the sixth month postnatal," she explained. "He wants to *barrage* that woman with impressions." The marketers' timeline was inching earlier by the decade, but it would take a technological breakthrough to make the leap to the first trimester.[41]

THE INTERNET AND BIG DATA PUSH
MARKETING EARLIER

That new technological day came with the popularization of the Internet and the ubiquity of e-mail. The Internet had become the place to go for information, of all kinds. Practically everyone had e-mail, and "spam" was the new name for junk mail. As BabyCenter.com and others discovered, it was not difficult to convince women to reveal their due dates, often immediately after a positive home pregnancy test. For many women, it seemed an acceptable trade in return for developmental updates via e-mail and useful coupons.[42]

While BabyCenter keeps its lists proprietary and tightly controls which "sponsors" send e-mails to BabyCenter members, many pregnancy websites compile lists for rent to anyone willing to pay. For example, the Little Miracle Prenatal list offers 240,000 addresses, including a subset of 50,000 specified as "first trimester moms," at a cost of $100 per thousand e-mails sent. Little Miracles explains how it collects all those addresses:

> Expectant moms glow with hope and joy when they first find out that there is a 'Little Miracle' growing inside of them. First, they want to share their excitement with the world, and as they seek information and sign up for pregnancy and parenting newsletters and fill out online surveys, their data is captured and brought to you on this list of self-reported expectant parents.

A couple of decades after *American Baby*'s Patricia Calderon dismissed the idea of marketing to women still suffering from morning sickness, Little Miracles touts the receptivity of these newly pregnant women: "They are not just in need of information on their coming babies and parenthood, they are also in need of baby products, furniture and supplies." For a little extra money, Little Miracles can target women even more finely, choosing by age, household income, geography, and ethnicity:

> This new database offers the unique selection of FIRST TIME MOMS so you can identify those folks who are starting from scratch to outfit their coming baby. They are very responsive to informational offers, parenting and pregnancy publications, LaMaze [sic], maternity apparel, self-pampering, beauty, baby care and feeding, diapers, nursing, cribs, and other baby necessities.[43]

Pregnant women were demonstrating their interest in sharing and shopping, and marketers were ready to encourage and inspire them to shop more and buy earlier.

Marketers like Little Miracles mail to women who volunteer the details of their lives. These women at least theoretically mean to share the information, even if in fact they often do not anticipate the ramifications of what they have done, or understand how widely their pregnancy status and other personal data will be shared. Some major marketers, however, have begun to make shrewd educated guesses about women's pregnancy status, even when women are not intending to share the news with them.

In 2012, investigative journalist Charles Duhigg showed how discount chain Target analyzed customers' purchasing patterns to predict when they were pregnant. Target's information technology specialists wrote sophisticated computer algorithms that analyzed prior purchasing patterns of customers who bought baby supplies, and then looked at other customers to see if these patterns matched. Even before a woman was looking at baby gear or diapers, her purchases could give away her pregnant condition. After some problematic incidents—in one case mailing baby ads to a teenager whose pregnancy was thereby "outed" to her family—Target maintained a soft sell. Ads for diapers and car seats were tucked in among more generic listings, so that a woman would feel that she had just happened across them, rather than suspecting that Target had become a creepy marketing stalker. Even a pregnant woman who consciously maintained a low profile and intended to wait to shop until her pregnancy seemed secure could face marketing enticement.[44]

Facebook, too, seemed like it might be looking for ways to reach pregnant women before those women necessarily wanted to be found. In 2012, journalist Cotton Delo reported for *Ad Age Digital* that Facebook appeared to be marketing baby products based on data mined from status updates. This certainly would be technologically possible. After all, women posted pictures of home pregnancy tests, phrases such as "morning sickness," and other clues that could easily identify likely targets. Facebook denied that the data mining they were doing was that direct. But they did sell ads for customer groups labeled as "expectant parents," and marketers working with Facebook told Delo that Facebook had said they were able to target them very precisely. Facebook may not exactly be reading status updates for "It's positive!" announcements next to pictures of pregnancy tests, but it is likely using algorithms in the same way as Target to compile lists of likely pregnant targets. Avoiding sign-ups at babycenter.com and its ilk does not guarantee escaping the consumer culture of pregnancy.[45]

MARKETING AFTER MISCARRIAGE

"It's been 16 months since my m/c [miscarriage], and I still get the 'this is the age/stage' your baby should be at flyers and coupons from the formula company. Sometimes it makes me want to scream, but I know it's my own fault because I had registered on the company's website to receive these free mailings . . . . I just can't bring myself to visit the site again to request they be stopped." In a 2008 babycenter.com forum thread, women who had miscarried gave each other sympathy and advice about how to cope with the marketing machines they had set into motion when they shared their due dates. "I did the same thing and signed whatever it was they wanted me to because no one says how common mc [miscarriages] are until you have one . . . . I lost my angel 12/31/07 and I STILL get the parenting Magazine (free) every month [a year later] even though I have sent a letter, email, and called them asking to stop. I told them that if I got one more that I was contacting a lawyer."[46] Another gave sympathetic advice. "(((((hugs)))) Next time you have a baby, do NOT sign that little sign up sheet they have for first time moms. Also, make sure anything you sign up for as far as child birth classes, online mother's groups, and hospital pre-registration will not sell your info."[47]

These women had happily and hopefully shared their news with marketers via pregnancy websites. The marketers boosted the hype for the joys of pregnancy ever higher to create a mood conducive to selling more stuff, earlier and earlier. But pregnancy is not remotely close to a sure thing in its early weeks. When these hoped-for pregnancies were lost, marketers' messages prolonged the pain.

* * *

American consumer culture boomed in the twentieth century, as more and more Americans had at least some disposable income. As parents had fewer children, they could lavish more on each child. As they increasingly focused on the emotional bond with each child, pregnancy purchases became gifts for an already beloved family member. Buying was fun, and purchasing cute clothes and gear for an expected baby was especially enjoyable.

It was also big business. As marketing came into its own as an industry, its practitioners targeted expecting parents—a particularly profitable segment of consumers—earlier and earlier in their pregnancies. They hyped the joys of pregnancy and babies from the moment of conception, hoping to beat out competitors in the race to shape new parent-consumers and their purchasing habits. There was little incentive to take the process slower or to acknowledge that early pregnancies are still tentative. While the most prominent websites and apps have recently taken steps to assist women who have miscarried in removing themselves from marketing lists, it is still far too easy for a miscarried pregnancy to electronically "live on" because of less scrupulous marketers who widely distribute women's contact information. And the problematic incentive remains: Marketers know that parents commonly remain loyal to their initial brand choices. So if ethical marketers wait, they lose out to those who are willing to deluge a pregnant woman with advertisements when she is newly pregnant. Marketers joined maternity care reformers in reaching out to pregnant women, urging them to invest even more in their pregnancies, in the context of a broader culture in which Americans' efforts to control their fertility outcomes came together with their desire to parent their unborn children lovingly from the very beginning.

CHAPTER 6

⚬〰⚬

Imagining the Baby

Debating Abortion

"I've been pro-choice since before I even understood what was at stake," explained writer J. J. Keith in a 2013 article for *Salon*, "and yet, when I chose to have a baby while still in my allegedly fertile late-20s, all I could produce were the kind of clots sucked out during a D&C. I chose baby. Where was my baby?"[1] Keith had three miscarriages before she gave birth to her two children. Like many Americans in the last several decades, she had grown up thinking of pregnancy in terms of abortion politics. Women had babies, or they had abortions if they chose to do so. Politically, you could be pro-life or pro-choice. But what happened when a woman lost a wanted pregnancy? Miscarriage was a silent repudiation to both sides—a denial of life and choice at the same time.

The pro-choice arguments Keith had taken for granted seemed facile and unfeeling in light of her frustrating struggle to have children. "The idea that some who could carry a baby to term would choose not to suddenly made me sad then angry then confused." They did not account for her feelings about her miscarriages after she had her children, either. "I would like to say that my son and daughter are the children always intended for me by some force that I don't understand and probably don't believe in; that those other pregnancies were just my real kids making RSVPs they couldn't keep, but that's just not how I feel. It doesn't make any sense to me, at least not intellectually, but I feel like I have five children—two born and three who were not born, which is a point-of-view that is hard to reconcile with being pro-choice."

Keith noted that neither she nor her religious, pro-life friends mourned her miscarriages as they would a stillbirth or the death of an already-born child. But they agreed that "what was lost was substantive." In trying to describe her feelings about her miscarriages, Keith ultimately concluded that "they are just wisps of evidence of a choice that doesn't go both ways, yet is fair. They are my never-borns."

It is clear in Keith's story that the language and arguments of the abortion debates profoundly shaped her understanding of pregnancy yet failed to offer a coherent or helpful way to understand miscarriage. Keith's 2013 essay offered readers a thoughtful way to remedy this disconnect between abortion debates and miscarriage experiences. It took five years for her to find the words to offer her perspective.

In the meantime, at the peak of her difficulties, while Keith was feeling torn apart by her losses, she was teaching a college seminar that addressed the ethics of abortion. At the time, she felt that her personal miscarriage experiences had no place in the public conversation about abortion. The class discussion the day she learned her third pregnancy was unviable and destined to miscarry was wrenching:

> That day in front of my class of college freshmen, my hands still smelling of the hospital-grade hand soap from my OB-GYN's bathroom and my never-to-be-baby still inside of me, I led that discussion about abortion that I planned back when I was going to be a mother, back when it wasn't going to be psychological torture to talk about pregnancy with a roomful of teenagers. I kept my face neutral as my students jumped in with their ideas about choice and freedom, their words both cautious and unscathed. We compared an embryo's right to keep growing to a woman's right to not be colonized by a force so mighty that it could kill her if it went wrong enough. We talked a lot about women *choosing* not to stay pregnant, but not at all of embryos being the ones to make the call.

In that miserable moment, it was clear to Keith how misleadingly incomplete abortion-related discussions of pregnancy were, and yet she felt required to employ the traditional terms of the abortion debate. Keith was understandably afraid that expressing her feelings might overwhelm a careful and rational class discussion. But she was also kept silent by the lack of any widespread public discussion of miscarriage that she might have been able to draw upon. As her students built their understandings of pregnancy and women's choices, even a teacher who understood all too well the precariousness of early pregnancy and the unpredictability of fertility could not find a comfortable way to share that knowledge.

The contemporary abortion debates, so critical to framing how Americans think about early pregnancy, are a misleadingly narrow lens through which to understand pregnancy. Activists and casual debaters alike have unwittingly contributed to the confusion and misery of those who miscarry wanted pregnancies.[2]

ABORTION BEFORE *ROE V. WADE*

Women and their health practitioners have always understood that pregnancies might be disrupted on purpose. Recipes for restoring the menses, or "emmenagogues," have long been a part of recorded medical practice, as have abortifacients, drugs that were intended to expel an embryo or fetus, often used after it died in utero and threatened the pregnant woman's health if retained. Until the nineteenth century, however, emmenagogues and abortifacients do not appear to have been a routine part of women's health practices. They were unreliable in small doses and dangerous when taken in amounts large enough to guarantee the expulsion of a fetus. Most of the time, women were aiming to have many children anyway, so they were not routinely trying to disrupt their pregnancies.

In the nineteenth century, middle-class couples' childbearing goals changed dramatically. Middle-class women and their husbands did everything they could to have carefully planned, intensively nurtured families with only three or four children. They did their best to prevent pregnancies, but they were also willing to interrupt pregnancies as long as it was before "quickening." Most people did not draw biological or ethical distinctions between contraception and abortion and saw both as means of preventing unwanted childbearing. Critics who were alarmed by shrinking middle-class families were no less discerning; they condemned the prevention of childbearing by any means.

Most of the vocal critics of fertility control in the nineteenth century were physicians who expressed their concerns in the pages of their medical journals. They traded reports of rising abortion rates in their communities. By the 1860s, observers estimated that 20 to 30 percent of pregnancies were aborted.[3] It is likely that in their alarm over abortion and their suspicion of women's motives, these physician-observers overestimated the true number of abortions. Since they believed that miscarriages generally had an external cause, and they understood that women who hoped to limit their family size welcomed early miscarriages, they may have counted all ended pregnancies as abortions. Even so, in the days before home pregnancy tests, the observed spontaneous miscarriage rate was likely about 12 to 15 percent, so a substantial number of pregnancies must have ended in induced abortion.

Abortion appears to have increased even as it was outlawed. "Irregular" physicians and patent medicine vendors advertised abortifacients in magazines, pamphlets, and newspapers, and abortion services were readily available in cities, even as abortion was gradually banned, state by state, between the 1840s and 1900.[4] Described as treatments to "restore the menses," abortifacient drugs and practices were widely accepted as long as they were used early in pregnancy by respectable, married women.

Even through the decades of its criminalization, abortion remained an open secret and a common practice for keeping one's middle-class American dream on track.[5] This was particularly evident during the Depression era. In 1939 the Maternity Center Association distributed a pamphlet, "How Does Your Baby Grow," in conjunction with its World Fair exhibit.[6] The last page exclaimed,

> Abortions are dangerous! Some young people get married and plan to have their babies when they can provide them with a comfortable home and the things that make life happy. But their plans are balked by an unexpected pregnancy. What to do? In their desperation, they turn to the professional abortionist—a discredited doctor. Little do they know what abortions do to people . . . . If you are thinking about an abortion—stop! Go to your family doctor. Talk it over with him. Remember, some women get pregnant only once in life. Don't make a move you'll regret.[7]

This remarkably honest and sympathetic treatment of abortion did not by any means favor the practice but may be somewhat less categorically opposed to abortion that it appears on the surface. Many doctors could be persuaded to provide abortions to their regular clients or to refer them to a trusted provider. The pamphlet author may have been thinking that a reader who was not dissuaded from abortion might at least manage to have one in a safe setting, to protect her health and future fertility. Through the 1930s, regular physicians often sympathized with longtime patients who were trying to build good lives for their families and quietly helped them obtain abortions.

In the 1940s and 1950s, enforcement of abortion laws intensified, making illegal abortions riskier and more expensive but no less central to American family building.[8] Doctors were frustrated because they saw women risking their lives to get abortions. These risky measures happened not only in extreme cases of rape or grave illness or when a woman was burdened with seven children and a disabled husband but also in cases where women saw their ambitions for a fulfilling middle-class lifestyle derailed by an unwanted pregnancy. Women sought abortions so that they could finish school or professional training, avoid marriage to a man they did not see as middle-class-husband material, help get their own or their husband's career or business off the ground, or space their children to avoid personal and financial depletion. Motherhood was a central part of most of their plans—so central that they wanted to do it exactly right. They wanted a husband who would be a true-life partner, secure finances, a nice home, and two or three children who arrived when everything was ready, spaced at reasonable intervals. This ideal was shared by both an established and an aspiring middle class. Motherhood was supposed to be a fulfilling and pleasurable vocation, and women took great pains, risking even life and limb, to arrange their lives according to this vision. A mistimed pregnancy could make all the difference.

Physicians were horrified to see their patients die of complications from unsafe illegal abortions and unable to persuade their patients to keep unwanted pregnancies. Frustrated to find their hands tied, criminalized if they provided abortions or referred patients to abortionists, doctors pushed back. The twentieth-century abortion debates began with a reform movement by physicians, starting in the late 1950s, to liberalize abortion laws and put judgment about abortion back in the hands of a woman's physician.[9] Ultimately, this was the right established in *Roe v. Wade* in 1973: the right of privacy surrounding decisions made by a woman and her doctor.

CHILDBEARING AFTER *ROE V. WADE*

Cultural norms and practices around abortion solidified in the decades after this landmark case. Far from being a challenge to existing norms, the Supreme Court's decision on abortion tended to reinforce de facto practices that had been established over the previous century or so. The reinforcement and exaggeration of the norms that had developed by 1973 can be seen in many of the ways Americans have used and debated abortion in subsequent decades.

Legalizing abortion reduced the risks involved in aborting and thereby reduced the pressure to compromise one's life plans. It was that much more possible to be in control of one's fertility and that much less acceptable to fall haphazardly into childbearing. Implicitly, women could feel required to either declare a pregnancy to be "wanted" or abort. Every unplanned pregnancy demanded a decision.

It could feel irresponsible to refuse abortion when circumstances were less than ideal. One woman explained her story to *New York* magazine in 1989:

> I got married at 20 and had my first at 21 and my second at 24. Then, when they were eight and ten, I found out I was pregnant. My husband is a locksmith and I was working as a receptionist, and I knew if I had the baby, I would have to quit my job. We were already having a tough time financially. I had two kids who I wanted to send to college, and I thought financially it would be a mistake. I used to stay up at night discussing it with my husband and crying. I felt it was wrong, but I also felt I wouldn't be able to give my first two kids what they needed. And God forbid our marriage didn't work out, I'd be stuck with three kids to raise. Those things go through your mind.

She went to an appointment at an abortion clinic but backed out at the last minute.[10]

One might expect, as Catholic theologians have posited, that this easy availability of abortion would lead to the cheapening of life: if abortion were legally and medically sanctioned, women might start to think that early pregnancy did not really "count." Paradoxically, legalization has produced almost the opposite effect. After *Roe v. Wade*, pregnancies that were not aborted demanded commitment, from the woman herself and preferably from her partner as well. Women had a decision to make in early pregnancy, so they thought hard about their pregnancies. And once they had decided to keep their babies, they felt attached to them. From this perspective, prenatal life appeared cheaper in the nineteenth century, when a woman with an unplanned pregnancy might take a wait-and-see attitude, knowing that accidents happen. After legalization, once a woman decided to keep a pregnancy, she and the people around her expected her to be committed to it and largely ignored the possibility of involuntary loss.

Legal abortion also increased the likelihood that the pregnancies women did choose to keep would be planned ahead and intensely desired. Sometimes these planned pregnancies were literally supported by previous abortions. In a series of online oral histories collected by historian Sarah Leavitt for the National Institutes of Health, one woman told the story of two positive pregnancy tests: the first, in 1991 when she was a new army recruit fresh out of high school, and the second, as a married woman twelve years later. The first time, she was embarrassed to be seen buying a home pregnancy test at the PX and was shocked and distressed at the result: "I was pregnant and not happy. I did what I felt was in my best interest at the time."

Her later positive test, as she told it, served to redeem her prior experience. "I am married and planned to get pregnant. . . . I was proud as I stood in the test aisle and took a great deal of time reading all of the boxes to see which one would give me the most accurate result. I tested three days before my period was due and I got two lines. I cried this time too but they were tears of joy. I was pregnant and happy. 12 years later, three college degrees, a husband and a much better result."[11]

But even when a particular woman's life course had not involved abortion, access to abortion indirectly supported women's wanted pregnancies by giving them confidence they would be free from childbearing while they carried out elaborate plans to put the rest of their lives into place first. This delayed childbearing would be heavily invested, planned, and anticipated for years (perhaps decades) ahead of the fact. As Katha Pollitt put it in a 1988 editorial in the *New York Times Magazine*, of herself and her friends who had their children in their late thirties, "No one had a baby before she was ready, wild to be a mother."[12] When those long-planned, heavily invested pregnancies miscarried, even early in pregnancy, it could be devastating.

This delayed childbearing tends to be considered a responsible choice. Americans celebrate the freedom to make life choices but at the same time praise choices that are considered thoughtful and responsible. Public health messages declare that responsible choices result in good lives. Women who delay childbearing until they feel fully ready to care for and enjoy children are praised. They may justifiably feel that everything is supposed to go as planned after they have conscientiously planned everything in advance. Ironically, women who responsibly delay childbearing may find themselves at increased risk for miscarriage, since miscarriage rates slowly rise after a woman's mid-twenties and more rapidly in her late thirties.

Abortion practices since legalization have framed pregnancy loss in another way as well: the most common procedure, suction abortion, has made the physical experience of abortion less like the physical experience of miscarriage. Prior to legalization, the majority of abortions were induced miscarriages. Only a regular physician was likely to perform a dilation and curettage (D&C), a fussy surgical procedure otherwise used to treat an incomplete miscarriage or various other uterine maladies. After legalization, D&C became the norm, soon replaced by suction evacuation of uterine contents. A woman went to an abortion clinic, had a five-minute procedure, and left not pregnant. She would have period-like bleeding for up to a couple of weeks but not the cramping, heavy bleeding, and passage of tissue that generally accompanies a miscarriage after about six or so weeks of pregnancy. In an earlier time, abortions were considered "induced miscarriages" and entailed a physical experience like miscarriage. In that earlier period, the opposite of "pregnancy" was "miscarriage" (whether involuntary or voluntary). After legalization, the opposite of "pregnancy" was "abortion," and miscarriage became invisible, an event that simply was not supposed to happen.[13]

Since legalization, women have had abortions earlier and earlier in pregnancy. In 1973, 38 percent of abortions were before eight weeks of pregnancy. By 2014, 67 percent of women who ended their pregnancies did so before eight weeks.[14] Women are not waiting to see if they miscarry; they abort as soon as they have made a choice, as early in pregnancy as possible. This means that a substantial proportion of abortions represent what would have been miscarried pregnancies in a previous generation. Therefore, a greater proportion of miscarriages are happening to wanted pregnancies. This contributes to the modern understanding of what differentiates abortion and miscarriage: abortion happens to unwanted pregnancies, and miscarriage happens to wanted pregnancies. Miscarriage, then, becomes an unambiguously bad thing, a derailing of an intended process rather than an expected and sometimes welcome part of reproductive life.

THE RHETORIC OF THE ABORTION DEBATES

At the same time that abortion practices frame miscarriage experiences, the abortion debates of the past several decades have given us much of the public language with which we talk and think about pregnancy and the meaning of embryos and fetuses. The debates have two almost entirely separate camps, with two sets of terminology and two frames for thinking about pregnancy. One camp is "pro-life," the other "pro-choice." For the most part the two framings of the abortion issue are not in direct opposition: "life" and "choice" are not actually opposites, except in what they are supposed to connote about abortion policy. Both contribute substantially to the feelings of the majority of Americans about pregnancy and pregnancy loss, even for most of those who put themselves firmly in one political camp or the other.

The abortion debates did not supplant some other way in which Americans routinely had public discussions about pregnancy; rather, they introduced the idea that everyone, whether or not they were pregnant, had ever been pregnant, or could possibly get pregnant, should have philosophically well-grounded opinions about the meaning of pregnancy. As the abortion law reform movement accelerated in the mid-1960s and began to impact state laws, it garnered substantial attention in the press. Newspapers, news magazines, women's magazines such as *Good Housekeeping, Redbook,* and *Mademoiselle,* and general-interest periodicals such as *Life, Readers' Digest,* and *People Weekly* gave regular, in-depth coverage to the abortion issue.

This attention has persisted, intensifying around elections, relevant legislative efforts, and violence aimed at clinics. Those events often served as a hook for a longer article about the current state of the abortion debates and public opinion. By the 1980s, books about the issue were published for middle and high school students and marketed to public libraries and schools.[15] In this way, abortion became the context in which young people learned to think and talk about pregnancy, until the stage when they are actually pregnant or trying to become pregnant, at which point other sources of discussion and advice also kick in. The abortion debates made pregnancy into something that ought to be considered, separate from one's own, actual pregnancy. It made the status of the embryo something one might contemplate and debate years, even decades, before considering becoming pregnant oneself.

The upshot of this is that pregnancy, and the meaning of an embryo or fetus, is first considered in the abstract and outside the experience of a particular pregnancy. This pregnancy-in-the-abstract does not have to be discovered via a home pregnancy test, morning sickness, or a blood test at the doctor's office; it simply exists, available for philosophical contemplation from the moment of conception. Unless the philosophical hypothetical has been qualified, it is like the pregnancies in the developmental timelines in prenatal educational materials: destined to unfold along an average developmental timeline, resulting in a healthy baby delivered exactly nine months after conception. The substantial possibility of pregnancy loss is nowhere to be found. This universalized abstraction of pregnancy most clearly grounds the pro-life side of the abortion discourse, but the way the debate has been framed, it demands consideration by everyone.

It is hard to reach childbearing age in contemporary American culture without having considered the meaning of early pregnancy and the moral status of the human embryo. This is evident, for example, in a 1986 *Life* magazine story of a fourteen-year-old girl who had a late second trimester abortion. She had delayed dealing with the pregnancy for a variety of reasons, including her own and her family's qualms about abortion. She reflected, "I used to think that I didn't like abortion, because it was like murdering some baby that didn't ever do anything. But when you're in this kind of situation yourself, and you're so young, abortion is better. . . .I don't want to be pregnant. I want to be normal."[16] At this young age, she already had a well-formed understanding of the meaning of pregnancy in the abstract, developed within the context of the abortion debates. When that understanding clashed so dramatically with the contingencies of her real-life pregnancy, she changed her mind. But this had required a reluctant change of heart. Her stepmother had urged her to keep the pregnancy: "Abortion was hard to accept because she was so far along. I was looking at it as being a real baby in there." For both of them, the meaning of this particular pregnancy was filtered through the lens and language of the abortion debates, a perspective they had both absorbed before there was a real pregnancy to consider.

When women get pregnant on purpose, this abstraction of pregnancy and embryo from the abortion debates hovers in the background, informing their understanding of the process, imbuing it with deep meaning from the first moment. And then, when desired pregnancies are lost, it is shocking, partly because the abstract model of pregnancy is a model of perfect development and inexorably unfolds to healthy birth unless willfully disrupted.

The specific terms of debate on each "side" have a profound influence as well. The terms "pro-life" and pro-choice" came into routine use in the popular media by around the late 1970s, though they were used earlier by activists. As *Time* magazine characterized it in 1979, "Across the country, the battle is turning increasingly political and is waged by men and women who offer no quarter. It is a fierce clash of fundamental beliefs in which name calling is considered as potent as reasoned argument. Thus the antiabortionists call themselves 'pro-lifers' and denounce their opponents as 'baby killers.' Those who support a woman's right to abortion call themselves 'prochoice' and deride the other side as 'compulsory pregnancy people.'"[17] Since that time, pollsters and politicians have regularly asked Americans to label themselves with one of these two categories.

As slogans, they have carried great rhetorical force. Put together, they almost sound the same as "life, liberty and the pursuit of happiness." And these are the slogans we have associated with pregnancy. A wanted pregnancy is an incredibly favored state of being, within the language of the abortion debates: a deliberately pregnant woman has both "life" and "choice." She fulfills both the feminist commitment to self-determination and the traditionalist elevation of home and family. When a woman with a wanted pregnancy miscarries, she is let down by both sides. It turns out you can choose whether or not to have an abortion, but you can't always choose whether or not to have a baby. And being "pro-life" does not guarantee that you get to "choose life," in the words of the slogan on pro-life billboards and license plates.[18]

Beyond the slogans, the political and cultural campaigns of the two sides have contributed mightily to our current experiences of early pregnancy loss. One of the most important components of the abortion debates, in terms of their impact on pregnancy loss, is the pro-life argument that human life, and therefore personhood, begins at conception. This argument did not begin with *Roe v. Wade*; in 1867 Harvard professor of medicine Horatio Storer declared that "physicians have now arrived at the unanimous opinion, that the foetus in utero is alive from the very moment of conception. . . . The first impregnation of the egg . . . is the birth of the offspring to life; its emergence into the outside world for wholly separate existence is . . . but an accident in time."[19] Nineteenth-century activist physicians pushed clergy to adopt this position, and many eventually did, including the Catholic hierarchy. In the mid-twentieth century, as liberal physicians and clergy agitated for abortion reform, this position became more firmly identified with the Catholic Church, and early organized efforts against abortion reform were Catholic led.

This argument, about personhood beginning at conception, was both a moral and a legal argument and eventually became an emotional argument as well: respect for life and a duty to protect persons became an obligation to love, or at least nurture, one's growing baby. A pro-life argument would not, theoretically, need to rely on an essential sameness between a fetus and an already-born child. In the Catholic tradition, all processes of generation were to be respected, and contraception, which frustrated the natural purpose of the marital union, was no more acceptable than abortion. But this continuity with the church's position on contraception was deemphasized, as the church fell further and further outside the mainstream in its insistence on the sinfulness of contraception. Catholicism's stand on abortion was taken out of theological context and re-packaged to make it palatable to a wider American audience. As Evangelicals joined Catholics in the anti-abortion movement in the 1980s, anti-abortion rhetoric deemphasized Catholic theology still further, focusing almost exclusively on the personhood of embryos.[20] Conception became a much brighter line. By the post–*Roe v. Wade* abortion debates, women were urged not just to respect life and generative processes but to nurture babies, and the starting point for this nurturing was supposed to be conception.

Pro-life political and cultural campaigns have created effective images and symbols to inspire Americans' emotional investment in early pregnancy, with the hope that it will lead them to support pro-life legislation. This has had unfortunate implications with regard to early pregnancy loss. Since the mid-1970s, predominant pro-life messages have highlighted the most babylike aspects of fetuses. A photo of the feet of an aborted ten-week fetus, taken in 1974, became a prominent symbol of the pro-life movement. The tiny feet stand in for the fetus; the viewer understands the fetus to be a tiny baby.[21] Other widely reproduced photos showed the face and hands of older fetuses, encouraging us to imagine this older fetus when we think about any pregnancy, at any stage.

Even when "the baby" does not look anything like a child yet, pro-life advocacy teaches the viewer imaginative strategies for connecting emotionally with it as such. In a 2006 campaign by a pro-life group on the Harvard campus, a blastocyst appeared to write its own narrative, with the scrawl and doodles of an especially refined five-year-old. "Hi! I am Elena! I might be just 30 hours old, but I already have my own 46 of what doctors call chromosomes making up my SPECIAL DNA" (see Figure 6.1). She quoted Dr. Seuss: "A person's a person, no matter how small." This compelling poster crucially obscures that Elena only has about a 30 percent chance of surviving to birth. Elena, in fact, is more likely to perish than to last long enough to be detected by a home pregnancy test.

In this series, though, created in the tradition of the developmental timeline in pregnancy manuals, Elena reappears at twenty-five days old (five and a half weeks since last menstrual period) with a beating heart. And like the child persona the imaginative narrative adopts, she already has a fantasy of her future calling: "Maybe I will be a racecar driver when I grow up." She would now be easily detectable by home pregnancy test, and the fact that she has a heartbeat is promising, though no guarantee,

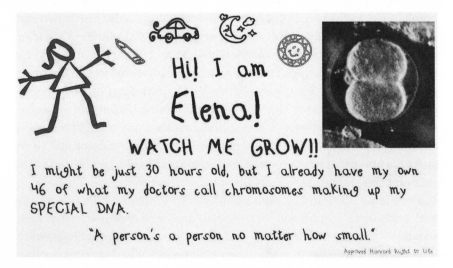

Figure 6.1 A pro-life poster from a 2006 Harvard student group. Images of the group's posters were shared across the Internet.

from the perspective of survival. Of course, many pregnancies that can be detected at five and a half weeks do not, in fact, contain viable embryos with beating hearts. It typically takes a woman's body several weeks to reabsorb or expel the remnants of an unsuccessful pregnancy, and hCG remains present as long as the uterus sustains the gestational sac, with or without an embryo. A woman comparing her own early pregnancy to the image on the poster, naming her baby and fantasizing about what she will be when she grows up, might be tragically mislead.

Despite these concerns, the central argument of the pro-life movement— that personhood begins at conception—is tremendously compelling to many people, and no matter how many pro-choice philosophers make logical and persuasive arguments otherwise, it seems to set the terms of the debate. This is perhaps partly because of its simplicity, but it is also because it is a clear moral argument that translates directly into a legal argument and a set of policy recommendations. If abortion is the killing of a person, it must be illegal to be consistent with current law, and public policy must work to suppress it.

While moral arguments made on the pro-choice side have been diverse and complicated, when it comes to the abortion "debates," or "wars," as they have been recently called, they have generally been defensively reduced to something like the "opposite" of the pro-life position: the fetus is not a person until viability, or perhaps birth. This simplified version of the pro-choice position is troubling to the many women who are politically pro-choice but mourn their miscarriages.

Given the lack of meaning attributed to embryos and fetuses in the pro-choice movement, the miscarriage support literature tends to borrow from pro-life language and imagery (see, e.g., Figure 6.2).[22] Women who look for support have lost pregnancies in a culture that has encouraged them to invest deeply in pregnancy very early on. The pro-life movement confirms that this investment was right and meaningful and that sorrow is appropriate because a baby has died. The use of this language does not necessarily mean that those offering support intend to promote a pro-life message.[23] The support literature is as likely to quote Khalil Gibran, a mystical poet celebrated by the 1960s counterculture, as the Bible. But the pro-life movement has created the public discourse that says that six-week embryos are babies, and so it is this discourse women often turn to when they are devastated by early losses, especially because so many of the promoters of investment in early pregnancy—the medical establishment pushing early prenatal care, the marketers of diapers and cord blood banking, the cheerfully scientific developmental timelines charting "your baby's growth"—seem to have nothing useful to say. In turn, the appropriation of pro-life imagery reinforces the idea that the only appropriate way to treat an early miscarriage is as the loss of a child.

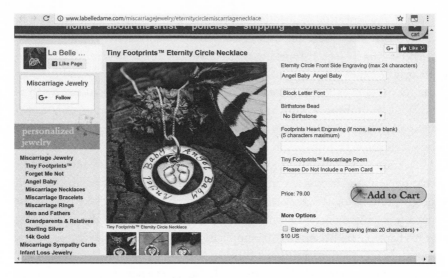

Figure 6.2 Miscarriage remembrance jewelry featuring the tiny feet that are a symbol of the pro-life movement.

A MIDDLE GROUND

Recently, there has been some discussion about "moving beyond" the pro-life and pro-choice terms of the abortion debate. Pollsters and reporters have pointed to the existence of a vast "mushy middle," representing the majority of Americans, since the contemporary abortion debate began. Only a small minority of Americans wants to outlaw all abortions or to legalize all abortions. Most agree that circumstances matter. Pollsters, however, have tended to ask Americans to put themselves in one camp or the other. And activists on both sides like to claim that most Americans agree with them. But according to an exasperated respondent to a recent poll, "There should be three [labels]. . . pro-life, pro-choice, and something in the middle that helps people understand circumstances. It's not just black or white—there's gray."[24]

When a polling organization finally framed the question differently, the results were illuminating. In 2011 the Public Religion Research Institute asked, "Please tell how well the following describe you. Pro-life: very well, somewhat well, not too well, not at all well, don't know." Then the same was asked for pro-choice. While 66 percent identified themselves at least "somewhat well" with the pro-life label, only 27 percent fully or mostly rejected the pro-choice label. In the other direction, 70 percent said the "pro-choice" label described them at least somewhat well, but only 31 percent fully or mostly rejected the pro-life identifier.[25] Clearly, many Americans think that abortion, and the meaning of early pregnancy, are more complicated than the terms of the abortion debate allow.

One reason most Americans do not see the issue as black and white is that, in practice, many people value pregnancy increasingly over the course of its development. Drawing on public opinion polls, interviews with activist organizers, and ethnographic accounts from inside abortion clinics, political scientist Jon Shields has shown that Americans across the political spectrum appear much less troubled by the destruction of early embryos than by abortions in mid-pregnancy. Pro-life leaders have mustered little energy from their base for banning or regulating *in vitro* fertilization based on the extra embryos it creates and discards. On the other side, a wide swath of politicians and their voters across the political spectrum supported the ban on late-term, dilation-and-extraction abortions. Many abortion providers, as committed as they are to women's right to choose, will only perform early abortions because they find the second-trimester procedure emotionally disturbing. Pro-life extremists have specifically targeted late-term abortion providers, such as George Tiller, David Gunn, and Barnett Slepian, for assassination. Pro-life and pro-choice sloganeering aside, in practice the majority of Americans are ambivalent. Many people see pregnancy as having a range of possible meanings, allow some pregnancies to carry more meaning than others, and see the emotional value of a pregnancy as increasing over the course of its development.[26]

* * *

Despite the firmly drawn lines of the abortion debates, many Americans are unwilling to think about abortion in absolute terms and in fact value pregnancies increasingly as they develop. We might be able to ease the burden of early miscarriage if we can explicitly capture this intuition. If we could define this middle ground in the abortion debates not as a "mushy" philosophical position but as a positive and beneficial way to think about early pregnancy, it might help us temper our attachment to still-tentative pregnancies and help us to moderate our feelings about early miscarriages.

CHAPTER 7

✺

Seeing the Baby

The Ultrasound Ritual

"Our first sonogram! How exciting! We were geeked and couldn't wait to see our baby. I mean, let's be real! We knew it would only be a tiny little black speck in her uterus, but it was OUR tiny little black speck that we have been waiting to create for months!" Sammie Mendez blogged the story of her wife Callie's 2014 pregnancy, the result of IVF, as "the chronicles of a non-belly mama: Thoughts from the Other 'Real' Mom." Because IVF pregnancies are closely monitored, their first sonogram was very early, at about six weeks' gestation.

The Mendezes had their sonogram in the office of their fertility specialist: "Our names are called. I spring to my feet, thanks to the 3 cups of coffee I've had in the past hour, and do my proud 'I'm gonna be a Mama' strut, protecting my lady and my unborn child from whatever dangers could present themselves in the 10 foot walk from chair to exam room." It was a moment of incredible anticipation. "I hold the door and in we go. We are about to see our little Poppy Seed."

What came next is a scene familiar to most Americans who have had a baby in the past three or four decades. "The nurse turns out the light and my eyes focus instantly on that black and white screen that only trained professional eyes can understand." The doctor was standing by, to interpret the image to the parents as much as to monitor the pregnancy. "I have no idea what I'm looking at, but as soon as the Dr. says, 'There's your baby!' I damn near lost it! My heart started racing, my palms started sweating, and I felt this surge of indescribable love for my Callie, laying there completely exposed, having been through so much just so we can have this incredible moment. I kiss her. I kiss her and I hold her hand and I admire her."

The doctor had a bit of surprising (though welcome) additional news: Callie was expecting twins. Sammie was over the moon:

> 2 gloriously chubby babies with 20 fingers for hand holding, 20 toes for tickling, 4 cheeks to kiss, 2 bellies for loud raspberries, 4 knees to kiss boo-boos, 4 eyes to show the wonders of this amazing world to. Oh man! It's 2! Our TWO Poppy Seeds growing in Mommy's belly. This adventure is going to be even more awesome than we anticipated. 2 little babies.

Sammie and Callie Mendez's ultrasound was a spectacular and special moment full of love for their growing family.[1]

Nutrition and lifestyle blogger Emily Malone shared a similar sense of excitement about her mid-pregnancy ultrasound during her first pregnancy in 2011. "We have had such a fun morning! I've been looking forward to our 20 week ultrasound since the day I found out I was pregnant." Malone described all the details of the exam conducted by a genial and knowledgeable sonographer and shared pictures. "I know I am clearly biased, but tell me—is this not the cutest little face you've ever seen? . . . I am on cloud nine after seeing our healthy little guy and hearing how big and strong he is." The baby's sex confirmed, Malone was also "excited to really dig into shopping for nursery things this weekend." Malone had anticipated that her mid-pregnancy ultrasound would be a truly special event and a time of intense bonding with her expected child, and indeed it was.

Malone's and Mendez's readers congratulated them just as enthusiastically. A commenter on Mendez's blog wrote, "This is the loveliest post. Made me tear up a teeny bit. Yay for you both—what a day that must've been!" Malone's readers shared their own reminiscences alongside their well wishes. "Wow, so neat that you can see all of that with the ultrasound. New life (and technology) is such a beautiful miraculous thing:) have fun picking stuff out!" Another exclaimed, "I never get sick of sonogram photos—could look at them all day!!" Several responded nostalgically. "Awww! It gets me all giddy because I remember how I felt seeing my own little ones on that screen." Another reflected, "It is truly an amazing experience and I felt the same rush of emotions and utter amazement at our 20-week ultrasound." A third sighed, "Ahhh I'm jealous—I remember all three times we had our 20 weeks sonogram and it was so special. Filled with lots of tears and smiles:)." Malone, Mendez, and their readers could as easily have been discussing a wedding or a baptism as an ultrasound exam.

All shared a sense of just how uniquely special, and yet universally meaningful, an ultrasound exam can be.[2]

Over the last few decades, Americans have built an elaborate ritual around
the ultrasound exam, with familiar features pregnant women and their
families can anticipate with pleasure. And like a wedding or a baptism, the
ultrasound exam ritual intensifies emotions, creates bonds, and prepares
its participants for important new family roles. This new ritual has had profound consequences for our experiences of pregnancy and pregnancy loss.[3]

FROM WAR TO OBSTETRICS

Ultrasound as a visualization technique originated in military technologies
of RADAR and SONAR and industrial technologies of metal flaw detection. In
the 1950s, capitalizing on wartime improvements in ultrasound technology,
medical researchers across Europe, Asia, and the United States experimented
with ultrasound as a visualization technique, attempting to use it to identify cancerous growths and structural issues in the brain, the eye, the bowel,
and the breast. In 1959 Glasgow obstetrics professor Ian Donald discovered
that ultrasound could give a clear, measurable image of the fetal head, and he
soon developed standards for measuring the age of the fetus based on the di-
ameter of the head. Researchers quickly found that fetuses were particularly
amenable to ultrasound imaging because of the dramatic contrast between
the structures to be visualized and the amniotic fluid which surrounded
them. By the early 1970s, Ian Donald's protégé Hugh Robinson had developed a technique for reliably detecting a fetal heartbeat by seven weeks' gestation, and the "crown-rump length" measurement, which remains the most
accurate method for measuring fetal age via ultrasound.[4]

Over the next two decades, ultrasound entered routine obstetric practice across Europe and the United States, and increasingly in other parts
of the world as well. While the United States does not keep official data
on ultrasound use, studies suggest that by 1987 a substantial majority of
women had at least one ultrasound, despite the fact that the American
College of Obstetrics and Gynecology consistently recommended against
routine scans done without a specific medical indication.[5]

DEVELOPING THE AMERICAN WAY OF SONOGRAPHY

While obstetric ultrasound is common in many parts of the world, it carries
different meanings in different places. For example, anthropologist Eugenia

Georges found that in Greece, ultrasounds are frequent but perfunctory, performed by obstetricians and rarely viewed by pregnant women. Women want them for reassurance that all is well with the pregnancy, and a basic diagnostic confirmation is typically all that obstetricians offer. In Israel, anthropologist Tsipy Ivry documented how obstetricians and patients search intensively for fetal defects in multiple ultrasounds throughout pregnancy, and women are discouraged from expecting a healthy outcome until the baby is born.[6] The emotional impact of ultrasound is not inherent in the technology. The ritual that American women, their families, and their medical caregivers have together built around the technology is what has made the ultrasound scan into a meaningful, connection-building experience.

This has become such an important ritual in North American culture that two anthropologists have conducted extensive studies to characterize it and probe its meaning. As Janelle Taylor and Lisa Mitchell have documented, by the early 1990s, sonographers and their clients had together developed a recognizable and reasonably consistent ritual around ultrasound scanning that pregnant women had come to anticipate. At that time, most women had a single mid-pregnancy scan, between eighteen and twenty weeks gestation, which is still considered the baseline sonogram for an uncomplicated pregnancy. At that exam sonographers generally consider their job to be twofold: checking thoroughly for medical problems in the fetus and placenta, and "showing the baby."

The ultrasound exam room is set up to facilitate both tasks. Women, and the partners, friends, or relatives they bring with them, expect to be able to view the monitor with the sonographer, or sometimes their own synchronized monitor. They anticipate listening to a narration that includes comments about fetal health, a "tour" of certain landmarks considered especially of interest to future parents, such as the heart, the spine, the profile, the fingers and toes, and the genitals, and a prediction of fetal sex. In turn, sonographers generally expect women and their significant others to express interest in the health-related information and excitement at "seeing the baby." When women or sonographers deviate from this script—for example, when a woman fails to show excitement or comment in ways which are understood to express parental concern, or when a sonographer is gruff and uncommunicative—the other party feels justified in complaining, though not necessarily directly. Women and their partners expect to be given an image or two to take home, or even a video, and sonographers build time and effort into the exam for capturing appealing, easy-to-read images.[7]

As obstetric ultrasound became routine, sonogram images escaped the bounds of doctors' offices. The images women took home from their exams became "baby's first picture," put up on refrigerators and pasted into baby books.[8] Sonographers made special efforts to give parents a "cute" view to keep, a sonographic slice that showed the fetal profile and the fingers, not, for example, a cross-section of the skull or the kidneys or the chambers of the heart. The clearest of these images made their way onto pro-life billboards and advertisements for cars and phone service, as culturally legible and emotionally compelling representations of "the baby inside."[9] Even when the images were blurry and the baby was hard to spot without coaching, pregnant women and their partners told anthropologists Taylor and Mitchell that they valued the images, showed them off to family and friends, and displayed them in their homes and offices.[10]

In a 2005 discussion on the conservative activist website Free Republic, commentator R. Scott described a young woman pulling out a bundle of ultrasound images to show her friends. He mused, "I have been aware of ultrasounds for a number of years, but only recently became aware of soon-to-be mothers carrying them around. She displayed a string of about a dozen pictures of her unborn girl. The women began exclaiming about her little face, hands etc. All I could make out was a series of blurs. Is interpretation of the pictures a woman's thing?" A woman answered him, "If you see the ultrasounds as the baby grows, and have more than one child, it becomes much easier to 'read them.' Trust me." Scott replied, "I'm beyond the age of looking forward to having more, so I don't look forward to gaining experience in reading ultrasounds—but if the pre-birth baby pictures keep being shown, I might learn."[11] Despite a lack of firsthand experience, Scott, like many Americans, was beginning to be coached in the viewing of ultrasound images. He was learning not only how to spot the baby but also how the images ought to be appreciated.

The ritual of obstetric ultrasound made its way onto the big screen as well, in popular movies such as *Nine Months* (1995), *Father of the Bride 2* (1995), and *Juno* (2007). By 2009, the popular TV series *Glee* could spoof the ultrasound ritual.[12] In one episode, Terri, who is faking a pregnancy, has blackmailed her doctor into conducting a sham ultrasound to "show the baby" to her husband Will. The obstetrician puts up a curtain between Terri and Will and places a DVD into the recorder, acceding to Will's request for a video because, as Will puts it, "My parents are going to kill me if I don't come home with a DVD." The physician waves the transducer around Terri's knees and corrects his previous "misreading" of the baby's sex, declaring the baby to be a girl. Will gazes at the screen on his side of the curtain in awe and begins to cry. Startled, Terri says, "Honey, I didn't know that having a boy was so important to you." Will replies, in a choked voice, "It isn't. I don't care what she is, she's all ours. I'm just so happy!"

It isn't clear whether the director expects viewers to interpret the image on the screen as Terri's knees or as the DVD from someone else's exam. Either way, they understand that the image on the screen, blurry as it is, will be seen by Will as his baby. And the TV audience understands that this is supposed to be an emotional, pleasurable ritual of bonding shared by the couple.

Expectations about the ultrasound exam and the emotional impact of the ritual surrounding it have become so powerful that it can be difficult and disturbing to question what we have created. In 2005, writer Gayle Kirshenbaum published a "My Turn" column in *Newsweek*, reflecting on her experiences of pregnancy, ultrasound, and her gradual and ambivalent journey into motherhood. She wrote,

> I expected to feel as excited about my first ultrasound as my friends had been about theirs. We were given our own printout of the squidlike creature we'd seen, magnified to fill the screen but in reality no bigger than a thumb. I stared at it and waited for a surge of maternal affection. What I felt was embarrassment at seeing what I might never have been meant to see--at having caught this entity in the act of becoming.[13]

Kirshenbaum recognized that her perspective was countercultural in the twenty-first-century United States. She wrote the column partly because she wondered whether women should abandon the emotional transition time of pregnancy and commit to motherhood at a stage when miscarriage is still a substantial possibility. It was a sensitive and difficult position to stake out: she had to question the assumptions of her sonographer, her prenatal yoga teacher, and her friends with sonograms displayed on their refrigerators—the assumptions built into the ultrasound ritual.

Indeed, Kirshenbaum was censured by some readers for her hesitation. One commentator, echoing the comments on Emily Monroe's blog posting, exclaimed, "when we saw ours, we both cried . . . we stared at the flimsy paper image for days in wonder, how can anyone look at something as magical as that and think . . . squid." Another judged her more harshly: "I remember the first time I saw my daughter on the ultrasound at ten weeks and it was amazing to see her little head, to see her move her small hands and legs. People who can't feel the awe in this and the sense of parenthood are sociopaths in my opinion."[14] Albert Mohler, president of the Southern Baptist Theological Seminary, called the column "a tragic portrait of motherhood."[15] While these comments were made by those with an explicitly conservative political perspective, with the abortion debates looming in the background, their expectations for the ultrasound ritual are shared to a large degree across the political spectrum. The ritual is supposed to be about bonding, and there is little room for ambivalence.

ULTRASOUND AT EIGHT WEEKS

Americans' ultrasound ritual was originally developed in the context of routine mid-pregnancy scans, conducted between eighteen and twenty weeks of gestation. At that stage, a routine scan in a low-risk pregnancy is unlikely to show any problems. At the same time, the scan is likely to feel particularly rewarding to the woman and her partner because the fetus is well-developed enough to be easily visualized in profile but not yet too big to be seen in a single image, and the fetal sex can generally be discerned. In the last fifteen years, this ritual has extended to an additional ultrasound exam commonly conducted between eleven and twelve weeks of gestation.[16]

More recently, many obstetricians have made eight-week ultrasound exams routine. Obstetricians have conducted early scans in cases of suspected ectopic pregnancy or miscarriage since the 1970s, but in the last decade many physicians have begun to use them to confirm and date the pregnancy.[17] Patients are generally told that the purpose is to date the pregnancy, and the substantial possibility of finding an unviable pregnancy is seldom mentioned. Early scanning has become increasingly common as obstetricians and hospitals try and date pregnancies more accurately in order to follow public health guidelines designed to stop doctors from inducing premature births.[18] And early and frequent scans are a routine part of *in vitro* fertilization procedures.

The ritual that pregnant women and their partners, relatives, and health-care providers developed in the context of the mid-pregnancy scan has been readily transferred to this very early ultrasound exam. While the ritual takes place in the private space of a doctor's office, people enjoy sharing it so much that there are hundreds of thousands of early ultrasound exam videos posted on YouTube. Some videos have been viewed more than a million times, though most appear to be intended for the enjoyment of family and friends. Rhea, a Philippina American from Los Angeles, was pregnant with the first of her three children when she posted a video of her early ultrasound. She and her husband, Mark, would eventually develop a business reviewing children's toys on YouTube, but her ultrasound video was an early amateur effort: it was more of a personal journal to share with family and friends than a professional production.

Rhea titled her video "My Ultra Sound. My Baby . . . 7 weeks and 4 days."[19] Viewers see Rhea laying on an exam table, looking sideways at the ultrasound screen as the sonographer runs the transducer over her abdomen. A female friend or relative is holding the video camera to film the scene. The sonographer affirms within seconds, "Oh yes, you're pregnant. First baby?" Rhea responds, "Yes, so happy!" The sonographer points to the screen, saying "there's your baby!" Rhea asks, "Oh, healthy?" The sonographer stumbles a bit, "Uh, I mean, like, I can't tell, but there it is." Rhea responds, "I see," and the sonographer reassures her with, "Wow, congratulations!"

Throughout, both women are laughing and smiling, and gazing together at the screen. The sonographer tells the friend with the video camera that she will let her know when to start taping, but the friend keeps taping throughout anyway. The sonographer assures Rhea that she will get plenty of keepsakes, because "I'll give you pictures, of course." As she conducts the exam, she continues with friendly chit-chat. "How old are you?" "I'm 27," Rhea responds cheerfully. "Oh, it's about time!" "Yes, so I'm so excited." The sonographer comes back to a profile image of the sac and embryo, saying, "Right there." Rhea looks, and exclaims, "Wow, perfect!" as the sonographer declares the current age and projected due date of the baby. "Seven weeks four days. So, May ninth." She returns to showing the baby, pointing to the screen: "That's the heart, right there." Rhea looks, and says wonderingly, "So you can see the heartbeat?" The sonographer explains, "This machine won't allow us to listen to the heart" ("I see," Rhea interjects) "but the heart rate is fine." Rhea concludes, "Great! As long as my baby is healthy. [giggle]." "Uh huh," responds the sonographer, non-committal but reassuring.

In this video, it is clear that Rhea came to the exam excited to "see the baby," with a friend or relative to record the exam and the image on the screen. The sonographer was happy to oblige and spent a fair amount of energy and extra scanning time "showing the baby." She was quick to clarify that she could not tell that the baby was healthy, but Rhea nevertheless expressed her satisfaction that she saw a healthy baby in her scan, especially after the sonographer pointed to the baby and demonstrated a healthy heartbeat. In the course of friendly chit-chat, the sonographer also affirmed the social appropriateness of Rhea's pregnancy, in discussing her age and intimating that the pregnancy was planned. Rhea, her guest with the video camera, and the sonographer worked together to locate a healthy, developing, socially desirable baby in the scan's images.

THE RITUAL MAKES IT REAL

While the resolution of scans has become high enough that an eighteen-week scan can show a quite clear image of a fetal profile, it becomes apparent from looking at take-home images of eight-week scans (six weeks after conception) that for many Americans the "baby-ness" of the baby does not depend solely on the resemblance between the ultrasound image and a newborn (compare Figure 7.1a and Figure 7.1b).[20] Ultrasound images have become quite sharp in recent years, and as the discussion on Free Republic demonstrates, Americans are becoming more and more sophisticated at reading them. We might persuade ourselves that the mapping we do to perceive a mid-pregnancy ultrasound image as essentially a picture of an almost-newborn is self-evident. But few people, even those who experience early ultrasound as a moment of profound bonding, would claim to be able to easily see the baby in an early scan. The power of it cannot reside in the recognition of tiny fingers and toes, or the shape of a face. The ritual itself, including the expectation all parties bring to it, is crucial.

Women are likely to come to eight-week scans ready to take part in this ritual. Court, a Houston-area vlogger and blogger with four children and over thirty-thousand YouTube followers, articulated in detail her expectations in her commentary before and after her first ultrasound as part of

(a)

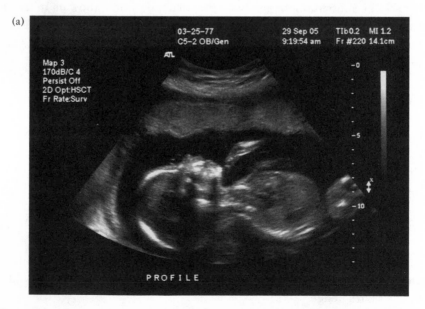

Figure 7.1a Ultrasound of a pregnancy at eighteen weeks gestation. iStock/jeffhochstrasser.

(b)

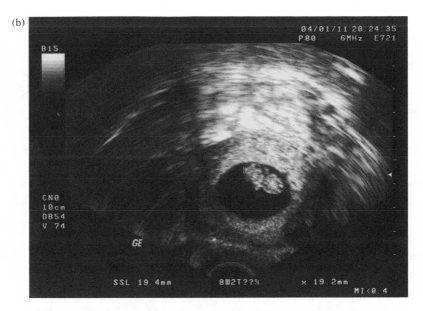

Figure 7.1b Ultrasound of a pregnancy at eight weeks gestation. iStock/pixalot.

her weekly ten-minute postings documenting her experience of her first pregnancy.

> 6-week vlog: I don't know if a lot of you ladies feel the same way, but I know with me, I'm super-excited, and really looking forward to everything that's going to happen, but I don't necessarily feel totally attached to the situation yet, and so I think whenever I see the picture or hear a heartbeat it's going to connect me in a much deeper way, and I'm really looking forward to that experience a lot. It's going to be awesome![21]
>
> 8-week vlog: [The ultrasound] was awesome! The only thing bad about it was the technician, she was just not into it at all. And I know that it's business for them, and they see it all the time, but you'd hope that in their field they could at least show a little bit of excitement. So that was kind of disappointing. She actually didn't even let me see the baby, or what she was doing, until the very end, and for maybe half a minute. She turned on the monitor and was like, "oh, here, you can look." And when she let me hear the heartbeat, (and my husband was there), she let us hear the heartbeat for about five seconds, I'm not kidding. So, I'm kind of annoyed, and definitely, the next time I get one, I won't let that happen, I'll speak up. But this time I just kind of was lying there, not sure what to expect, and I just let it happen. But regardless of that, the actual ultrasound was so awesome. When we heard the heartbeat, both of us were like, 'oh, wow, that is amazing." And it was definitely as cool seeing the little baby, even though

it kind of looked like a blob [laugh]. It was definitely as cool as everyone said it was.[22]

Even without the possibility of spotting little fingers and toes, there are still multiple points along the way when "seeing the baby" and bonding with it may be enacted by the participants in the ultrasound ritual.[23] A woman and her partner may come to the exam with specific expectations about what they will see and feel, which they may already have articulated in terms of seeing and bonding. Even if they have not, it can happen during the exam. The sonographer may begin the exam by suggesting, "Let's take a look at the baby." Even if she is more circumspect, as many sonographers deliberately are before they have confirmed a heartbeat, a woman who approaches the exam more cautiously may find herself drawn into that set of language and expectations once she is in the exam room looking at a screen set up to accommodate her viewing. She may start to ask a question and find herself asking about "the baby," since she may feel awkward trying to use the language of "embryo" or "fetus." As anthropologist Lisa Mitchell has shown, in mid-pregnancy exams women and their partners find themselves reprimanded if they speak about "my fetus."[24] We are comfortable talking about "the fetus" as an objective, scientific term for fetuses in general, or even for a given fetus when we regard it as detached from a woman, but the construct "my fetus" sounds inappropriate. So discussion about what is on the screen, if it is named at all, is quite likely to be named as a "baby." In sum, even before the sonographer demonstrates a heartbeat and points to the screen, saying, "there's the baby," the participants in the ultrasound ritual have already begun the process of seeing and bonding with a baby.[25]

MAKING PREGNANCIES "REAL" MAKES LOSSES REAL, TOO

Given the expectations that women and their partners bring to ultrasound exams, and the organization of the ritual itself, it is easy to understand how devastating the discovery of a miscarriage can be. And there is a substantial chance that a baby and a miscarriage will be discovered at the same time in the context of an eight-week ultrasound. If the exam reveals a healthy heartbeat, and the woman has not been previously diagnosed with repeated pregnancy loss, the pregnancy has around a 98 percent chance of going to term.[26] However, if the pregnancy is destined to miscarry, as around 20 percent of confirmed pregnancies are, there is a good chance she will find out at an eight-week ultrasound. Miscarriages generally do not begin immediately after an embryo has died. It may take a couple of weeks, sometimes many weeks, for the placenta to stop developing and hormonally maintaining the pregnancy. At eight weeks' gestation, these pregnancies are likely to appear as empty gestational sacs, the embryo having already been reabsorbed by the woman's body. Or the exam might reveal an embryo with no heartbeat, or embryo with a heartbeat that is too slow to remain viable.

While many readers criticized Gayle Kirshenbaum, the journalist who was reluctant to put her sonogram printout on her fridge, for her failure to embrace the ultrasound ritual, some seconded her caution from bitter experience. One letter, published in *Newsweek* the following week, described the painful consequences of discovering a miscarriage during the ultrasound ritual.

> Thank you so much for publishing an article about pregnancy, and the vulnerability inherent in it. The idea that we are supposed to be ecstatic about the life inside us is sometimes damaging if the idea that that life can end so fast is not also considered. I was incredibly excited to see evidence of the little life inside me for the first time, when my first ultrasound was scheduled at eight weeks. My mother came with me to share in that joy. We were absolutely stunned when the ultrasound operator could not find the heartbeat that was a sign of the life blossoming within my body. So instead of going home with my baby's first picture, I was kept in a hospital to take care of what my body had not yet done for itself when my baby's heart stopped beating. Five years later, my pain has barely receded. On average, one of every three pregnancies ends in miscarriage, often before the mother even knows it. So why do so many women proclaim their motherhood at five weeks? An ended pregnancy, by choice or not, is never something you want to share with all those people you so hopefully shared the news with just a few weeks before. I can barely look at sonogram pictures without a feeling of loss and sadness. I hope, for every woman's sake, that these first pictures never become a source of regret and sadness for them as well.
>
> J. West
> Kent, Wash.[27]

J. West embarked on her eight-week ultrasound exam with the expectations so evident in Rhea's YouTube posting and Court's vlogs, expectations extended from the ritual anthropologists have consistently found associated with mid-pregnancy exams. At the same time that she saw this as a moment when the pregnancy was supposed to become more "real," she did not go in seriously considering the possibility that this would not happen. And indeed, the ultrasound did confirm the "realness" of the pregnancy for her, just not in the way she anticipated: rather than bringing her joy, it brought her sorrow, representing the baby and its death in the same moment.

This exam could be read as one in which the participants would conclude, "I guess we were wrong, she was not pregnant after all." That is one legible interpretation of the statement she presumably heard from the sonographer: "I can't find a heartbeat." While the letter doesn't detail this, it is quite possible that the sonographer detected evidence of a pregnancy that never developed to the point of having a heartbeat in the first place. But in the context of the ritual as it has been constructed, the sonographer's pronouncement is most readily heard as, "the baby's heart has stopped beating. The baby has died."[28]

The visual evidence is equally open to different readings. It takes a fair amount of training on the part of the sonographer, and coaching on the part of the woman and her partner, to see a baby in an eight-week ultrasound. If the ritual were different, the sonographic image might be taken as evidence that there was no baby there in the first place or at least not yet a baby there. This might be especially true when, as commonly happens in early miscarriages, the exam revealed an empty gestational sac (what the obstetrician or sonographer may call a "blighted ovum").[29] But in the current ritual, the sonographic image represents a baby who has died, and as West so poignantly describes, it can become a focus of intense and lasting pain.

When a desired pregnancy is successful, the rituals developed around the technologies of early pregnancy allow us to celebrate sooner, "bond" sooner, joyfully anticipate the arrival of a baby sooner, shop for a layette and set up a nursery sooner. Vlogger Court and her husband prepared carefully for the anticipated moment of hearing their baby's heartbeat at the eight-week ultrasound, and she recorded her elation in detail as a special memory to eventually share with her child.

At the same time, the first two months are when pregnancies are most vulnerable to miscarriage and, in fact, are quite likely to be lost. And when a pregnancy is not destined to result in a baby, the effects of our rituals are troubling. J. West experienced lasting sorrow after the shock of discovering her miscarriage at her eight-week ultrasound exam, in the midst of what she had anticipated as a celebratory ritual of new life and a growing family. The ultrasound ritual is not organized to accommodate the substantial possibility of early pregnancy loss. We want our technology to give us certainty. But the sense of certainty it gives us is false, and we often feel betrayed. We want to use our technology to deepen our joy and expand our horizon of parental bonding. But much of the time our technological rituals sharpen our losses and bring sorrow.

These are not failings of the technology per se, but rather the result of the ways in which we use them and interpret them. While ultrasound is central to our pregnancy monitoring practices, there is nothing inherent in it that dictates our current uses or interpretations of the images and objects it produces. We could anticipate the eight-week ultrasound (or the ten-week Doppler scan) as an exam that shows whether or not the pregnancy we suspect is actually going to develop. We could use our technology to help us let pregnancy unfold gradually in the way that the slow accumulation of physical symptoms of pregnancy once did.

CHAPTER 8

cVo

Detecting the Baby

The Home Pregnancy Test

" 'I cried like a baby,' said Heather, and for K. B. it was the 'best feeling in the world.' Keisha did her 'happy dance' when she got the good news." In 2014, BabyCenter surveyed a thousand pregnant women about their experiences with home pregnancy tests. "Just over half of the women surveyed were so thrilled they saved their positive test, and 38 percent of pregnant women and moms say they *still* feel excited every time they look at it." Like ultrasounds, home pregnancy tests have become a ubiquitous celebratory ritual of pregnancy.

While about half the women surveyed were with their spouses when they took the test, a number of others found ways to make their pregnancy announcements unique and memorable. Babycenter highlighted special and sentimental stories, in women's own words.

Dayna wrote her partner a poem in which the first letter of each sentence spelled out 'We're pregnant.' Linden 'wrote on my belly telling him there was a baby inside,' and LMK 'bundled my four pregnancy tests into a bouquet and told him he was going to be a daddy.' 'I . . . gave the positive test to my toddler to hold and asked my husband to change his diaper,' remembered L. MacDonald. Steffi 'bought a T-shirt for my 11-month-old saying "I'm the big sister," put it on her, and let my husband notice it!' . . . Several moms-to-be took advantage of the holidays to tell their partner. 'It was very close to Christmas, so I wrapped up a slip of paper with my due date and let him unwrap it,' wrote J.P. Jennifer M. 'made the test a Christmas ornament and hung it on the Christmas tree.'[1]

Many women used the physical test itself as a key part of their pregnancy announcement. But even when they did not, the test's positive result made women feel confident memorializing their news with a T-shirt, a poem, or an ornament. It was the first moment in an expected child's life that a woman could preserve for posterity, and many did so with enthusiasm.

PREGNANCY DIAGNOSIS BEFORE THE HOME PREGNANCY TEST

Until the invention of a laboratory test for human chorionic gonadotrophin (hCG) in 1927, women and their doctors did not expect to be able to diagnose pregnancy with any great certainty until they could detect fetal movement and a fetal heartbeat, around the middle of the second trimester. Interest in early diagnosis began growing, though, long before the invention of the lab test.

During the nineteenth century, as the modern field of gynecology emerged, physicians began to express greater urgency about being able to diagnose pregnancy. They were developing new therapies for women's reproductive ills, but they needed to know when it was appropriate to apply them. In medical journals and textbooks of obstetrics and gynecology, they warned each other of the perils of misdiagnosing a pregnancy as illness and vice versa. They shared hints and tips about how to avoid the humiliation of having a supposed tumor pop out as a baby. More darkly, they cautioned about women pretending to be ill in order to obtain illicit abortions from naïve doctors who thought they were treating menstrual suppression.[2]

At first, the long lists of signs and symptoms of pregnancy that nineteenth-century doctors shared with each other were simply compilations of popularly understood and long-documented wisdom. An educated doctor could run systematically through the lists in his medical textbooks and make sure he did not miss anything. But it was no great improvement on what a woman could learn from her family and friends and her own prior experiences.

Doctors began slowly making headway in diagnosing pregnancy when they adopted what was an innovative practice at the time: visually examining and touching patients' bodies to understand what was wrong. Before the nineteenth century, doctors predominantly diagnosed illness and prescribed treatment based on patients' descriptions of their symptoms and their medical history, rather than by examining their bodies. Male physicians diagnosed and treated female patients' reproductive issues without necessarily looking at them or touching them, especially in their "secret" parts.[3] A potentially pregnant woman would tell a doctor if she felt her belly growing and noticed movement, rather than the doctor trying to touch her body to feel it himself. During the nineteenth century, as physicians' authority grew and their mode of examination shifted from primarily history-taking to viewing and palpating the body, they constructed new knowledge of physical signs of pregnancy.

Visual- and touch-based knowledge of pregnancy signs developed gradually over decades. At first, these newly defined "objective" pregnancy signs gave no certainty about pregnancy to the outside observer any earlier than quickening would for the pregnant woman. They reflected more of a mistrust that pregnant women were able and willing to diagnose themselves than any superior ability to make a diagnosis.

Charles D. Meigs's 1856 edition of *Obstetrics: The Science and the Art* gives a sense of this continued feeling of uncertainty despite physicians' increasing access to potentially pregnant women's bodies. Meigs, a prominent obstetrician and professor at the prestigious Jefferson Medical College in Philadelphia, began his discussion of pregnancy signs by describing the timeline of a woman's own suspicion and confirmation of her pregnancy. He pointed out that while a missed menstrual period would lead a married woman to suspect she might be pregnant, there were many other likely causes of amenorrhea. A second missed period, "especially if it be not accompanied with any signs of depraved health, renders the suspicion still more valid; while after a third and fourth omission, the change of form, and at last the perceptible motion of the embryo put all doubt to flight." He acknowledged other long-recognized signs of early pregnancy, including nausea, breast and areolae changes, increased salivation and urination, gastric disturbances, and food cravings, but designated these as signs "to be noted after pregnancy is fully ascertained," not signs that could be "depended on as sure evidences of its existence."[4]

Meigs described two innovative methods a physician could use to detect pregnancy but was unwilling to grant them certainty until the stage of pregnancy at which a woman would likely have quickened. "By means of the Touch, pregnancy may be doubtfully ascertained, before quickening has taken place, but not surely. By the Touch, we can readily learn that the womb is enlarged, altered in form, and contains something; but I do not see how any physician can absolutely aver what that something is, unless he can perceive a spontaneous motion in it."[5] And if the physician perceived a spontaneous motion, the pregnant woman would almost certainly have begun to perceive those motions as well.

Meigs preferred a second novel diagnostic practice: auscultation, with either stethoscope or "the direct application of the ear to the abdomen of the woman," to detect the fetal heartbeat. "The sounds of the foetal heart need never be mistaken."[6] While this method was exciting for the level of certainty it gave the physician in making a differential diagnosis between pregnancy and an illness imitating pregnancy, "to look for [the heart-beat] earlier than the fourth month is, however, in general, merely to lose one's time and find a disappointment."[7] Meigs described pregnancy signs that could be detected by an outside observer independent from the pregnant woman's perceptions or narrative of her bodily history, but these signs were only reliably available after a pregnancy would normally have quickened.

Toward the end of the nineteenth century, as a coterie of prominent researchers in the United States and Europe established themselves as experts in women's reproductive systems, those new gynecologists established somewhat more reliable ways of diagnosing pregnancies earlier in gestation. They codified the signs of early pregnancy, describing them and claiming them by name. "Hegar's Sign," described in 1895 by German gynecologist Ernst Ludwig Alfred Hegar, was a softening of the uterus that could be detected between four and twelve weeks of pregnancy. To feel it the physician put two fingers of one hand in the woman's vagina, his other hand on her abdomen, and palpated the uterus between them. "Chadwick's Sign" was a visible change in color of the cervix, vagina, and labia, made blueish by an increase in blood flow starting around six weeks of pregnancy.[8] "Goodell's Sign," named for prominent nineteenth-century Philadelphia gynecologist James Goodell, was a softening of the cervix that could be felt by around six weeks of pregnancy. None of these signs were certain. But taken together they were a helpful supplement to the traditional signs of missed periods, nausea, and breast tenderness.

The newly codified gynecological signs of pregnancy were not intended for routine use. They were all intimate and invasive, requiring penetration of the vagina, and women and their physicians thought of them as useful primarily for differential diagnosis. If a woman seemed ill, and she and her physician were trying to figure out whether the problem was pregnancy discomfort, some other illness that might require immediate treatment, or a combination, a visual and hands-on examination of the woman's genitalia might seem in order. Otherwise, it was standard practice to simply wait a few months for confirmation.[9]

THE DEMAND FOR EARLIER PREGNANCY DIAGNOSIS

In her 1922 pregnancy guide *Getting Ready to Be a Mother,* Carolyn Conant Van Blarcom urged her reader to start seeing a doctor from the very beginning of her pregnancy. The problem of pregnancy diagnosis was a stumbling block, though: "I am sorry to have to admit, at the outset, that making this important discovery is far from being a simple matter." Exasperated, she continued, "One would suppose, after all these ages, during which countless babies have been born and countless pregnancies have been observed by doctors and others, that there would be some known way of finding out definitely, at an early date, whether or not a baby was coming." Reflecting the common wisdom of her era, she assured her reader that once she had missed two periods (i.e., around nine or ten weeks of pregnancy), she could assume that she was most likely pregnant, especially if she also had nausea and breast tenderness.[10] She spent several pages describing what all the possible symptoms might feel like, to help her conscientious reader figure out whether she should see a doctor. As *Better Homes and Gardens'* 1943 publication *Baby Book: Prenatal to Six Years* put it: "If you miss two periods, it's fairly certain. If you have gone over your period and start losing your breakfast, or begin to urinate frequently, lady, your doctor wants to see you!"[11]

In the same years that modern prenatal care was making its debut, physicians and scientists were laying the groundwork for a lab test for pregnancy. During the late nineteenth and early twentieth centuries, researchers began to realize that chemical messages from glands in the brain and gonads regulated physiological processes, including reproduction. If these chemical messages regulated ovulation and menstruation, surely they could be measured to evaluate a woman's pregnancy status. Simultaneously, laboratory tests became an increasingly important part of modern medicine.[12] One early attempt at a pregnancy test was modified from the Wasserman test for syphilis.[13] The Wasserman test, invented in 1906, was quickly becoming a requirement for obtaining a marriage license in many states. Laboratory tests were coming into common use in clinical medicine, in public health efforts, and even in government surveillance, so it made sense that scientists around the world were trying to invent one for pregnancy.[14]

The first truly successful pregnancy lab test, referred to as the "rabbit test," was the Ascheim-Zondek test for human chorionic gonadotrophin (hCG). It was introduced in 1927, though it would never become routine for uncomplicated pregnancies. It was such an involved and expensive test that it was only used in cases where differential diagnosis was important. In the original version, five mice were injected with an extract of the woman's urine twice a day for three days. The mice were then dissected, and the woman was diagnosed as pregnant if any of the mice showed evidence of ovulation. Zondek's illustration showed a dissected mouse with her belly peeled open and her limbs pinned to a table, a martyr to the cause of pregnancy diagnosis. Whether the test was done with mice, rabbits, or, later, frogs, it was a destructive process many physicians did not want to order routinely.[15]

Diverse historical developments pushed women and their doctors to want to diagnose pregnancy earlier and pulled new science into pregnancy care faster than some scientists and obstetricians entirely intended. Public health educators like Van Blarcom urged women to seek prenatal care. By 1930 the widely distributed United States Children's Bureau pamphlet *Prenatal Care* urged women to have a complete medical check-up, including an internal exam to diagnose pregnancy, as soon as they believed they were pregnant.[16] Home pregnancy guides gave a bevy of diet, exercise, and sleep recommendations they urged women to follow from the beginning of pregnancy to ensure a healthy baby. Marketers began to see pregnant women as valuable customers and encouraged them to buy for the baby. Women began to hope their physicians would do better than informing them that they might just be pregnant, and time would tell.

Anticipating that some women would ask for the test, mid-century pregnancy manuals explained that lab tests were only done in special cases and that women should trust their doctors and be patient. Humorist Jean Littlejohn Aaberg, in her 1944 *ABC for Mothers-to-be*, noted that "It is often a matter of extreme annoyance to the inexperienced patient that her doctor will not say for certain that she is pregnant when she knows full well she is. So does he, usually, but technically a physician can say with certainty that a patient is pregnant only after the condition is well advanced."[17] In Eastman's *Expectant Motherhood*, first published in 1940, the A-Z test was dismissed as "expensive. . . quite unnecessary in most cases, and is generally performed only when the physician finds some medical reason for haste in making the diagnosis."[18] The U.S. Children's Bureau 1949 pamphlet included a revision to address women's interest in pregnancy testing. "All that is needed is a little patience, for time will soon tell whether a baby is on the way. Your doctor may not think it is necessary to do a pregnancy test on you and if he doesn't, don't urge him. They are expensive and usually have to be done in a special laboratory."[19] Women were given a frustratingly mixed message: they were supposed to take special care of themselves from the very first moment of pregnancy, and yet they were supposed to relax and let the passage of time bring certainty as to their pregnancy status.

Social and medical revolutions of the 1960s and 1970s brought more intensity to women's desire for an early pregnancy test. Reliable birth control, in the form of the Pill, encouraged the expectation that one could and should plan one's family precisely. The legalization of abortion in 1973 meant that a woman might really need to know sooner rather than later that she was pregnant. Middle-class women routinely began prenatal care in the first trimester. Women were less and less willing to tolerate the uncertainty of a possible early pregnancy.

Laboratory pregnancy tests grew cheaper, easier and more reliable. From 1927 through the 1950s, physicians were reluctant to routinely use expensive and slow animal-based tests and to kill so many animals if it would not have clinical benefit. But in the 1960s and 1970s, new and continually improving immunoassays made testing cheaper, more reliable, and increasingly more sensitive, detecting hCG as early as four weeks after conception (about two weeks after the missed period).[20] By 1972, the technology that would be incorporated into home pregnancy tests was already available in labs and hospitals.[21] Women expected to be able to get pregnancy diagnoses from their doctors within a few weeks after a missed period, even if it was not strictly medically necessary. Pregnancy testing had become routine, if not yet a do-it-yourself technology.

Routine pregnancy testing at the doctor's office within a few weeks after a missed period changed the typical experience of the first months of pregnancy. It condensed an experience that had typically entailed months of suspecting and monitoring into a few weeks of wondering followed by an abrupt moment of certainty. Before the availability of the test, a woman, her partner, and her doctor kept track of the accumulation of pregnancy signs and gradually came to a sense of certainty that the woman was, indeed, pregnant. The baby's kicking made it a sure thing. A pregnancy was not something discovered all at once; it arrived with a much more diffuse sense of realization. By the time a woman announced her pregnancy, she had been gradually growing more used to the idea and more confident in its reality over the course of months. Over those same months, the pregnancy itself grew more stable and less likely to miscarry. The pregnancy test compressed what had been a gradual evolution into a brief moment of intense feeling, detached from the biological reality of the fragility and tentativeness of early pregnancy.

Once the technology to make a home pregnancy test was well established, there was one last barrier to overcome: the stigma attached to pregnancy tests by their association with abortion. Some physicians preferred not to perform lab tests for pregnancy even in their offices because they wanted to withhold the information from women who may have sought an abortion. Many who opposed abortion did not want women to be able to circumvent their physicians with over-the-counter pregnancy tests. Given the strength of the anti-abortion movement in the 1970s, pharmaceutical companies were hesitant to market a home pregnancy test because they feared being accused of abetting abortions. Women were reluctant to demand the tests because of their association with the stigmatized practice of abortion. As a result, the introduction of the home pregnancy test was delayed in the United States until the late 1970s.[22]

THE PREGNANCY TEST COMES HOME

The over-the-counter pregnancy test was approved by the Food and Drug Administration in 1976 and was widely marketed beginning in 1978.[23] Historian Sarah Leavitt has gathered several hundred oral histories for the National Institutes of Health about home pregnancy testing from women and their partners, revealing how Americans have experienced home pregnancy testing from the late 1970s until the mid-2000s.[24] When the home pregnancy test first came on the market, it was quite literally a lab test wrapped in an over-the-counter package, resembling a home chemistry set. One respondent described her memory of a test she took in 1988. "I had to pee in a cup and use a dropper to add the urine to a vial along with some sort of reagent and my hands were shaking so violently that I almost dropped it." Another recalled, "It was NOT easy to use. I remember buying the cheapest one, because we were just starting out and broke. You pretty much felt like a chemist when you did this particular test. There were droppers to put drops of urine into a tube, you had to shake it up and then put this stick with little white beads in the end into the tube and wait something like 10 or 15 mins. If it turned bluish or greenish, it was positive." It might have been quicker and more private than going to a doctor, but it was still an elaborate process.

The fact that the test was offered over the counter meant that it could be advertised free of the pharmaceutical industry norms that reined in direct-to-consumer prescription drug advertising at the time. In widespread advertising, first in magazines and later on television, home pregnancy test manufacturers offered their vision of what home pregnancy tests could and should mean to the women who used them.

The first ads, arriving in 1978 at the height of the feminist movement, not surprisingly emphasized women's empowerment. "The E.P.T. In-Home Early Pregnancy Test is a private little revolution any woman can easily buy at her drugstore. At last, early knowledge of pregnancy belongs easily and accurately to us all."[25] As Sarah Leavitt and anthropologist Linda Layne have pointed out, in retrospect it does not actually appear all that revolutionary. One way or another, a positive pregnancy test quickly led a woman to a doctor's office. And yet, in the context of the women's health movement, in which activist women learned to do self-examinations and demonstrated for reproductive rights, knowledge itself was widely viewed as empowering, even when it could not be acted upon.[26]

Advertisers also played up the importance of pregnancy testing to pre-natal care. They pointed to new understandings of teratogens—drugs or other exposures that disrupt fetal development—and public health efforts to get women prenatal care as soon as possible. One of E.P.T.'s earliest ads explained, "The first 60 days are critical in fetal development. Improper nutrition, cigarettes, alcohol, even commonly used household medications can be harmful in these crucial first 60 days before most women even know for sure that they are pregnant. Now with E.P.T. you can know. Now, when you call your doctor, you have the results of your test to report. And time is on your side at last."[27]

More evocative than the public health message was the emotional mes-sage. In television ads, manufacturers promoted the joy of the positive test. E.P.T. ran a series of commercials that showed couples finding out their preg-nancy status on camera.[28] That precious, intense moment of discovering a pregnancy, compacted into an instant and caught on film, recalled a movie marriage proposal or the birth of a baby. The commercials showed how con-firmation of pregnancy could become one of those meaningful experiences that punctuate a person's life course, rather than a series of maybe-could-be moments that coalesced blurrily into relative certainty.[29]

That moment of emotional intensity was not a theatrical conceit; it reflected a common experience of pregnancy testing. Journalists Susan Lapinksi and Michael deCourcy Hinds described their experience in their joint journal of the journey to parenthood. It was 1979, so the pregnancy test they used required "carefully mixing the potions and placing the test tube in its mirrored holder." The two of them "sat back on the edge of the bed, cheering each reddish-brown speck that floated down and joined its circle of friends. A doughnut shape meant a baby, a smudge meant nothing, according to the directions. We were supposed to wait for two hours, but within half an hour, there was no doubt. We were pregnant! *'We're going to have a baby!'* we kept telling each other, but the thought didn't sink in. It kept floating to the surface, like the bubbles in our champagne."[30] Another woman explained, "When I got married, then I wanted to be pregnant! The stick kind was so easy. My husband waited downstairs and when I saw the positive result I thought, 'What have I done!?' I was scared and excited at the same time. I went to tell him and he got sick. We were both scared and excited!" Another described how she "cried tears of joy when the test came up positive." Yet another woman described an incredible cascade of emotions: "My initial reaction was utter disbelief followed by giddiness followed by regret and anxiety followed by excitement followed by more fear and ultimately resulting in what I might call happy resignation."[31]

Commercials also illustrated cute and memorable ways a woman could announce the result to her spouse. In a 1987 commercial for EPT, actress Nancy Travis sang snippets of pop songs to her TV husband as they snuggled in bed: "Baby, I'm a want you, Baby, I'm a need you!" "Rock-a-bye baby!" until her husband got the picture. Her husband lit up, asking, "Are you serious?" They hugged gleefully, Travis singing a raucous "Hello my baby, hello my darling" until her husband rolled her over on the bed, suggestive of a celebratory romp. The voiceover concluded, "It's the nicest way to find out if you're having a baby, or not."[32]

Memorable pregnancy announcements were treasured in real life, as well. One woman explained in her oral history, "I took the test alone right before I jumped in the shower to get ready for work—completely confident I was NOT pregnant! sure enough, once I popped out of the shower to check the pink strip it was a little pinker than I had imagined it would be! A blood test two hours later confirmed the test! I surprised my equally thrilled and excited husband with a stork bouquet!"[33]

The certainty of the emotional pregnancy announcement appeared, misleadingly, to be bolstered by the remarkable reliability of the test. In its early ads, E.P.T. claimed that in clinical tests (meaning that a doctor administered the test), it was 97 percent accurate for positive results. Women at home got similar results. The ad explained that it was less accurate for negative results; a substantial number of women who got negative results would retest a week later and find that they were, indeed, pregnant. What was not well explained was the meaning of an "accurate result." "Accurate" meant that it was the same result that would be obtained from a blood test. It did not mean that a woman had a 97 percent chance of carrying a baby to term. A competing brand, Predictor, claimed a 98.9 percent accuracy rate, with no qualifications. These statistics misleading conveyed that "positive for pregnancy" means "will have a baby in nine months." The reality was that with either of these brands, if a woman tested as instructed, nine days after the beginning of her expected period, she would have a 12 to 15 percent chance of miscarrying a detected pregnancy.[34]

With its promise of a sweet, emotionally intense, definitive beginning to pregnancy, home pregnancy testing quickly became ubiquitous. By 1987, a third of American women in a large national survey had gotten over whatever hesitation they might have felt about setting up a chemistry set in their bathrooms and used a home pregnancy test. More than half of the most highly educated women had used one at some point.[35] Usage would continue to rise. Home pregnancy tests were becoming big business.[36]

RITUAL AND SOUVENIR

In 1988, Unilever introduced a one-step test, allowing women to pee on a stick to get results.[37] This version of the home pregnancy test was much easier to use, gave quicker results and, as a by-product, generated a souvenir. With the widespread adoption of the one-step test by the early 1990s, home pregnancy testing became entrenched as a key moment of pregnancy. Like ultrasound, it symbolized much more than a simple test. A positive result for a wanted, planned pregnancy took on the status of a happily-anticipated rite of passage.[38]

Once the test carried so much meaning, many women created unique ways to memorialize it. One woman described, "On Valentine's Day 1999 I secretly took a home pregnancy test and got a big positive. I presented the test to my husband as a V. Day gift. We were so happy." She found herself tempted to try to make her next pregnancy announcement as special as the previous one. "As I type this, a box of HPTs [home pregnancy tests] is menacing to me from my medicine cabinet upstairs. I am currently 8 days past ovulation and have been charting my BBT [basal body temperature]. My period is due Dec. 29. The test instructions state you can test four days before your expected period. That would be tomorrow—Christmas Day! I am unsure how to proceed. Test and have the most fantastic Christmas present or wait, lest a negative impact our day."[39] Beginning in the 2000s, bloggers, some of whom built successful advertising-supported "Mommy Blogs" dedicated to enhancing women's experience of childbearing and rearing, posted lists of cute and inspiring ways for women to announce and memorialize their positive results.[40]

Anna Prushinskaya, who wrote about her pregnancy for *The Atlantic*, described joining several online communities to share her hopes and worries about pregnancy starting as soon as she was "trying to conceive." One of the communities was dedicated to helping its members read pregnancy test results. "I joined this site because I wanted to 'catch' my pregnancy as soon as it happened. My cycles were irregular, and I didn't want to miss it and keep drinking my daily couple glasses of wine. Really I was peeing on all these sticks because I am neurotic, and this Internet community was perfect for letting my anxiety about pregnancy, birth, and becoming a mother run wild. It was great to see that I was not alone." Prushinskaya took pleasure in joining in as the women in the group announced their positive tests and congratulated each other. She was looking forward to her turn, but "I was in Northern Michigan without phone reception when I got my big fat positive ('BFP'), and so I never got the chance to get the epic 'up' vote for it . . . I must admit, I was disappointed. I took a photo of the test anyway."[41] Prushinskaya was not just looking forward to having a baby; she was anticipating experiencing a specific celebratory moment in that journey with her online community.

The ritual pleasure of taking and sharing a home pregnancy test was not necessarily secondary to its medical results. It carried so much meaning, it could feel worth taking even when the pregnancy was already confirmed. Explained one oral history respondent,

> In the spring of 2000 when I was 34, my husband and I had just finished our 2nd IVF cycle (in NYC). I had gone to the clinic in the morning for a blood pregnancy test and found out I was pregnant. For 3 years, every single month, we had found out that I wasn't pregnant so we really couldn't believe that it was different this time. After an evening of grinning at each other, my husband went across the street and bought a pregnancy test so that we could see this miracle for ourselves. . . . We cheered when we saw the lines appear and we hung up the little piece of cardboard on our bulletin board (where it still hangs).[42]

For this couple, there was no expectation or pretense that the test would actually provide information. Rather, they took the test so they could take part in the same rite of passage that Prushinskaya was celebrating with her online friends.

This couple was not alone in keeping the positive test or a representation of it. One respondent saved both of her positive pregnancy tests, the first from 1990, when she was twenty-nine years old. While she was not willing to completely rely on the home test until it was confirmed by a test at the doctor's office, "The sticks became treasured items and are on the first page of each child's baby book." Another reflected as she wrote her home pregnancy test story, "I wish I had saved the wand, as my first memento of my son, announcing his future arrival."[43]

For many people, the pregnancy test stick serves as a material representation of the child inside. In baby blogs and Facebook posts, couples sometimes announce their pregnancies by sharing photos in which the test wand stands in for the expected child in a family portrait. For example, one couple shared on their blog a photo of the positive home pregnancy test cupped jointly in both of their right hands, their wedding rings evident in the background. Another showed a couple embracing, with the home pregnancy test held up between them. On a Mothering.com pregnancy forum like the one Prushinskaya had joined, one woman urged another, "Are you planning on uploading a photo? I'd love to see your BFP [big fat positive]!!!" When the second woman posted a photo, she responded, "congrats! what a beautiful test!! 😉"[44] She added a winking emoji, perhaps acknowledging that these words were more appropriate for a photo of a newborn than a photo of a pregnancy test, and yet, the reference was clear. A couple of decades ago, observers exclaimed at how ultrasound images were becoming "baby's first pictures." Today, home pregnancy tests are beginning to take on a similar valence, even earlier in pregnancy. The genre of newborn family portraits has been extended, not only to maternity photos displaying a pregnant belly but to anticipatory family pictures with a positive home pregnancy test (compare Figure 8.1a, Figure 8.1b, and Figure 8.1c).[45]

SO SENSITIVE

As the size of the market for home pregnancy tests became apparent, competitors challenged E.P.T.'s dominance with more sensitive tests that gave results earlier and faster. E.P.T.'s first generation of tests from the late 1970s could begin to detect hCG and therefore generate positive results as early as nine days after the expected menstrual period. At that point, a woman would have definitely missed her period and was reasonably likely to have felt some other symptoms of pregnancy. She needed to do the test with her first morning urine, so that it would be relatively concentrated, and it took about two hours to get results. Even then, the package insert made it clear that a test would miss many pregnancies that would only be evident a week or two later, and she would likely need to re-test.[46]

By 1982, Ortho Pharmaceutical's Daisy 2 test could produce results within an hour, a short enough time that a woman could test in the morning and get a result before she needed to leave for work.[47] In 1985, Tambrand Inc.'s First Response test advertised that it was "the most sensitive ever perfected . . . based on breakthrough technology from the maker of Tampax tampons." Three times more sensitive than its competitors, it could be used as early as the day after an expected period, it took only twenty minutes to show results, and it was easier to read than other tests. Rather than looking for doughnut-shaped sediment that could be disrupted by shaking hands, the user simply needed to observe whether the test liquid turned blue.[48] The quest for ever-earlier and simpler tests continued in the one-step test era.

(a)

(b)

(c)

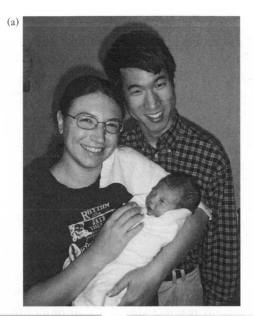
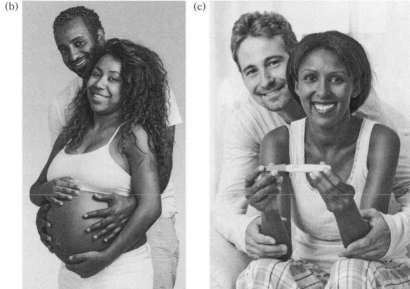

Figure 8.1 Family portraits, with a new baby, a pregnant belly, and a home pregnancy test. Photo credits: 8.1a: John Freidenfelds (Lara Freidenfelds personal collection); 8.1b and 8.1c: iStock/RusianDashinsky.

For two decades obstetric textbook authors resisted incorporating these tests that would displace obstetricians' specialized diagnostic skills. By 1999, *Danforth's Obstetrics and Gynecology* finally admitted that the hCG test outperformed the doctor. "Evaluation of the signs and symptoms associated with the presumptive diagnosis of pregnancy, while a useful adjunct, has largely been superseded by the widely available urine pregnancy test."[49] The hCG tests could confirm pregnancies before any other signs or symptoms could be detected. They were cheap, reliable, and ubiquitous, routinely used as part of lab work and hospital screening for women of childbearing age. No one saw any reason to look for or trust traditional signs of pregnancy anymore.

By the mid-2000s, home pregnancy tests could detect hCG at such miniscule concentrations that testing had nearly reached its biological limit. Tests could detect more than half of pregnancies five days *before* an expected menstrual period and most of the rest by the day after the expected period. The most basic traditional sign of pregnancy, the missed menstrual period, was no longer a woman's first inkling that she might be pregnant.

This super-sensitivity carried a number of consequences. Marketers saw that women would buy a lot more tests if they used them every month while they were "trying," not just when they had actually missed a period. They had done market research showing that those who wanted a positive result bought more tests than those hoping for a negative.[50] If it took on average three months for a sexually active woman to become pregnant, manufacturers could triple their sales if they could convince women to take the tests early and sell even more if they could persuade women to test repeatedly until they got their periods or got a positive test. Test manufacturers heavily promoted the sensitivity of the tests and reiterated their longtime argument that the earlier a woman knew about her pregnancy, the better she could take care of herself and her baby.

Women cooperated with marketers' urging to buy lots of pregnancy tests, but manufacturers did not profit as much as they might have anticipated because women learned to buy them on the cheap. By 2010, cut-rate pregnancy tests were available on line in bulk, at dollar stores, and in affordable drug store generics. Anyone could buy a no-frills pregnancy test for less than a cup of coffee. In earlier years, the typical $10 price tag might have kept a woman from throwing away money on tests before she had missed a period and suspected a pregnancy, but once she could pick up a pack of two for a dollar, there was no financial reason to hold off.

Over-the-counter ovulation kits, which copied the pee-on-a-stick format in a test that pinpoints the day of ovulation, gave women more certainty as to which day they could start testing for pregnancy. Because ovulation is hormonally linked to the menstrual period following it rather than the one preceding it, a woman who does not have absolutely regular periods cannot be sure which day ovulation has happened, and therefore at what point a pregnancy test might yield a positive result. With the knowledge from the ovulation kit, she can start testing exactly nine days after she has ovulated (five days before the expected period), which is the first day she might be able to register a positive test.

Ovulation kits were originally understood to be a technology for addressing infertility; a woman would not have thought to use one unless she had been having trouble getting pregnant and needed to confirm that she was ovulating and having intercourse at the appropriate time. In recent years, ovulation kits have also become popular among women who do not have a history of infertility but who are simply eager to get pregnant as soon as possible and inclined to monitor their fertility. They are stocked in drug stores next to the home pregnancy tests and cost about $10 for a month's supply, even less on line and in bulk. Women who use ovulation kits learn about their pregnancies earlier than anyone could have imagined just a few decades ago.

With all of this early testing came the frequent problem of faint results that were hard to interpret. While tests are not meant to be eyeballed for estimates of hCG levels, a greater concentration of hCG does produce a darker and clearer result. It takes several days after the embryo implants in the uterus for hCG levels to rise enough to get a robust reading. Some women, like Prushinskaya, consulted websites dedicated to puzzling over faint lines, "tweaking" them with filters to discern the lightest positives. Like ovulation kits, these online communities originally served women struggling with infertility but now have a wider audience.

As Prushinskaya explains,

> How this site works is one person posts a photo of a pregnancy test, and the other users on the site vote on whether it looks positive, negative, or not clear. Pregnancy test results seem like they should be obvious. But in fact, there is a window of time, before the concentration of the hormone human chorionic gonadotropin (HCG) surpasses a pregnancy test's sensitivity, when one can get the coveted second line, but that line is very faint.

The woman on the Mothering.com forum who received congratulations on her "beautiful" test had, earlier in the day, fretted, "I know there are a million threads like this. I know, because I have read back on most of them! But I am 12 dpo [days past ovulation], I took a test this morning (FRER [First Response Early Result]) and there is only a faint pink line. With my first it was dark so fast there was never a doubt. I can't stand this definite maybe. I guess I just have to be patient and wait a few days? What do you think? Just some support would help! 😊"[51]

Web forums of like-minded women were, indeed, a good source of support. Prushinskaya found that she "couldn't ask my husband his opinion; he'd say, 'Well, clearly that's negative,' instead of staring at the strips like I did, looking for that ghost of a line. Other women on the site found their husbands similarly stoic. These women understood me." It was hard to be patient and wait a few days to re-test, even if that was the obvious solution. It was too tempting to pour time and energy into puzzling out a result.

Fellow web forum participants "used high-contrast and black-and-white filters (built into the site's interface) to get a better read on the tests."[52] Some of the women who ran these web forums or regularly volunteered to read results gave detailed instructions for how to take apart the test and photograph the inner test strip. When these sites began several years ago, they were very much do-it-yourself efforts, but recently a number of tweaking apps for smartphones have become available. A user uploads a photo of her test, and the app automatically applies filters to give her a likely positive or likely negative result.[53]

Alternatively, beginning in the mid-2000s some women turned to digital tests, which display a textual readout of "pregnant" or "not pregnant," to get a definitive answer. As one advocate of digital tests joked, "You know a man designed the line kind. No woman in her right mind would have decided to purposely torture all women by searching for that second line every cycle!"[54] The digital readout was not an innovation in the test chemistry, just in the display; a chromometer makes the test determination and translates color depth beyond a certain threshold as a positive result, eliminating pale lines that unsettle test users.

Digital tests also put the diagnosis into words. The test itself provides the translation from visual lab result into clinical meaning rather than requiring the test taker to make that translation. It removes one source of human error or uncertainty, making the test seem more definitive. As Jennifer, one oral history respondent, described, "I had several positives over a few days, and I got the digital because a recent Miscarriage had me scared I would miscarry this time as well. My friends suggested I get the digital because seeing the word might make it feel 'real.'" Jennifer's friends were right, in a way. The words did heighten the impact of the test, though not in the direction she expected. "Sadly I saw Not Pregnant, and started to miscarry the next day."[55] Jennifer wanted to believe that a definitive-sounding diagnosis would mean that she had a definite pregnancy, but her concern about the precariousness of early pregnancy was well founded. A positive test one day does not guarantee another positive test the next day.

Jennifer was far from alone in registering a pregnancy that soon miscarried. Books and websites about pregnancy estimate that between 12 percent and

20 percent of recognized pregnancies miscarry. These are underestimates. They are generally based on what are called "clinically recognized pregnancies," meaning that a woman has been diagnosed by her doctor. Most doctors are unwilling to test for pregnancy until a woman is at least two weeks overdue for her period, so they do not count any miscarriages that happen before six weeks' gestation. A woman who uses a home pregnancy test at the earliest possible moment actually has about a 30 percent chance of discovering later that she has lost the pregnancy.[56] Current home pregnancy tests are so sensitive that they are highly misleading. It is true that they are "99 percent accurate" in detecting hCG. Yet they are only 70 percent accurate in predicting the chance of having a baby in nine months.

PREGNANCIES KNOWN BY PREGNANCY TESTS ALONE

Pregnancy tests are often the only indicator of pregnancies destined to miscarry early. These pregnancies generally do not produce as much hCG, so they are less likely to produce noticeable pregnancy symptoms such as tender breasts and nausea, even if they last past the expected menstrual period. A clinical study has shown that "late periods" that are actually early pregnancy losses, if they arrive by six weeks after the previous period (i.e., six weeks' gestation), are indistinguishable from normal periods.[57] When pregnancies miscarry by the time of the expected menstrual period, even the most basic symptom of a late period is missing.

Given the availability of pregnancy tests so sensitive that they can register a pregnancy even before a missed period, it is easy for a woman to discover a pregnancy and then a miscarriage before she has any sign of pregnancy aside from the test result. For example, one woman, responding to a posting on Babycenter.com asking for advice about how early one could start trying to get pregnant again after a miscarriage, wrote,

> wow. . . I also had a miscarriage on Aug. 16, 2007. I just got chills realizing how many of us were going through the same thing that day. Honestly, I don't know if this is good advice but I'm not going to wait. If I hadn't taken a pregnancy test 4 days before I would have never known I was pregnant and would have kept trying the next month as usual. I never imagined that I would be so absolutely devastated. I hope it happens for both of us soon. Good luck!![58]

As this woman found, even a miscarriage that she knew would have been unrecognizable without a test could come with profound emotional consequences.

Lots of testing can turn a typical healthy woman's childbearing experience into one that appears fraught with difficulties. Andee's oral history narrated her test experiences, starting in 1996, through six pregnancies, three of them ending in miscarriage and one in partial miscarriage of a twin.

> My best friend bought it for me, I believe it was an EPT early pregnancy test. A double pack. I was 17 and lived in Washington and tested at her house. I was about 6 weeks pregnant and the line showed up within seconds. This was my second pregnancy. I didn't test with my first one, which ended in miscarriage. . . . We wanted it to be positive. My finacee and I were elated. . . . With my third pregnancy . . . I took one test. It came up positive within seconds. It took us two months to get pregnant. With my fourth pregnancy. . . I took about two tests. I got very faint lines each time. . . and I miscarried at 5 weeks. With my fifith [sic] pregnancy I took 8, yes . . . . 8 tests. The lines seemed to get fainter and [sic] the days went on and this pregnancy again ended in miscarriage at 5 1/2 weeks. With my sixth pregnancy I got a positive pregnancy test at 11 dpo [days past ovulation]. . . . it showed up within seconds. When I had a blood test done at the dr's it showed my hcg numbers very very high. I started bleeding and thinking I was miscarrying again. . . .but my numbers stayed high. Turns out I miscarried a twin early. But I was still very pregnant. Baby boy was born in May 02.[59]

Through Andee's reproductive life, she monitored her fertility more and more closely, though not because she had any difficulty getting pregnant. Over the years, as tests grew more sensitive, she moved the time of first testing earlier and earlier. With her first pregnancy, she did not test at all; with the second one, she tested about two weeks after her missed menstrual period. The testing time is unclear with her third pregnancy. With her fourth pregnancy, she was aware of a miscarriage at five weeks, which is approximately one week after the beginning of her missed menstrual period, and she had already taken two pregnancy tests. With her fifth pregnancy, she had already taken eight tests by the time she miscarried a week and a half after her missed period, which means that she probably began testing within a day or two of her missed period. With her sixth pregnancy she was monitoring her ovulation and tested at the first possible moment recommended at that point by the test manufacturers, three days before her expected menstrual period.

Without pregnancy tests, Andee would almost certainly have believed that she had had four pregnancies, one of which miscarried. With pregnancy tests, she experienced six pregnancies. From her narrative, she appears to have experienced two miscarriages solely through the reading of the tests, and one from the tests plus other medical technology. The loss of a twin in her sixth pregnancy was inferred via a range of technology, starting from her early home pregnancy test, and including hCG levels monitored at her doctor's office starting early in pregnancy and most likely an ultrasound. Early pregnancy testing can create complicated and distressing reproductive histories from experiences that, as recently as a few decades ago, would have looked like relatively smooth and easy childbearing.

CHEMICAL PREGNANCY

Physicians, who know just how frequently early pregnancies miscarry, have come up with a label to distinguish very early losses: the "chemical pregnancy." By "chemical," they mean that the pregnancy registers on an hCG test but does not show up on an ultrasound. This label is meant to help women see the pregnancy as not altogether "real," a label many women find reassuring.[60] The label also has clinical meaning, since pregnancies that end before a gestational sac can be visualized on an ultrasound do not "count" for medical purposes, for example in IVF clinic statistics.

Online advice givers, though, often undermine physicians' efforts to distinguish chemical pregnancy from clinical pregnancy and therefore from miscarriage. For example, on one health information website, a woman posed the question, "Does a chemical pregnancy mean I had a false positive pregnancy test?" The expert answered, "Although the term sounds like it was a false pregnancy, a chemical pregnancy is actually a very early form of miscarriage. In a chemical pregnancy, a conception did actually occur, but the loss happened before the pregnancy had developed far enough to be confirmed clinically (such as by ultrasound)."[61]

The language and concepts for talking about very early pregnancy, and early pregnancy loss, are still developing. Medical and popular advice givers will undoubtedly continue to negotiate the terms used to describe reproductive processes that were invisible until very recently. Many women might, in practical terms, want to consider a chemical pregnancy to be a type of "false positive."

EVEN EARLIER?

While a positive hCG test is currently the first viable indicator of pregnancy, hCG is not in fact the first substance a woman's body produces in response to fertilization. Within a couple of days after fertilization, and before implantation, a protein called "early pregnancy factor" can be detected in the blood of a woman who has conceived.[62] Right now, there is no practical way to measure early pregnancy factor. The test for it is involved and expensive, only usable in scientific studies.[63] Based on current knowledge about fertilization and early pregnancy, a test for early pregnancy factor would reveal many more pregnancies destined to miscarry than to become babies. Only about 30 percent of fertilized eggs successfully implant and develop into term pregnancies and live births. The other 70 percent perish, about half before implantation, and many more during the first weeks after implantation. It is hard to imagine how this information would be useful to us, outside of diagnostic testing related to fertility treatment. Perhaps this is why no one has yet pursued a commercial version of the test. If a test for early pregnancy factor did become available, we would need to re-think, yet again, how we understand a "positive" result for pregnancy. Does a test make a pregnancy "real?"

* * *

Since their introduction on the American market in 1978, home pregnancy tests have become ubiquitous and increasingly sensitive. They promise the opportunity to start caring for a pregnancy and bonding with a baby soon after conception. Their material form can seem to concretely represent the baby inside. They appear to give greater assurances of early certainty about pregnancy, with their promises of "99 percent accuracy." But paradoxically, the more sensitive they get the less accurately they predict the birth of a baby in nine months, and the more likely they are to create the experience of a miscarriage.

Conclusion

At the end of October 2017, a year and a half after she and her husband decided to "try" for their third child, blogger Emily Malone announced with joy and relief that she was several months pregnant. It had been a rough road. She had already shared the details of two early miscarriages in a blog post in April and suffered one more early pregnancy loss after that. "All of the emotional ups and down[s] put a huge stress on our family and my marriage."[1]

It was not only the miscarriages themselves that were difficult; it was also the stress of what "felt like years of limbo and lack of any long term planning in our lives."[2] The stress was worst when they were "actively trying for another pregnancy," to the point that "there were a few stretches where we decided to take a break from trying in order to focus [o]n physical and emotional healing."

The successful pregnancy came shortly after Malone and her husband had made their peace with remaining a family of four and stopped actively trying. "I had a third miscarriage in June, and at that point we said *enough*. We had an awesome summer. We healed as a family. We felt more grateful than ever for our two amazing boys and all the fun they bring to our lives." And that was when "we were both surprised and excited when I realized I was pregnant yet *again* in late August."[3]

While Malone had given up on "trying," she had not yet given up her habits from over a year of monitoring her pregnancy status. "I think because we've been through this so many times, I've gotten used to just taking those early test strips whenever it was even a remote possibility. Casey didn't believe me this time until I went out and bought one of those digital ones that said 'pregnant!'" As a result, "We have known for a while now—from as early as one can possibly know!" That made for a long and difficult wait before she felt confident that the pregnancy was viable and was comfortable sharing the news with her blog readers.

If it weren't for the home pregnancy tests she had taken, and the follow-up blood work and ultrasounds triggered by those tests, Malone might have interpreted her experiences during her year of trying to have a third child quite differently. Miscarriages at six weeks are often indistinguishable from menstrual periods, and Malone did not have pronounced pregnancy symptoms with the pregnancies she miscarried.[4] She had previously experienced a frustrating year of extra-long menstrual cycles and infertility before her first pregnancy; without the home pregnancy tests, she might have interpreted this year of irregular, heavy cycles in the same light. It still would not have been an easy year. She would have been through the physical challenges and hormonal ups and downs, and she would still be disappointed not to be expecting a baby. But the technology, along with the expectations of modern pregnancy, made the year into one of repeated, emotionally exhausting grief.

In the moments when Malone stopped "trying" and planning, she was much more able to enjoy her life and appreciate her family. And in the end, the successful pregnancy came when it was going to come, with or without her hyper-conscious efforts. Once it arrived, it felt like the right and destined path all along. The history that has shaped modern childbearing has made it difficult to imagine or accept this more relaxed and fatalistic attitude toward pregnancy. But it might do us good. Knowing the history, how might we envision a happier future? How might we tweak our metaphors and reshape our culture so that we can appreciate our blessings while we accept the inevitable imperfections of childbearing?

RETHINK OUR METAPHORS FOR CHILDBEARING: FROM "PLANNED" TO "PREPARED"

Emily Malone reflected that part of her distress over her miscarriages was that she was unable to plan her family life when her fertility was unpredictable. The metaphors of birth "control" and family "planning" have a long history, beginning with the nineteenth-century impulse to limit family size and growing into the twentieth-century development and adoption of effective and legal contraception. Progressive era and mid-century reformers chose modern metaphors of "planning" and "control" to describe their intentions.

But what if we chose a different metaphor to describe our use of contraception? What if we talked about "Prepared Parenthood" rather than "Planned Parenthood"? What if we asked whether a pregnancy was "welcomed" rather than whether it was "intended"? The "prepared childbirth" movement of the mid- and late-twentieth century was based on an explicit acknowledgment that birth is not predictable, especially if the doctor and hospital do not intervene to force it into a specified pattern. It empowered women and families, not by assuring them that they had control and could plan the birth, but by helping them to be ready for what might happen. We could call on a notion of "Prepared Parenthood" to describe using contraception until a woman and her partner are ready to care for children, and then being open and ready to receive children when they arrive. We could maintain the benefits of modern contraception, while leaving room for the exigencies of unpredictable human reproductive processes.[5]

RETHINK OUR METAPHORS FOR CHILDBEARING: FROM "BONDING" TO "NURTURING"

As most of the purposes and meanings women and their families once attached to childbearing—obedience to God, financial security in old age, continuity of a patriarchal family line—have fallen away over the centuries, the emotional relationship with a child has remained the one culturally agreed-upon reason to have a baby. "Attachment" and "bonding" have become the central metaphors for the loving relationship that has been at the heart of modern parenting since the mid-twentieth century. Simultaneously, expectations for building a parenting relationship moved earlier and earlier into pregnancy, to almost the moment of conception.

Given this trajectory, what if we talked about "nurture" instead of "bonding," at least at the beginning of the parenting journey? During pregnancy especially, the "bonding" can only flow in one direction, from parent to child, in any case. Emily Malone found this to be a helpful way to think about the early, tentative stages of her final pregnancy, explaining that "other than obviously trying to take care of myself as best as possible, I refused to allow myself to go down any emotional paths, for fear of what could potentially happen."[6] While some might see this as a lack of bonding, Malone was, in fact, nurturing her potential baby. Her way of showing and experiencing love is appropriate for this stage of pregnancy, and no less worthy than a relationship we might call "bonding." Emphasizing "nurture" could also be a helpful precedent for parenting babies and older children: there are times when children are difficult and parents do not feel loving and "bonded" with them, and yet they can be good and loving parents by acting in nurturing ways toward their offspring.

PUSH BACK ON EVERYONE WITH ULTERIOR MOTIVES

Besides revising our central childbearing metaphors, it would also be helpful to identify the ways in which the various "experts" who have congregated around childbearing women over the past century or so may not always have had women's best interests at heart when they encouraged deep attachments to newly formed pregnancies. Over the course of the twentieth and twenty-first centuries, marketers, public health advocates, anti-abortion activists, parenting gurus, and pharmaceutical companies have increasingly jumped on the early pregnancy bonding bandwagon, with various goals in mind. To the degree that they are misleading women about the likelihood and normalcy of miscarriage in order to persuade women to behave according to their wishes, they are acting unethically. Each of these groups ought to consider how they might craft new messages that are sensitive to the possibility of miscarriage. Women and their partners can push back on each of these groups with skepticism toward unrealistic claims and assumptions about pregnancy, and redirect their attention and spending toward those who discuss pregnancy and miscarriage honestly.

Push Back on Marketers and Advertisers

As Americans became avid consumers, advertisers and marketers developed sophisticated methods for reaching their audiences and delivering emotionally compelling appeals. New and expecting parents were prime targets, and marketers learned to deliver their appealing and sentimental messages to potential customers earlier and earlier in their pregnancies. In recent decades, marketers have figured out how to reach women so early that many of the women in their target audience will miscarry.

Newly pregnant customers need to understand that they are being groomed into enthusiastic parent-consumers through baby gear advertisements and baby name lists, when marketers sell their names and due dates. As consumers, we would be wise to exercise caution about sharing our due dates until we are confident we want to unleash an unstoppable advertising torrent. Marketers have spent the past half-century learning to out-compete each other by making their pitches ever earlier in pregnancy, with increasingly sentimental messages meant to encourage our investment in our pregnancies. Their goal is that we get attached to their brands; their method is to encourage us to get attached to our pregnancies.

PUSH BACK ON PUBLIC HEALTH MESSAGES

Over the last century, Americans increasingly went to doctors for regular, preventive care during pregnancy, and physicians and public health nurses and activists alike promised that medical care would keep women and their growing pregnancies safe and healthy. Widely distributed developmental timelines seemed to imply that pregnancy would inevitably progress to the birth of a healthy child, so long as the pregnant woman followed doctor's orders. The timelines were intended to bolster a woman's emotional connection to her expected child so as to inspire her to follow prenatal care guidelines, as least as much as to teach her about the science of development.

Public health advocates have not given women enough credit for their desire to have healthy pregnancies. At my talks for medical and public health professionals, some have suggested that telling women the truth about the commonness of early pregnancy loss would lead them to be less careful about taking care of their pregnancies. Better, they say, to encourage women to bond with their early pregnancies so that the pregnancies that do succeed will be healthier. This approach is emotionally coercive and demeaning to women, while unlikely to have any great positive impact. Women who are dealing with addiction or abusive living situations cannot simply turn their lives around no matter how much they love their children or form attachments with their pregnancies; they need social support so that they are able to take care of their pregnancies. Women who have the resources to take care of themselves will put information on pregnancy self-care to good use even if they understand that miscarriages are common; there is no need for misleading public health messages. Falsely encouraging women to believe they have more control over outcomes than they actually do leaves women who miscarry with undeserved feelings of guilt and anxiety that affect them and their future parenting.

Push Back on Anti-Abortion Rhetoric

Over the centuries abortion has gone from an occasional and largely unremarked upon practice for protecting a woman's health, to a frequent and eventually criminalized method of reducing family size, to a legal, if highly contested, way for women to end unwanted pregnancies. Public debates about abortion shape how we think about early pregnancy, and pro-life and pro-choice arguments alike give a misleading picture of how much control anyone has over early pregnancy. Pro-life depictions of early pregnancy have tended to inform the pregnancy loss support literature, as counselors look for ways to acknowledge many women's feelings of deep loss even very early in pregnancy.

Like public health advocates, anti-abortion activists ought to be honest about the biological reality of pregnancy loss when they craft their messages. Around 70 percent of conceptions cannot become babies, no matter how much we wish it. Biologists describe human reproduction as "inefficient"; our species is sustained by a reproductive process in which the majority of conceptions are not viable.[7] We may decide that those conceptions nonetheless deserve special spiritual recognition and inherently have a unique dignity as the inception point of human life. We may not in good conscience suggest to women and their partners that each conception is already a fully formed, viable baby. Some will become babies; many more will not. Messages from those who take a theological, moral, or legal stance against abortion by encouraging women and their partners to love blastocysts just like they love their babies inflict great suffering on those who are destined to miscarry.

Push Back on Parenting Advice

Parenting gurus who have developed the philosophy of "attachment parenting," and more recently "attachment pregnancy," also need to inform their philosophical stance with a dose of biological reality.[8] If early pregnancy loss is so common, maybe women aren't meant to bond with their pregnancies in the first eight weeks. There is no evidence that very early attachment results in better birth or parenting outcomes. It clearly backfires in cases where women become attached early, miscarry, and then are anxious and fearful during subsequent pregnancies. Worse, those same gurus heap on the guilt when women who are anxious and fearful of another loss find themselves unable to attach early to the next pregnancy. A less absolutist philosophy of bonding and attachment would clearly make for more humane pregnancy advice and might lay the groundwork for more realistic and forgiving parenting advice as well.

Push Back on Pharmaceutical Companies and Their
Pregnancy Tests

As women established greater control over their fertility and pregnancies, home pregnancy testing became a ritual of pregnancy, confirming the implantation of an embryo even before a missed period. Yet, a large portion of the pregnancies detected so soon do not, in fact, result in the birth of a baby.

Pharmaceutical companies that sell home pregnancy tests and ovulation kits need to recognize that their products can create distressing side effects and adjust their marketing accordingly. Seeking to sell more tests, they encourage women to test for pregnancy before they even miss menstrual periods, effectively turning the home pregnancy test into something to be used every month rather than only when a pregnancy is suspected. The increasingly elaborate tests created by pharmaceutical companies to encourage ever-more heightened monitoring of pregnancy status can be welcome tools for confirming a woman's ability to conceive, but it is important to recognize that these companies are in the business for profit, not to promote women's health. Many women would do better with less testing. A woman who waits until she is a week or two overdue for her period will spend less money on tests and is less likely to be diagnosed with a chemical pregnancy.[9]

CREATE NEW NARRATIVES FOR PREGNANCY THAT
INCLUDE MISCARRIAGE

Changing how we think about early pregnancy is not just a matter of removing or ignoring damaging advice and aggressive sales pitches; we need to substitute alternate ways to think and talk about conception and early pregnancy that take early pregnancy losses into account. There are a number of opportunities for sharing a re-crafted narrative: in developmental timelines, in home pregnancy test inserts, on websites and in apps, in the general media, and at doctors' offices.

In textbooks and pregnancy guides, development is illustrated on a timeline, as if there is a single and universal story for how every pregnancy unfolds. We need a new picture of pregnancy that includes the 70 percent of conceptions that do not make it to nine months. Pregnancy manuals could include a pregnancy timeline that shows how only a minority of pregnancies complete the whole trajectory. In their daily and weekly updates, pregnancy apps could add a filter that shows early embryos as translucent—not all "there"—and gradually becoming more opaque as the days and weeks progress. If this new and more accurate representation of human development is incorporated into sex education and biology textbooks, pregnancy manuals, and pregnancy websites and apps, many more people will go into pregnancy with a realistic expectation of how it is likely to unfold.[10]

Home pregnancy test inserts offer another opportunity for better explaining how pregnancy really works. Inserts should clarify that the test is a very accurate measure of the presence of hCG but that the presence of hCG is not an accurate indicator of a viable pregnancy until well past a missed menstrual period. Inserts can present this information in an encouraging light, explaining that hCG detection followed by a menstrual period indicates a chemical pregnancy, which means that the test taker should be reassured that she is ovulating and able to get pregnant. Insert text can suggest a follow-up test at eight to ten weeks to provide a more certain confirmation of pregnancy, if the test taker has not yet consulted her physician.

Websites and apps can adjust their narratives about early pregnancy so as to help and not hurt when someone is destined to miscarry. Apps commonly encourage women to take weekly "baby bump" pictures starting from the beginning of pregnancy to create a time lapse video of the pregnancy as a cute memento. They ask women to fill out a profile page when they first download the app, which includes information such as the expected baby's nickname, which may really be more appropriate for a later stage of pregnancy. Since the apps ask for a woman's last menstrual period date or due date up front, they could easily be programmed to wait until eight or ten weeks before they cue these sentimental investments in pregnancies that are not yet secure. They could offer realistic versions of the developmental timeline and refrain from encouraging women to establish daily bonding rituals until the second trimester. Most of them have a pre-pregnancy section, where readers can be advised that early miscarriages are a common and expected part of the process of getting pregnant and having a baby.

Women's magazines and general newspapers publish frequent articles about fertility and childbearing; reporters who cover these topics could more regularly note that for many women, part of the process of having children includes having an early miscarriage or two along the way. If this expectation were built into the timeline that people take for granted when they prepare for their pregnancies, it could inform how women approach apps, websites, baby gear stores, and the rest.

Doctors and midwives, like Emily Malone's practitioners, can also be part of the solution, though they often do not get a chance to offer their perspective very early in the process. They can be an important source, though, when miscarriages happen. First, it is important for practitioners to be cautious about how they decide to reassure their patients when the situation is not entirely clear. Emily Malone's midwife gave her an upbeat, "congratulations, Mom!" shortly before Malone had her second miscarriage following some bleeding. Optimism is fine, but practitioners need to choose their words carefully.

Second, when a doctor finds bad news on an ultrasound, she should describe the situation first and ask the patient if she wishes to see it, rather than making assumptions. Over the last few decades we have developed the ultrasound exam into an elaborate ritual of "seeing the baby," but not every ultrasound needs to follow this script. Malone may have preferred not to see and hear the slowing heartbeat when she miscarried. On the other hand, if the ultrasound shows an empty gestational sac, a woman may feel comforted to see that her body has already reabsorbed the embryo and that it does not look like the more-developed embryo on that day's developmental update on her pregnancy app.[11] If physicians set expectations for first trimester ultrasounds differently from later ones, it would help differentiate early scans from the later ritual of meeting the baby.

Third, health care providers have a particularly important role in reassuring women that early miscarriages are common and normal, that they are generally unpreventable and not the woman's fault, and that they do not mean that a woman has any greater chance of miscarrying her next pregnancy. Health-care providers can reach women with this message at preconception appointments, during early prenatal care appointments, and in pregnancy guides.[12]

None of this is an argument for trying to educate women about everything that can go wrong in pregnancy. It is important to distinguish between bad things that are likely to happen and those that are relatively rare. Something like early miscarriage, which happens in about a fifth of confirmed pregnancies, is something we need to anticipate and prepare for accordingly. The long list of much rarer childbearing complications that tend to be lumped in with miscarriage, on the other hand, does not need to be given the same treatment. Trying to learn about and anticipate all of the various possibilities leads to much worry relative to the potential benefit. It is enough to learn a short list of warning signs that indicate a call to the doctor, without delving into the details. We can be realistic and still decide not to borrow trouble, a good lesson for years of child-rearing to come.[13]

CREATE ALTERNATIVE NARRATIVES FOR MISCARRIAGE

Whether we are health care practitioners, on-line advice-givers, or well-meaning family and friends, we need to offer a range of ways for women to understand their miscarriages and respect different ways of thinking about them. Some miscarriages represent a woman's last chance to have a child, while others are brief and temporary setbacks in a family's formation. Circumstances matter. So do individuals' philosophical and religious beliefs. It can be insensitive for people to assume that "it was early" and "you can always have another one;" likewise, it can also be insensitive for friends, neighbors, and advice writers to assume, as the Nurture app does, that for every pregnancy loss "it really doesn't matter how far along the pregnancy was when the miscarriage occurred, you and your partner are still going to feel upset, and the woman, especially, will have to go through the stages of grief before feeling more balanced again."[14] If advice writers and counselors prescribe this kind of grief, more women will suffer than might otherwise, and those who do not grieve in this way may feel guilty for not feeling the "right" amount of motherly love.

The most recent edition of *What to Expect When You're Expecting* helpfully acknowledges that there are a range of possible and legitimate responses to early pregnancy loss. Previous editions had told women that "losing a baby, even this early, is tragic and traumatic . . . allow yourself to grieve, a necessary step in the healing process. Expect to be sad, even depressed, for a while."[15] An explanation of miscarriage published on the WhatToExpect.com website between book editions insisted that "no matter how early in pregnancy you lost your baby, you'll feel that loss deeply. Even if you never saw your baby, you knew that he or she was growing inside of you, and you formed a bond; however abstract the attachment, you felt it. . . . You may have trouble sleeping and eating—and accepting. And you may cry. A lot. These are all natural, healthy responses to the death of a loved one (and you loved your baby, even if you never had a chance to know your baby), something you're enduring right now." The 2016 print edition, modified from the website, describes this kind of grieving first, but it also recognizes that "[s]ome couples approach an early pregnancy loss matter-of-factly, easily accepting that this pregnancy wasn't meant to be, ready to move on, and eager to try again."[16] These edits, which identify a range of legitimate responses to early pregnancy loss, are an important course correction.

During pregnancy, the baby becomes "real" not only through biological development, but also through all the ways in which we give it social and cultural recognition. Anthropologist Linda Layne has argued that this is the kind of "realness" that matters, and this is what needs to be recognized and honored when a woman miscarries. In the miscarriage support groups Layne studied, women and their partners found comfort in acknowledgment by family, friends, and each other that they had really lost babies and that their grief was therefore warranted.[17]

Other women may come to terms with their miscarriages differently. Some women deliberately delay announcing their pregnancies until after the first trimester, partly because they realize that saying this news out loud will make it more "real." Well-wishers will offer congratulations and send baby gifts. Consciously or unconsciously, women may prefer to postpone social recognition of their pregnancies because they know that if they lose a pregnancy, they would rather it not seem as "real" in the first place.[18]

Still other women may handle early pregnancy losses by retrospectively reconsidering what the positive pregnancy test really meant. Layne describes the process by which pregnancies become socially "real," but she does not address the possibility that this process could be reversed. In fact, people have considerable capacity for reconsidering their feelings, reinterpreting past events, and coming to new understandings of what has happened to them. No one should be made to feel guilty for deciding retrospectively that a pregnancy that was lost in its early stages was not "real" in the same way as a full-term pregnancy.

A miscarriage may be seen in a different light after a successful pregnancy. Once blogger Emily Malone felt secure enough to share the news of her final pregnancy, she reflected on her winding journey. "A sweet baby girl to complete our family next May. We truly cannot believe it. Our hearts are so full and it feels like the long road that led us here brought us to where we were meant to end up all along." That spring, Malone joyfully announced her little girl's arrival. Commenting on Malone's pregnancy announcement, Haley shared a similar story. "Once you have this baby you will be amazed at how she really was meant to be. It still makes me so emotional when I remember that if I had not had my miscarriages, I wouldn't have ended up with the baby I did."[19] Miscarriages are rightly seen as a part of the journey to building a family.

SUPPORT CHILDBEARING AND TREAT INFERTILITY

An important part of the reason we continue to seek more precise control of childbearing is that in contemporary American society, families' financial security and long-term prospects often depend on couples being able to have children exactly when they intend. This is too much pressure to put on a biological process that simply isn't that precise or predictable. Even without any specific fertility issues, it takes anywhere from nine months to two years to make a baby. A woman might get pregnant immediately and have a baby in nine months, or she might "try" for six months, get pregnant, miscarry, recover, "try" again for six months, and then have a baby. Both of these scenarios are typical and healthy. Even beyond this range, plenty of people need more time, and perhaps some medical assistance, to have their children. And yet they can have the families they desire if they have the social support it takes to be open to children whenever they arrive.

When couples face unresolved infertility, we should recognize the profundity of that problem for many people's lives. It should not require a miscarriage for them to be permitted to mourn the unattainability of the family they so desire. While advice on popular websites, in prominent pregnancy advice books, and on pregnancy apps tends to treat every miscarriage as the same kind and degree of problem, for many couples, it is not a miscarriage per se that is devastating, but the loss of what may be a last chance to have a child. As a society, we need to recognize the gravity of permanent infertility to people's aspirations for their lives and consider providing public support to those who need treatment for infertility, whether or not that infertility takes the form of early miscarriages.

EXPECT AND ACCEPT CHILDBEARING AND PARENTING IMPERFECTION

The history that reshaped pregnancy and miscarriage experiences in fact reconfigured childbearing and parenting more broadly. Parents increasingly strive for perfect control, not just over the spacing of pregnancies but over the entire process of childbearing and over the education and development of their children as well.[20] The increasingly emotional focus of the parent-child relationship has intensified every pleasure and every disappointment in that relationship, from pregnancy onward. Parents have found themselves with ever-increasing caretaking responsibilities, between the consumer culture that swirls around families and encourages the purchase of childhood-enhancing goods, and the increasing influence of medical practitioners who urge precise and demanding caretaking responsibilities upon parents. New knowledge and new technologies seem to hold out the guarantee of safety and happiness for our children, if only parents apply them meticulously enough. And, as with early pregnancy, parents feel anxious and guilty when they inevitably fall short of perfection.

One of the most critical historical lessons of this book is that we need to give ourselves reasonable leeway for imperfection across the entire enterprise of bearing and raising children. Our history of ever-increasing success in controlling reproduction has led us to mistakenly assume that this trajectory can culminate in perfect control. In fact, assuming most of us continue to reproduce the old-fashioned way, we are bumping up against natural limits on our ability to have children exactly when we want them. Once children arrive, parents continue to have less control over their children's development than they might wish.

Our history has set us up to feel like we should try to control everything about childbearing out of an intense love for our children and a desire to protect them. But this is often counterproductive. When our standards for ourselves as parents are perfectionist, we inevitably fail. If failures make us anxious and even more determined to prevent them, we set up a vicious cycle. If we respond to the possibility, or the reality, of an early pregnancy loss by trying even harder to control something that we cannot in fact control, we are setting ourselves up for a parenting experience that will be, at best, a paradox of "all joy and no fun," as journalist Jennifer Senior has cogently observed—and one in which anxiety may frequently overshadow joy.[21]

With an understanding of the history, we can reset our expectations to serve us better—to help us anticipate and tolerate the inevitable imperfections of childbearing and childrearing. This, in turn, can allow us to appreciate and enjoy the blessings of modern childbearing culture, including a remarkable level of control over birth control and family planning, a high regard for the emotional relationship between parents and children, effective medical care, and a bountiful consumer culture that has provided tremendous parenting resources. If we approach childbearing with the assumption that there will be an abundance of unexpected and unavoidable bumps and byways in our parenting journey, we give ourselves a chance to relax and appreciate the good parts, set aside undeserved guilt and regret in the moments when fate is less kind, and cultivate compassion for ourselves and our fellow parents.[22] In understanding and even accepting miscarriages as part of childbearing, we can more fully embrace this most human of endeavors.

NOTES

INTRODUCTION

1. Emily Malone, "You Must Have Been a Beautiful Baby," *Daily Garnish*, March 7, 2011, http://www.dailygarnish.com/2011/03/you-must-have-been-a-beautiful-baby.html; Lara Freidenfelds, ""Cherish Every Moment" of Parenting?," *Lara Freidenfelds: Historian of Health, Reproduction, and Parenting in America*, April 7, 2015, http://larafreidenfelds.com/2015/04/07/cherish-every-moment-of-parenting/.
2. Malone, "Beautiful Baby," http://www.dailygarnish.com/2011/03/you-must-have-been-a-beautiful-baby.html.
3. "Week 9: My Pregnancy Journey," *Daily Garnish*, March 16, 2011, http://www.dailygarnish.com/2011/03/week-9-my-pregnancy-journey.html.
4. "Dealing with Pregnancy Anxiety," *Daily Garnish*, March 9, 2011, http://www.dailygarnish.com/2011/03/dealing-with-pregnancy-anxiety.html.
5. Ibid.
6. "The Newest Malone," *Daily Garnish*, March 11, 2011, http://www.dailygarnish.com/2011/03/the-newest-malone.html.
7. "Love and Loss," *Daily Garnish*, April 5, 2017, http://www.dailygarnish.com/2017/04/love-and-loss.html.
8. Ibid.
9. Ibid.
10. For relatively recent examples of this perspective see Elizabeth M. Whelan, *Pregnancy Survival Guide* (New York: American Baby Books, 1978), 69: "Medical treatment is available for heading off a threatened miscarriage, but when it cannot be prevented, it is most often interpreted as a lost opportunity rather than a lost baby—and the couple is eager to start a new pregnancy as soon as possible." Also, first-person narrative of miscarriage experiences in Judy Carter, "A Waiting Time," *Redbook* 152, no. 3 (January 1979). For changing representations in popular magazines, see Leslie J. Reagan, "From Hazard to Blessing to Tragedy: Representations of Miscarriage in Twentieth-Century America," *Feminist Studies* 9, no. 2 (Summer 2003).
11. Malone, "Love and Loss," http://www.dailygarnish.com/2017/04/love-and-loss.html.
12. A. J. Wilcox et al. "Incidence of Early Loss of Pregnancy," *New England Journal of Medicine* 319, no. 4 (July 28, 1988).
13. Allen J. Wilcox, *Fertility and Pregnancy: An Epidemiologic Perspective* (New York: Oxford University Press, 2010), 145; N. S. Macklon, J. P. Geraedts,

and B. C. Fauser, "Conception to Ongoing Pregnancy: The 'Black Box' of Early Pregnancy Loss," *Human Reproduction Update* 8, no. 4 (July–August 2002); Gavin Jarvis, "Estimating Limits for Natural Human Embryo Mortality," *F1000Research* 5, no. 2083 (August 25, 2016); A. J. Wilcox, C. R. Weinberg, and D. D. Baird, "Time of Implantation of the Conceptus and Loss of Pregnancy," *New England Journal of Medicine* 319 (June 10, 1999).

14. Wilcox, *Fertility and Pregnancy*, 185.

15. Kirsten Duckitt and Aysha Qureshi, "Recurrent Miscarriage," *American Family Physician* 78, no. 8 (October 15, 2008).

16. Anne-Marie Nybo Andersen et al., "Maternal Age and Fetal Loss: Population Based Register Linkage Study," *British Medical Journal* 320, no. 7251 (June 24, 2000); K. A. O'Connor, D. J. Holman, and J. W. Wood, "Declining Fecundity and Ovarian Ageing in Natural Fertility Populations," *Maturitas* 30, no. 2 (October 12, 1998).

17. In this book many examples are drawn from BabyCenter.com, both because it is by far the dominant online forum for discussing pregnancy and because it is demographically well documented. Its users are strikingly similar to American demographic breakdowns as a whole, with racial minorities slightly over-represented, high-income individuals somewhat under-represented, and Democrats somewhat (but not dramatically) over-represented (Quantcast, 2017). If there is an online space that could be said to represent the mainstream, where discussion is generally peaceful but nonetheless reveals a range of strong opinions on topics from abortion to breastfeeding to co-sleeping, this is it. BabyCenter forums are a reasonable proxy for the broad American middle and aspiring-middle class primarily addressed. These types of online forums are widely used across the Global North (Deborah Lupton, Sarah Pedersen, and Gareth Thomas, "Parenting and Digital Media: From the Early Web to Contemporary Digital Society," *Sociology Compass* 10, no. 8 (August 2016); Deborah Lupton, "The Use and Value of Digital Media for Information About Pregnancy and Early Motherhood: A Focus Group Study," *BMC Pregnancy and Childbirth* 16, no. 171 (July 19, 2016).

18. See works cited throughout the book. Recent influential scholarship includes Shannon Withycombe, *Lost: The Meaning of Miscarriage in Nineteenth-Century America* (New Brunswick, NJ: Rutgers University Press, 2018); Jacqueline Wolf, *Cesarean Section: An American History of Risk, Technology, and Consequence* (Baltimore: Johns Hopkins University Press, 2018); Jessica Martucci, *Back to the Breast: Natural Motherhood and Breastfeeding in America* (Chicago: University of Chicago Press, 2015); Johanna Schoen, *Abortion after Roe* (Chapel Hill: University of North Carolina Press, 2017); Janet Golden, *Babies Made Us Modern: How Infants Brought America into the Twentieth Century* (New York: Cambridge University Press, 2018); Ilana Lowy, *Imperfect Pregnancies: A History of Birth Defects and Prenatal Diagnosis* (Baltimore: Johns Hopkins University Press, 2017) among many others.

For an interpretation of the contemporary cultural landscape of miscarriage based on ethnographic fieldwork in pregnancy loss support groups, see Linda L. Layne, *Motherhood Lost: A Feminist Account of Pregnancy Loss in America* (New York: Routledge, 2003). See also subsequent related scholarship, including "Some Unintended Consequences of New Reproductive and Information Technologies on the Experience of Pregnancy Loss," in *Women, Gender and Technology*, ed. Mary Frank Fox, Deborah G. Johnson, and Sue V. Rosser (Urbana: University of Illinois Press, 2006); Linda Layne, "Designing a Woman-Centered Health Care Approach to Pregnancy Loss: Lessons from Feminist Models of Childbirth," in *Reproductive Disruptions: Gender, Technology, and Biopolitics in the New Millennium*, ed. Marcia C. Inhorn (New York: Berghahn Books, 2007); Linda L. Layne, "The Home Pregnancy Test: A Feminist Technology?," *Women's Studies Quarterly* 37, no. 1–2 (Spring/Summer 2009); "Why the Home Pregnancy Test Isn't the Feminist Technology It's Cracked up to Be and How to Make It Better," in *Feminist Technology*, ed. Linda L. Layne, Sharra Louise Vostral, and Kate Boyer (Urbana: University of Illinois Press, 2010).

19. See argument about class and menstruation in Lara Freidenfelds, *The Modern Period: Menstruation in Twentieth-Century America* (Baltimore: Johns Hopkins University Press, 2009), and similarly about pregnancy in Ziv Eisenberg, "The Whole Nine Months: Women, Men, and the Making of Modern Pregnancy in America" (PhD diss., Yale University, 2013).

On the embrace of "intensive parenting" and "concerted cultivation" parenting strategies across socioeconomic groups, see Patrick Ishizuka, "Social Class, Gender, and Contemporary Parenting Standards in the United States: Evidence from a National Survey Experiment," *Social Forces* (December 22, 2018). On guilt and blame when poor mothers struggle to meet middle-class norms, see Kelly Ray Knight, *Addicted.Pregnant.Poor* (Durham, NC: Duke University Press, 2015), 157–158; Molly Ladd-Taylor and Lauri Umansky, eds., *"Bad" Mothers: The Politics of Blame in Twentieth-Century America* (New York: New York University Press, 1990); Linda C. Fentiman, *Blaming Mothers: American Law and the Risks to Children's Health* (New York: New York University Press, 2018).

Slightly more than half of pregnancies are planned. While this rate may be dismayingly low by the standard of public health advocates, in historical terms it is an astounding achievement. For the approximately two-thirds of women whose income is above 200 percent of the poverty line—about $50,000 for a family of four—the figure is even more striking: 70 percent of pregnancies are intentional (Lawrence B. Finer and Mia R. Zolna, "Declines in Unintended Pregnancy in the United States, 2008–2011," *New England Journal of Medicine* 374, no. 9 (March 3, 2016); "Distribution of the Total Population by Federal Poverty Level (above and Below 200 percent Fpl)," Henry J. Kaiser Family Foundation, https://www.kff. org/other/state-indicator/population-up-to-200-fpl/?currentTimeframe=0&sort Model=%7B%22colId%22:%22Location%22,%22sort%22:%22asc%22%7D.).

CHAPTER 1

1. The Holyoke Diaries, 1709–1856, (Washington, DC: Library of Congress, 1911), http://archive.org/stream/holyokediaries00dowg/holyokediaries00dowg_djvu. txt.
2. Ibid.
3. Ibid.
4. Also see Michelle Marchetti Coughlin, *One Colonial Woman's World: The Life and Writings of Mehetabel Chandler Coit* (Amherst: University of Massachusetts Press, 2012), xxiv, on emotional and introspective reserve in early diaries.
5. The best scholarly reconstructions of ordinary colonial-era women's lives include Laurel Thatcher Ulrich, *Good Wives: Image and Reality in the Lives of Women in Northern New England, 1650-1750* (New York: Knopf, 1982), and *A Midwife's Tale: The Life of Martha Ballard, Based on Her Diary, 1785-1812* (New York: Knopf, 1990), Mary Beth Norton, *Founding Mothers and Fathers: Gendered Power and the Forming of American Society* (New York: Knopf, 1996), and *Liberty's Daughters: The*

Revolutionary Experience of American Women, 1750-1800 (Ithaca, NY: Cornell University Press, 1980), and Cornelia Hughes Dayton, *Women before the Bar: Gender, Law, and Society in Connecticut, 1639-1789* (Chapel Hill: University of North Carolina Press, 1995). For the primary source that comes closest to a robust record of the intimate life of an individual, see Elaine Forman Crane, ed. *The Diary of Elizabeth Drinker* (Boston: Northeastern University Press, 1991). Drinker seldom mentioned her pregnancies and did not describe her births, but she kept a diary for much of her adult life and recorded many useful details for the history of childbearing.

6. Judith Walzer Leavitt, *Brought to Bed: Childbearing in America, 1750 to 1950* (New York: Oxford University Press, 1986), 14–16; Marie Jenkins Schwartz, *Born in Bondage: Growing up Enslaved in the Antebellum South* (Cambridge, MA: Harvard University Press, 2000), 4–5; Peter Kolchin, *American Slavery, 1619-1877* (New York: Hill and Wang, 1993), 44.

7. Susan E. Klepp, *Revolutionary Conceptions: Women, Fertility, and Family Limitation in America, 1760-1820* (Chapel Hill: University of North Carolina Press, 2009), 206–207. While abstention was commonly advised by medical writers, historian Valerie Fildes does not believe that abstention was commonly practiced (Valerie Fildes, *Breasts, Bottles and Babies: A History of Infant Feeding* (Edinburgh: Edinburgh University Press, 1986), 105). For an eighteenth-century New England example of conception likely triggering weaning: Rose Lockwood, "Birth, Illness and Death in 18th-Century New England," *Journal of Social History* 12, no. 1 (Autumn 1978): 123.

8. "The Amazing Baby Boom of Billerica, Mass.," http://www. newenglandhistoricalsociety.com/amazing-baby-boom-billerica-mass/.

9. Ulrich, *Good Wives*, 157–161; Steven Mintz and Susan Kellogg, *Domestic Revolutions: A Social History of American Family Life* (New York: The Free Press, 1988), 49; Nancy Schrom Dye and Daniel Blake Smith, "Mother Love and Infant Death, 1750-1920," *Journal of American History* 73, no. 2 (September 1986): 334–35.

10. Schwartz, *Born in Bondage*, 4.

11. Karin Calvert, *Children in the House: The Material Culture of Early Childhood, 1600-1900* (Boston: Northeastern University Press, 1992), 19–24; Schwartz, *Born in Bondage*, 43.

12. Ulrich, *Good Wives*, 29–30.

13. Calvert, *Children in the House*, 31–36.

14. Klepp, *Revolutionary Conceptions*, 64, 66; "Revolutionary Bodies: Women and the Fertility Transition in the Mid-Atlantic Region, 1760-1820," *Journal of American History* 85, no. 3 (December 1998): 910.

15. Ulrich, *Good Wives*, 146–147, 59.

16. Catherine M. Scholten, *Childbearing in American Society: 1650-1850* (New York: New York University Press, 1985), 25–27; Norton, *Founding Mothers and Fathers*, 222–223; and Ulrich, *Good Wives*, 126–135. For an in-depth description of very similar birth and lying-in practices from seventeenth century England, see Adrian Wilson, "The Ceremony of Childbirth and Its Interpretation," in *Women as Mothers in Pre-Industrial England*, ed. Valerie Fildes (New York: Routledge, 1990). Example of father's exclusion from birth chamber and thankful prayers: Lockwood, "Birth, Illness and Death in 18th-Century New England," 121.

17. Norton, *Founding Mothers and Fathers*, 225–227; Rebecca J. Tannenbaum, *The Healer's Calling: Women and Medicine in Early New England* (Ithaca, NY: Cornell University Press, 2009), 48.

18. Schwartz, *Born in Bondage*, 9 and 123.
19. Klepp, *Revolutionary Conceptions*, 70–71.
20. Elaine Tyler May, *Barren in the Promised Land: Childless Americans and the Pursuit of Happiness* (Cambridge, MA: Harvard University Press, 1995), 26; Klepp, *Revolutionary Conceptions*, 70.
21. Schwartz, *Born in Bondage*, 191.
22. Linda A. Pollock, "Embarking on a Rough Passage: The Experience of Pregnancy in Early-Modern Society," in *Women as Mothers in Pre-Industrial England*, 46; William Buchan, *Domestic Medicine*, eleventh ed. (Edinburgh: Printed by Balfour Auld and Smellie, 1790 (1st edition 1769)), 530.
23. Leavitt, *Brought to Bed*, 13–35.
24. Laurel Thatcher Ulrich, "Vertuous Women Found: New England Ministerial Literature, 1668-1735," *American Quarterly* 28, no. 1 (Spring 1976): 31; Nancy Cott, *The Bonds of Womanhood: "Woman's Sphere" in New England, 1780-1835* (New Haven, CT: Yale University Press, 1977), 127–128.
25. Coughlin, *One Colonial Woman's World: The Life and Writings of Mehetabel Chandler Coit*, 41–44.
26. Scholten, *Childbearing in American Society: 1650-1850*, 15–16; Ulrich, *Good Wives*, 136–41; Norton, *Liberty's Daughters*, 73. For the antebellum South, Sally G. McMillen, *Motherhood in the Old South: Pregnancy, Childbirth, and Infant Rearing* (Baton Rouge: Louisiana State University Press, 1990), 40–41. McMillen explains that even well-off women were not expected to rest or stop normal activity during pregnancy and could not realistically do so. For Europe, Jacques Gelis, *History of Childbirth: Fertility, Pregnancy and Birth in Early Modern Europe* (Boston: Northeastern University Press, 1991), 76.
27. Scholten, *Childbearing in American Society: 1650-1850*, 15–16; Schwartz, *Born in Bondage*, 31.
28. Ulrich, *Good Wives*, 136–38.
29. Schwartz, *Born in Bondage*, 20–27.
30. For example, Buchan, *Domestic Medicine*, 532; Alexander Hamilton, *A Treatise on the Management of Female Complaints and of Children in Early Infancy* (New York: Samuel Campbell, 1795), 135-137; Thomas Ewell, *The Ladies Medical Companion* (Philadelphia: William Brown, 1818), 118–121. On imported home medical guides, Charles E. Rosenberg, ed. *Right Living: An Anglo-American Tradition of Self-Help Medicine and Hygiene* (Baltimore: Johns Hopkins University Press, 2003), 2–3.
31. Buchan, *Domestic Medicine*, 7, 531–34; Hamilton, *A Treatise on the Management of Female Complaints and of Children in Early Infancy*, 61, 78, 106–135.
32. New England Historical Society, "Over and Over, Mary Vial Holyoke Suffers the Heartache of Losing a Child," http://www.newenglandhistoricalsociety.com/mary-vial-holyoke-suffers-heartache-losing-child/.
33. Mary Fissell, "When the Birds and the Bees Were Not Enough: Aristotle's Masterpiece," *Public Domain Review* (2015), http://publicdomainreview.org/2015/08/19/when-the-birds-and-the-bees-were-not-enough-aristotles-masterpiece/; *Aristotle's Masterpiece* (New York: Published for the Trade, 1846), https://archive.org/details/8709661.nlm.nih.gov.
34. Gelis, *History of Childbirth*, 46.
35. Quoted in ibid., 47.
36. David Cressy, *Birth, Marriage, and Death: Ritual, Religion and the Life-Cycle in Tudor and Stuart England* (Oxford: Oxford University Press, 1997), 43.

37. Pollock, "Embarking on a Rough Passage: The Experience of Pregnancy in Early-Modern Society," 43–44.
38. Barbara Duden, *The Woman Beneath the Skin: A Doctor's Patients in Eighteenth-Century Germany* (Cambridge, MA: Harvard University Press, 1991), 111.
39. Ibid., 157–170; Freidenfelds, *The Modern Period*, 24–27.
40. Patricia Crawford, "The Construction and Experience of Maternity in Seventeenth-Century England," in *Women as Mothers in Pre-Industrial England*, 17. For an example of an experienced mother who announced a suspected pregnancy to her husband within six weeks of conception of her eighth child in eighteenth-century New England see Lockwood, "Birth, Illness and Death in 18th-Century New England," 122.
41. See description of heavy period/miscarriage at ten weeks in Laura Gowing, *Common Bodies: Women, Touch and Power in Seventeenth-Century England* (New Haven, CT: Yale University Press, 2003), 143, testimony from England in 1650; Duden, *Woman Beneath the Skin*, 163–164. For examples of the uncertainty even experienced mothers could feel about amenorrhea, early pregnancy, and early miscarriages, see Mary Poor's diaries and letters in Janet Farrell Brodie, *Contraception and Abortion in Nineteenth-Century America* (Ithaca, NY: Cornell University Press, 1994), 10–25.
42. "Whites": Duden, *Woman Beneath the Skin*, 130–131; nutritional amenorrhea: Alexandra Lord, "'The Great Arcana of the Deity': Menstruation and Menstrual Disorders in Eighteenth-Century British Medical Thought," *Bulletin of the History of Medicine* 73, no. 1 (Spring 1999): 43; malaria: Darrell B. Rutman and Anita H. Rutman, "Of Agues and Fevers: Malaria in the Early Chesapeake," *The William and Mary Quarterly* 33, no. 1 (January 1976).
43. Cathy McClive, "The Hidden Truths of the Belly: The Uncertainties of Pregnancy in Early Modern Europe," *Social History of Medicine* 15, no. 2 (August 2002): 226. An 1865 letter from Mary Adams to her sister Eliza records a case of a neighbor who thought she was pregnant for over a year and had even hired a "girl and nurse" to help at and after the birth but then "gave it up" as a "false conception." Parker Family Letters, in the possession of Marianne Parker Brown, Berkeley, CA, published with permission.
44. Shannon Withycombe, "Slipped Away: Pregnancy Loss in Nineteenth-Century America" (PhD diss., University of Wisconsin at Madison, 2010), 48–49.
45. Pollock, "Embarking on a Rough Passage: The Experience of Pregnancy in Early-Modern Society," 57–58.
46. Duden, *Woman Beneath the Skin*, 174; Buchan, *Domestic Medicine*, 531.
47. For example, Hamilton, *A Treatise on the Management of Female Complaints and of Children in Early Infancy*, 128–29; Buchan, *Domestic Medicine*, 531–32.
48. Pollock, "Embarking on a Rough Passage: The Experience of Pregnancy in Early-Modern Society," 49–52.
49. Katharine Park, "Birth and Death," in *A Cultural History of the Human Body in the Medieval Ages*, ed. Linda Kalof (Oxford: Berg, 2010), 22; Gowing, *Common Bodies*, 112.
50. Shannon Withycombe, "From Women's Expectations to Scientific Specimens: The Fate of Miscarriage Materials in Nineteenth-Century America," *Social History of Medicine* 28, no. 2 (2015); Withycombe, *Lost*, 44–52.
51. Park, "Birth and Death," 21.
52. Mark Jackson, "'Something More Than Blood': Conflicting Accounts of Pregnancy Loss in Eighteenth-Century England," in *The Anthropology of Pregnancy*

Loss: Comparative Studies in Miscarriage, Stillbirth and Neonatal Death, ed. Rosanne Cecil (Oxford and Washington, DC: Berg, 1996), 203–204.

53. Pernille Arenfeldt, "Betrayed by the Body: 'Miscarriages' in Sixteenth Century Germany" (paper presented at the Berkshire Conference on the History of Women, Minneapolis, MN, 2008): Elisabeth to Anna, 9 January 1582. Used with permission.

54. McClive, "The Hidden Truths of the Belly: The Uncertainies of Pregnancy in Early Modern Europe," 223.

55. Withycombe, "From Women's Expectations to Scientific Specimens," 4–6. See also Gowing, *Common Bodies*, 121.

56. Barbara Duden, "The Fetus on the 'Farther Shore': Toward a History of the Unborn," in *Fetal Subjects, Feminist Positions*, ed. Lynn Marie Morgan and Meredith W. Michaels (Philadelphia: University of Pennsylvania Press, 1999), 19–20.

57. Quoted in ibid., 21. Also see Klepp, *Revolutionary Conceptions*, 69: "The woman remained at the center of the images of pregnancy, and process was stressed over end; the future child was an uncertain, hazily conceptualized possibility. Even after birth, women's offspring were frequently referred to only as 'my little flock'—the undifferentiated, but now animate, products of fruitfulness."

58. Park, "Birth and Death," 23.

59. Sara M. Butler, "Abortion by Assault: Violence against Pregnant Women in Thirteenth-and Fourteenth-Century England," *Journal of Women's History* 17, no. 4 (Winter 2005).

60. McClive, "The Hidden Truths of the Belly: The Uncertainies of Pregnancy in Early Modern Europe," 216.

61. The same practices were followed in England until a major legal reform in 1803, which specifically criminalized the administering of "poison or some other destructive or noxious and destructive substance. . . with intent to procure miscarriage or abortion where the woman may not be quick with child at the time, or it may not be proved that she was quick with child" (https://en.wikisource.org/wiki/Lord_Ellenborough%27s_Act_1803); James Mohr, *Abortion in America: The Origins and Evolution of National Policy* (New York: Oxford University Press, 1978), 24.

62. We cannot know whether tightly-spaced births were the specific cause of Holyoke's stillbirths, but we do know that tightly spaced births correlate with stillbirth in modern populations: Maureen Norton and James D. Shelton, "Stillbirth and Healthy Timing and Spacing of Pregnancy," *Lancet* 378 (September 3, 2011).

63. Susan E. Klepp, "Colds, Worms, and Hysteria: Menstrual Regulation in Eighteenth-Century America," in *Regulating Menstruation: Beliefs, Practices, Interpretations*, ed. Etienne Van de Walle and Elisha P. Renne (Chicago: University of Chicago Press, 2001). Compare with anthropologist Caroline Bledsoe's description of West African women who use modern birth control to space pregnancies in order to preserve their health and thereby increase fertility. Caroline Bledsoe, *Contingent Lives: Fertility, Time, and Aging in West Africa* (Chicago: University of Chicago Press, 2002). Enslaved colonial Americans may also have used abortion to space pregnancies: Schwartz, *Born in Bondage*, 41–42.

64. Cornelia Hughes Dayton, "Taking the Trade: Abortion and Gender Relations in an Eighteenth-Century New England Village," *The William and Mary Quarterly* 48, no. 1 (January 1991).

65. Brodie, *Contraception and Abortion in Nineteenth-Century America*, 43.

66. Duden, *Woman Beneath the Skin*, 163–164; Klepp, "Colds, Worms, and Hysteria," 32–35; Brodie, "Menstrual Interventions in the Nineteenth-Century United States," in *Regulating Menstruation*, 39.

67. Steven Mintz, *Huck's Raft: A History of American Childhood* (Cambridge, MA: The Belknap Press of Harvard University Press, 2004), 14–15.

68. Crane, *The Diary of Elizabeth Drinker*, 420, March 13, 1784.

69. Quoted in Dye and Smith, "Mother Love and Infant Death," 332 and 335. See also Ulrich, *A Midwife's Tale: The Life of Martha Ballard, Based on Her Diary, 1785 - 1812*, 40–46; Lockwood, "Birth, Illness and Death in 18th-Century New England," 111–15.

70. William Bradford Reed, *The Life of Esther De Berdt, Afterwards Esther Reed, of Pennsylvania* (Philadelphia: C. Sherman, 1853), 168.

71. G. J. Barker-Benfield, "Stillbirth and Sensibility: The Case of Abigail and John Adams," *Early American Studies: An Interdisciplinary Journal* 10, no. 1 (Winter 2012): 19–25. Adams quote from L. H. Butterfield, et al., ed. *Adams Family Correspondence* (Cambridge, MA: Belknap Press of Harvard University Press, 1963–2011), 2:308, Abigail Adams to John Adams, August 12, 1777.

72. Crane, *The Diary of Elizabeth Drinker*, 99, 139.

73. Stewart Mitchell, *New Letters of Abigail Adams 1788-1801* (Boston: Houghton Mifflin Company, 1947) p. 244, Phil, Apr 7, 1800; (http://records.ancestry.com/Anna_Greenleaf_records.ashx?pid=32096201).

CHAPTER 2

1. Jennifer Borget, "The Big Goal," (June 20, 2009), http://www.babymakingmachine.com/2009/06/the-big-goal.html.

2. William Bradford Reed, *The Life of Esther De Berdt*, 171, quoted in Klepp, *Revolutionary Conceptions*, 83. Historian Susan Klepp's *Revolutionary Conceptions* deeply and persuasively lays out the relationship between revolutionary ideology and women's beliefs and actions, building on arguments suggested by Mary Beth Norton in *Liberty's Daughters: The Revolutionary Experience of American Women, 1750-1800* (Ithaca, NY: Cornell University Press, 1980). I rely on her analysis for the revolutionary era and early Republic.

3. Quoted in *Revolutionary Conceptions*, 122.

4. Ibid.

5. Quoted in ibid., 92.

6. Norton, *Liberty's Daughters*, 235.

7. Quoted in Klepp, *Revolutionary Conceptions*, 105.

8. Quoted in ibid., 116.

9. Ibid., 195.

10. Janet Farrell Brodie, "Menstrual Interventions in the Nineteenth-Century United States," in *Regulating Menstruation*, 118–119.

11. Both quoted in Klepp, *Revolutionary Conceptions*, 210.

12. Quoted in ibid., 97. Wollstonecraft would later die at age thirty-eight of septicemia caused by birth complications. Also examples from Scholten, *Childbearing in American Society: 1650-1850*, 14 and Norton, *Liberty's Daughters*, 232–233.

13. Quoted in Klepp, *Revolutionary Conceptions*, 206–207.

14. "Colds, Worms, and Hysteria: Menstrual Regulation in Eighteenth-Century America," 25.

15. Brodie, *Contraception and Abortion in Nineteenth-Century America*, 24–25.

16. Klepp, *Revolutionary Conceptions*, 187.

17. Quoted in ibid., 117.

18. Brodie, *Contraception and Abortion in Nineteenth-Century America*, 57–86.

19. Mohr, *Abortion in America*, 46–50.

20. Shannon Withycombe, "Unusual Frontal Developments: Negotiating the Pregnant Body in Nineteenth-Century America," *Journal of Women's History* 27, no. 4 (Winter 2015): 174.

21. Andrew S. London and Robert A. McGuire Cheryl Elman, "Fertility, Economic Development, and Health in the Early Twentieth-Century U.S. South," *Journal of Interdisciplinary History* 46, no. 2 (2015).

22. Herbert S. Klein, *A Population History of the United States* (New York: Cambridge University Press, 2004), 133–34.

23. Lara Freidenfelds, "The Historical Development of Modern Distinctions between Contraception and Early Abortion" (paper presented at the American Association of the History of Medicine annual meeting, Baltimore, MD, 2012).

24. On the weighing of options, Brodie, "Menstrual Interventions in the Nineteenth-Century United States," 47; Linda Gordon, *The Moral Property of Women: A History of Birth Control Politics in America* (Chicago: University of Illinois Press, 2007), 30–31.

25. Mohr, *Abortion in America*, 46–50.

26. Brodie, *Contraception and Abortion in Nineteenth-Century America*, 224–231; Mohr, *Abortion in America*, 97.

27. Mohr, *Abortion in America*, 46–50; Brodie, *Contraception and Abortion in Nineteenth-Century America*, 189–190.

28. Sharla M. Fett, *Working Cures: Healing, Health, and Power on Southern Slave Plantations* (Chapel Hill: University of North Carolina Press, 2002), 65.

29. For example Horatio Robinson Storer, *Why Not? A Book for Every Woman* (Boston: Lee and Shepard, 1867), 28–34.

30. Thomas L. Nichols, *Esoteric Anthropology* (Malvern, UK: T. L. Nichols, 1873), 87. Originally published in 1853, followed by several re-printings by the author. See also Edwin Hale, cited in Shannon Withycombe, *Lost: The Meaning of Miscarriage in Nineteenth-Century America* (New Brunswick, NJ: Rutgers University Press, 2018), 66.

31. Nichols, *Esoteric Anthropology*, 136.

32. John Harvey Kellogg, *Plain Facts for Old and Young* (Burlington, IA: I. F. Segner, 1881), 271. Originally published 1880.

33. On Kellogg's understanding of menstruation, see Freidenfelds, *The Modern Period*, 45, 78, 79.

34. Hannah Sorensen, *What Women Should Know* (Salt Lake City: George Q. Cannon & Sons Company, 1896), 80. See Withycombe, "Unusual Frontal Developments: Negotiating the Pregnant Body in Nineteenth-Century America," 11–15 for examples of welcome miscarriages revealed in nineteenth century women's letters.

35. "Slipped Away: Pregnancy Loss in Nineteenth-Century America," 2.

36. Parker Family Letters, in the possession of Marianne Parker Brown, Berkeley, CA, published with permission.

37. Withycombe, "Slipped Away: Pregnancy Loss in Nineteenth-Century America," 36–38.

38. Withycombe, *Lost*, 20–21, 82–88.

39. As an African American journalist, Borget was sensitive to how easily women could be unfairly accused of sexual irresponsibility: Lisa Rosenthal and Marci Lobel,

"Stereotypes of Black American Women Related to Sexuality and Motherhood," *Psychology of Women Quarterly* 40, no. 3 (September 2016).

40. Jennifer Borget, untitled, (March 20, 2011), http://www.babymakingmachine.com/2011/03.
41. Brodie, *Contraception and Abortion in Nineteenth-Century America*, 255–258.
42. William J. Robinson, *Sex Knowledge for Women and Girls: What Every Woman and Girl Should Know* (New York: The Critic and Guide Company, 1917), 149.
43. Carole R. McCann, *Birth Control Politics in the United States, 1916-1945* (Ithaca, NY: Cornell University Press, 1994), 23–24, 74–75, 185.
44. Ibid., 11.
45. Ibid., 37.
46. Andrea Tone, *Devices and Desires: A History of Contraceptives in America* (New York: Hill and Wang, 2001), 151–200.
47. Reagan, "From Hazard to Blessing to Tragedy," 132–139; for example of early twentieth-century homemade pessaries successful in child spacing: Andi Powers, "Bitter Lessons," *High Altitude History* (2017), https://historymsu.wordpress.com/2017/03/08/bitter-lessons-andi-powers/.
48. Rose Holz, "Nurse Gordon on Trial: Those Early Days of the Birth Control Clinic Movement Reconsidered," *Journal of Social History* 39, no. 1(Fall 2005): 116.
49. On high rates of childbearing (only 8 percent of women born in the early 1930s never had children) see Steven Mintz, *Huck's Raft*, 421 fn 4. Paula Fass describes the baby boom as a period "in which children were valued as children, and when the perceived rewards of childrearing provided mothers with a form of personal satisfaction. Childhood itself seemed to have become a national resource." Paula Fass, *The End of American Childhood: A History of Parenting from Life on the Frontier to the Managed Child* (Princeton, NJ: Princeton University Press, 2016), 185.
50. Margaret Marsh and Wanda Ronner, *The Empty Cradle: Infertility in America from Colonial Times to the Present* (Baltimore: Johns Hopkins University Press, 1996), 183–188.
51. Ziv Eisenberg, "Clear and Pregnant Danger: The Making of Prenatal Psychology in Mid-Twentieth Century America," *Journal of Women's History* 22, no. 3 (September 2010).
52. Lara Freidenfelds, "The History of Women in Biomedical Research," in *The Teaching Hospital: A History of Brigham and Women's Hospital*, ed. Peter Tishler, Christine Wenc, and Joseph Loscalzo (New York: McGraw Hill, 2013), 235–36.
53. Borget, "The Big Goal."
54. William F. Pratt and Christine A. Bachrach, "What Do Women Use When They Stop Using the Pill?," *Family Planning Perspectives* 19, no. 6 (November-December 1987); Tone, *Devices and Desires*, 204–231.
55. Robin C. Nelson, "The Pill," *Printer's Ink* (August 26,1966), 49.
56. Martha J. Bailey, "More Power to the Pill: The Impact of Contraceptive Freedom on Women's Life Cycle Labor Supply," *The Quarterly Journal of Economics* 121, no. 1 (February 2006) and "Momma's Got the Pill: How Anthony Comstock and *Griswold V. Connecticut* Shaped U.S. Childbearing," *American Economic Review* 100, no. 1 (March 2010).
57. Rebecca M. Kluchin, *Fit to Be Tied: Sterilization and Reproductive Rights in America, 1950-1980* (New Brunswick, NJ: Rutgers University Press, 2009), 50–72.
58. Charles F. Westoff and Elise F. Jones, "Contraception and Sterilization in the United States, 1965-1975," *Family Planning Perspectives* 9 (July-August 1977).

59. L. Peterson, "Contraceptive Use in the United States, 1982-1990," in *Advance Data from Vital and Health Statistics* (Hyattsville, MD: National Center for Health Statistics, 1995).

60. Martha J. Bailey, Melanie Guldi, and Brad J. Hershbein, "Is There a Case for a 'Second Demographic Transition?': Three Distinctive Features of the Post-1960 Fertility Decline," in *Human Capital and History: The American Record*, ed. Leah Platt Boustan, Carola Frydman, and Robert A. Margo (Chicago: Chicago University Press, 2014).

61. John E. Anderson, "Planning Status of Marital Births, 1975-1976," *Family Planning Perspectives* 13, no. 2 (March-April 1981): 62. As an example of the shift in expectations, in 1979 Jean Collins described her experience of pregnancy: "When I tell some of my non-work friends, they ask if the baby is planned—wanted. My mother says such questions were unheard of a generation ago." (Jean E. Collins, "Working and Pregnant: What It's Like to Be Really Happy About Both," *Glamour*, November 1979, 104).

62. Barbara Seaman, *The Doctors' Case against the Pill* (New York: P. H. Wyden, 1969), 19, quoted in Tone, *Devices and Desires*, 245.

63. Pratt and Bachrach, "What Do Women Use When They Stop Using the Pill?"

64. Planned Parenthood Federation of America, "The Birth Control Pill—a History," (PPFA, 2013), 4: Enovid had 10,000 micrograms of progestin and 150 of estrogen; in around 1998 low-dose pills had 150 mg of progestin and 20–50 mg of estrogen.

65. Sarah S. Brown and Leon Eisenberg, eds., *The Best Intentions: Unintended Pregnancy and the Well-Being of Children and Families* (Washington, DC: National Academies Press, 1995), p. 3.

66. The unintended pregnancy rate continues to fall among all income groups, but large disparities remain: Lawrence B. Finer and Mia R. Zolna, "Declines in Unintended Pregnancy in the United States, 2008–2011," *New England Journal of Medicine* 374, no. 9 (March 3, 2016).

67. Jennifer Borget, "Timing," (March 23, 2011), http://www.babymakingmachine. com/2011/03.

68. Borget, "How Far Apart to Space the Kiddos?" (August 25, 2011), babymakingmachine.com.

69. Borget, "Getting Pregnant (Again)" (October 11, 2011), babymakingmachine. com.

70. Borget, "Baby #2?: He Says/She Says," (March 21, 2012), babymakingmachine. com.

71. Borget, "Kiddo Fashion for TWO + Diaper.com Giveaway" (May 22, 2012), babymakingmachine.com.

CHAPTER 3

1. http://www.whattoexpect.com/forums/november-2010-babies/archives/ hard-time-bonding-with-the-baby-due-to-previous-miscarriage.html, accessed January 7, 2013.

2. Laurel Thatcher Ulrich, ""The Living Mother of a Living Child": Midwifery and Mortality in Post-Revolutionary New England," *The William and Mary Quarterly* 46, no. 1 (January 1989).

3. Dye and Smith, "Mother Love and Infant Death, 1750-1920," 338.

4. Ibid., 339.

5. Ibid.

6. Quoted in Mohr, *Abortion in America,* 87.

7. Sylvia Hoffert, *Private Matters: American Attitudes Toward Childbearing and Infant Nurture in the Urban North, 1800-1860* (Urbana: University of Illinois Press, 1989), 39–42. Nineteenth-century women and their physicians did not regard miscarried fetuses as stillborn babies until about seven months' gestation (the time of viability in that era): Withycombe, "Slipped Away: Pregnancy Loss in Nineteenth-Century America," 146–175.

8. Scholten, *Childbearing in American Society: 1650-1850*, 50–51, 88–89; Cott, *The Bonds of Womanhood*.

9. Dye and Smith, "Mother Love and Infant Death," 338–340.

10. Rebecca Jo Plant, *Mom: The Transformation of Motherhood in Modern America* (Chicago, IL: University of Chicago Press, 2010), 9–10, 46–47.

11. Scholten, *Childbearing in American Society: 1650-1850*, 66.

12. Dye and Smith, "Mother Love and Infant Death," 330, 43–44.

13. "Several shared realities cut across the boundaries of class, ethnicity, gender, or region, especially a high incidence of child mortality. As late as 1895, 18 percent of children—one in six—died before their fifth birthday. While mortality was greatest among the poor, most affluent families with five or six children experienced the death of at least one child." Mintz, *Huck's Raft*, 134.

14. Scholten, *Childbearing in American Society: 1650-1850*, 71.

15. Mintz, *Huck's Raft*, 20–21.

16. Viviana Zelizer, *Pricing the Priceless Child: The Changing Social Value of Children* (New York: Basic Books, 1985), 25–27.

17. Hoffert, *Private Matters*, 169–177; Carol Sanger, *About Abortion: Terminating Pregnancy in Twenty-First-Century America* (Cambridge, MA: Belknap Press of Harvard University Press, 2017), 136–140.

18. On continued economic importance of children, especially outside of urban middle class, see Mintz, *Huck's Raft*, 135.

19. On late twentieth-century intensive parenting, see Sharon Hays, *The Cultural Contradictions of Motherhood* (New Haven, CT: Yale University Press, 1996). On colonial American extensive parenting, see Ulrich, *Good Wives*, 61.

20. Zelizer, *Pricing the Priceless Child*, 5–6.

21. Hays, *The Cultural Contradictions of Motherhood*, 43 citing Lynn Y. Weiner, *From Working Girl to Working Mother: The Female Labor Force in the United States, 1820-1980* (Chapel Hill: University of North Carolina Press, 1985).

22. Zelizer, *Pricing the Priceless Child*, 189–195.

23. Golden, *Babies Made Us Modern*, 7–41; Zelizer, *Pricing the Priceless Child*, 169–95. This pattern accelerated during the baby boom: Wayne Carp, ed. *Adoption in America: Historical Perspectives* (Ann Arbor: University of Michigan Press, 2002), 127, 60–61.

24. Richard A. Meckel, "Levels and Trends of Death and Disease in Childhood, 1620 to the Present," in *Children and Youth in Sickness and in Health*, ed. Janet Golden, Richard A. Meckel, and Heather Munro Prescott (Westport, CT: Greenwood Press, 2004), 16–17. See also Fass, *The End of American Childhood*, 96–99, and Samuel H. Preston and Michael R. Haines, *Fatal Years: Child Mortality in Late Nineteenth-Century America* (Princeton, NJ: Princeton University Press, 1991).

25. Irvine Loudon, "Maternal Mortality in the Past and Its Relevance to Developing Countries Today," *American Journal of Clinical Nutrition* 72 (Suppl) (July 2000).

26. Plant, *Mom*, 118–145.

27. Rima Apple, *Perfect Motherhood: Science and Childrearing in America* (New Brunswick, NJ: Rutgers University Press, 2006).

28. Cited in Ann Hulbert, *Raising America: Experts, Parents, and a Century of Advice About Children* (New York: Knopf, 2003), 32: Ellen Key, *The Century of the Child* (New York: J. P. Putnam's Sons, 1909).

29. Plant, *Mom*; Marga Vicedo, *The Nature and Nurture of Love: From Imprinting to Attachment in Cold War America* (Chicago: University of Chicago Press, 2013), 33–36. On 1950s child-centered homes and 1950s anxieties about child-rearing, see Mintz, *Huck's Raft*, 276–283.

30. Historian Marga Vicedo has described this history in perceptive and fascinating detail, and I rely on her analysis here. Vicedo, *Nature and Nurture of Love*.

31. Ibid., 60–67.

32. In ibid., 65, picture from *Life*, August 22, 1955, 73.

33. Ibid., 57–60.

34. Ibid., 39–40, 69–72.

35. Ibid., 73–81.

36. Apple, *Perfect Motherhood*.

37. Plant, *Mom*, 113–15; Vicedo, *Nature and Nurture of Love*, 71.

38. On new emphasis on personal fulfillment in the 1960s and 1970s, and the challenges this posed to family life: Mintz and Kellogg, *Domestic Revolutions*, 205–207.

39. Kluchin, *Fit to Be Tied,* 33–34; Matthew Connelly, *Fatal Misconception: The Struggle to Control World Population* (Cambridge, MA: Harvard University Press, 2008), 7–8; Paul Ehrlich, *The Population Bomb: Population Control or Race to Oblivion?* (New York: Ballantine Books for the Sierra Club, 1968).

40. "A New Movement Challenges the U.S. To Stop Growing," *Life*, April 17, 1970, https://books.google.com/books?id=lFUEAAAAMBAJ&pg=PA32&source=gbs_toc_r&cad=2#v=onepage&q&f=false.

41. "One Man's Answer to Overpopulation," *Life*, March 6, 1970, https://books.google.com/books?id=dVAEAAAAMBAJ&pg=PA3&dq=life+march+6+1970&hl=en&sa=X&ved=0CC4Q6AEwAmoVChMI7PGXsY3yxgIVgUc-Ch2sVQNU#v=onepage&q=life%20march%206%201970&f=false.

42. The Sierra Club advocated closing the US border as well as limiting US population growth. In the 1990s the membership voted down this stance. https://en.wikipedia.org/wiki/Sierra_Club.

43. Clyde Haberman, "The Unrealized Horrors of Population Explosion," *New York Times*, May 31, 2015, https://www.nytimes.com/2015/06/01/us/the-unrealized-horrors-of-population-explosion.html.

44. Ehrlich, *The Population Bomb*, 140, 74. "It is the behavior of [the middle and affluent classes] which causes the greatest symptom of overpopulation in the U.S.—environmental deterioration. Minority groups usually are the prime victims of this and related symptoms, such as unemployment and rising crime rates. And until recently, the poor were largely denied even the means to limit their families. If first responsibility to reduce birth rates rests with any one group in the U.S. it rests with the affluent."

45. Betty Friedan, *The Feminine Mystique* (New York: W.W. Norton, 1963).

46. Shulamith Firestone, *The Dialectic of Sex: The Case for Feminist Revolution* (New York: William Morrow and Company, 1970); quote: https://en.wikipedia.org/wiki/Shulamith_Firestone.

47. Mintz and Kellogg, *Domestic Revolutions*, 207–208.

48. Sara M. Evans, "Sons, Daughters, and Patriarchy: Gender and the 1968 Generation," *American Historical Review* 114, no. 2 (April 2009): 336–37.

49. Thomas Gordon, *Parent Effectiveness Training: The Tested New Way to Raise Responsible Children* (New York: David McKay Company, 1970). Historian Paula Fass traces this approach to a much longer pattern of American parents expecting that their children would have new and different lives than their own and therefore cultivating independence and self-determination as a part of childrearing in a way that was not typical of their European forebears. See Fass, *The End of American Childhood*, 9.

50. Elizabeth M. Whelan, *A Baby? Maybe. . . a Guide to Making the Most Fateful Decision of Your Life* (New York: Bobbs-Merrill, 1975).

51. "Republican Party Platform of 1976," American Presidency Project, http://www.presidency.ucsb.edu/ws/?pid=25843.

52. Daniel K. Williams, *God's Own Party: The Making of the Christian Right* (New York: Oxford University Press, 2010), 235–244.

53. Mintz and Kellogg, *Domestic Revolutions*, 233–235.

54. Marshall H. Klaus and John H. Kennell, *Maternal-Infant Bonding: The Impact of Early Separation or Loss on Family Development* (New York: Mosby, 1976).

55. Richard W. Wertz and Dorothy C. Wertz, *Lying-In: A History of Childbirth in America* (New Haven, CT: Yale University Press, 1989), 254–56; John Vitello, "John Kennell, Advocate of Infant Bonding, Dies at 91," *New York Times*, September 22, 2013, https://www.nytimes.com/2013/09/22/health/john-kennell-advocate-of-infant-bonding-dies-at-91.html.

56. This was the approximate ratio I found in examining all popular articles on bonding listed in the readers' guide beginning in the late 1970s.

57. Freidenfelds, ""Cherish Every Moment" of Parenting?".

58. For example, L. Josten, "Prenatal Assessment Guide for Illuminating Possible Problems with Parenting," *American Journal of Maternal-Child Nursing* 6 (March–April 1981). For a review including critical commentary by R. T. Mercer see Mary E. Muller, "Development of the Prenatal Attachment Inventory," *Western Journal of Nursing Research* 15, no. 2 (April 1993).

59. William Sears, *Creative Parenting: How to Use the New Continuum Concept to Raise Children Successfully from Birth Through Adolescence* (New York: Everest House, 1982), 47.

60. Kara Swanson, *Banking on the Body: The Market in Blood, Milk, and Sperm in Modern America* (Cambridge, MA: Harvard University Press, 2014), 200–226; W.W. Watters and J. Sousa-Poza, "Psychiatric Aspects of Artificial Insemination (Donor)," *Canadian Medical Association Journal* 95 (July 16, 1966).

61. "The Babies I Thought I Could Never Have," *Redbook*, May 1969, 20 and 26.

62. Hays, *The Cultural Contradictions of Motherhood*. Intensive parenting was most accessible to middle-class women but not confined to them. See, for example, Sinikka Elliot and colleagues' sociological research on working-class black women: Sinikka Elliott, Rachel Powell, and Joslyn Brenton, "Being a Good Mom: Low-Income, Black Single Mothers Negotiate Intensive Mothering," *Journal of Family Issues* 36, no. 3 (2015).

63. William Sears and Martha Sears, *The Baby Book: Everything You Need to Know About Your Baby from Birth to Age Two* (New York: Little, Brown, 1993).

64. On mid-twentieth-century psychiatrists and attachment theorists' openness to bottle feeding, see Jessica Martucci, *Back to the Breast: Natural Motherhood and Breastfeeding in America* (Chicago: University of Chicago Press, 2015), 34–44. On continuing pressure for intensive mothering in the decades following Hays's

publication, see essays in Linda Rose Ennis, ed. *Intensive Mothering: The Cultural Contradictions of Modern Motherhood* (New York: Demeter Press, 2014).

65. Garey Ramey and Valerie A. Ramey, "The Rug Rat Race" (Washington, DC: Brookings Papers on Economic Activity, 2010).

66. Madeline Walker, "Intensive Mothering, Elimination Communication and the Call to Eden," in *Intensive Mothering: The Cultural Contradictions of Modern Motherhood.*

67. Jennifer Senior, *All Joy and No Fun: The Paradox of Modern Parenthood* (New York: Ecco, 2014).

68. Its appearance cannot be traced directly to the academic social sciences literature on bonding. I examined the first page of Google searches on "bonding during pregnancy" and "prenatal bonding" limited to a single, specific year for a sampling of years between 1990 and 2015. Before 2001, I found few relevant results, and they were links to academic database abstracts. Beginning in 2001, they were increasingly relevant and increasingly non-academic articles located on pregnancy and parenting websites. The first few I found were authored by more marginal writers, advocating ideas about pre-conception spiritual connections to future children. Within a few years, these articles were written by mainstream freelance health writers. They mostly did not cite academic research on the topic, but rather wrote from their own experience or from interviews with mothers. They appeared to be drawing on a common, colloquial language of "bonding," rather than a psychological definition.

69. "Your Pregnancy: 9 Weeks," http://www.babycenter.com/6_your-pregnancy-9-weeks_1098.bc, accessed April 27, 2018: "Activity: Start a daily ritual to connect with your baby. It's not too early to start bonding with your baby! Start by setting aside some time each day to connect with your little one. Just after waking up and/or before going to sleep works well for many expectant moms. During these times, sit quietly and gently rest your hands on your belly. Focus on your breathing and start thinking about your baby (your hopes and dreams, your intentions as a parent, etc.). It's a great way to focus on the miracle unfolding inside you and to plan for the kind of parent you want to be." For a discussion of the challenge of bonding before feeling movement and a long list of ways to bond nevertheless, see Luschka, "Six Ways to Bond with Your Unborn Baby," *Natural Parents Network* (2012), http://naturalparentsnetwork.com/ways-to-bond-unborn-baby/ A commenter points out that it's hard to bond before quickening, and yet there is pressure to do so.

CHAPTER 4

1. Glow Nurture has been used by hundreds of thousands of women: Davey Alba, "Does Glow's App Help Women Conceive? The Data's Tricky," *Wired*, October 28, 2015, https://www.wired.com/2015/10/does-glow-fertility-app-really-help-women-get-pregnant/.

2. Apps for menstrual cycle monitoring and fertility are increasingly popular: Brian Dolan, "Report Finds Pregnancy Apps More Popular Than Fitness Apps," Mobihealthnews, http://www.mobihealthnews.com/20333/report-finds-pregnancy-apps-more-popular-than-fitness-apps; Alba, "Does Glow's App Help Women Conceive? The Data's Tricky," https://www.wired.com/2015/10/does-glow-fertility-app-really-help-women-get-pregnant/.

3. http://community.babycenter.com/post/a53011240/glow_nurture_app accessed June 14, 2016.

4. Katie Dupuis, "Best Pregnancy Apps for First-Time Mamas," *Huffington Post* (2016), https://www.huffingtonpost.ca/2016/06/02/best-pregnancy-apps_n_10263974.html.

5. Lara Freidenfelds, "When More Care Means More Pain: The Development of Early Prenatal Care and Its Impact on Early Pregnancy Loss" (paper presented at the Bates Nursing History Center Seminar, University of Pennsylvania, 2014).

6. Linda K. Kerber, *Women of the Republic: Intellect and Ideology in Revolutionary America* (Chapel Hill: University of North Carolina Press, 1980).

7. Quoted in Cott, *The Bonds of Womanhood*, 99.

8. Mary Fissell, *Vernacular Bodies: The Politics of Reproduction in Early Modern England* (New York: Oxford University Press, 2005), 46–47; Ulrich, *Good Wives*, 129.

9. Nancy Cott, "Passionlessness: An Interpretation of Victorian Sexual Ideology, 1790-1850," *Signs: Journal of Women in Culture and Society* 4, no. 2 (Winter 1978): 227–228.

10. Jan Lewis and Kenneth A. Lockridge, "'Sally Has Been Sick': Pregnancy and Family Limitation among Virginian Gentry Women, 1780-1830," *Journal of Social History* 22, no. 1 (Autumn 1988): 12; Klepp, *Revolutionary Conceptions*, 66.

11. Lewis and Lockridge, "Sally Has Been Sick," 12.

12. Both cited in ibid., 7.

13. Wertz and Wertz, *Lying-In*, 94.

14. Leavitt, *Brought to Bed*, 36–63; Loudon, "Maternal Mortality in the Past and Its Relevance to Developing Countries Today".

15. Jacqueline Wolf, *Deliver Me from Pain: Anesthesia and Birth in America* (Baltimore: Johns Hopkins University Press, 2009), 13–43.

16. Wertz and Wertz, *Lying-In*, 77–94.

17. Ulrich, *Good Wives*, 135.

18. Leavitt, *Brought to Bed*, 175–176.

19. Wertz and Wertz, *Lying-In*, 102–103.

20. Ibid., 79–80; Sylvia Hoffert, *Private Matters*, 30–31. According to Hoffert, in 1860, women were just beginning to consider removing themselves from society, and it was after this that "confinement" began to mean the months before birth as well as after. She says it was the result of pressure for women to prioritize motherhood and doctors telling women that they were delicate.

21. Arlene Eisenberg, Heidi Eisenberg Murkoff, and Sandee Eisenberg Hathaway, *What to Expect When You're Expecting* (New York: Workman, 1984). The book has been issued in several more best-selling editions and remains in print.

22. Emma F. Angell Drake, *What a Young Wife Ought to Know* (Philadelphia: Vir, 1902), 125.

23. Elisabeth Robinson Scovil, *Preparation for Motherhood* (Philadelphia: Henry Altemus, 1896), 20.

24. Leslie J. Reagan, *When Abortion Was a Crime: Women, Medicine, and Law in the United States, 1867-1973* (Berkeley: University of California Press, 1997), 57–58. Women doctors continued to fight this assumption in the twentieth century, for example as documented in Edith Eugenie Johnson, *Leaves from a Doctor's Diary* (Palo Alto, CA: Pacific Books, 1954).

25. For example, Alice B. Stockham, *Tokology, a Book for Every Woman*, 29th ed. (Chicago: Sanitary Publishing, 1885), 249–250.

26. Withycombe, *Lost*, 16–30, 82–88.

27. Sara Dubow, *Ourselves Unborn: A History of the Fetus in Modern America* (New York: Oxford University Press, 2010), 25–27; Withycombe, *Lost*, 72–82.

28. Withycombe, *Lost*, 125–161. See also Sanger, *About Abortion*, 76–81.

29. Shannon Withycombe, "Changing Bodies, Changing Behaviors: The Development of Prenatal Care in the U.S.," presented at *History of Women's Health Conference* (Philadelphia 2013); Withycombe, "Unusual Frontal Developments," 173–174; Thomas L. Nichols, *Esoteric Anthropology* (Malvern, UK: T. L. Nichols, 1873), 128; Seth Pancoast and William Wesley Cook, *Pancoast's Tokology and Ladies' Medical Guide: A Complete Instructor in All the Delicate and Wonderful Matters Pertaining to Women* (Chicago: Stanton and Van Vliet, 1903), 257–264; Stockham, *Tokology*, 34.

30. Wertz and Wertz, *Lying-In*; Ziv Eisenberg, "The Whole Nine Months: Women, Men, and the Making of Modern Pregnancy in America" (PhD diss., Yale University, 2013), 57–59, 221; Plant, *Mom*, 118–127; Molly Ladd-Taylor, *Raising a Baby the Government Way: Mothers' Letters to the Children's Bureau, 1915-1932* (New Brunswick, NJ: Rutgers University Press, 1986), 151; Golden, *Babies Made Us Modern*, 18–19.

31. See, for example, the disapproving account of one obstetrician who thought that prenatal care would "relieve many mothers of that mental depression fostered by depressing tales of sorrow and suffering that is frequently told her by gossiping friends." Armstrong Taylor, "Influence of Medical Work in Obstetrics," *California and Western Medicine* 22, no. 9 (September 1924): 442.

32. Mrs. Max West, *Prenatal Care* (Washington, DC: Government Printing Office, 1913), 21.

33. Lydia Pinkham, "Help for Mothers," (Lynn, MA: Lydia E. Pinkham Medicine Company, 1920), 31.

34. Carolyn Conant Van Blarcom, *Getting Ready to Be a Mother: A Little Book of Information and Advice for the Young Woman Who Is Looking Forward to Motherhood* (New York: Macmillan, 1922); Carolyn Conant Van Blarcom, *Obstetric Nursing: A Text-Book on the Nursing Care of the Expectant Mother, the Woman in Labor, the Young Mother and Her Baby* (New York: Macmillan, 1922).

35. Freidenfelds, *The Modern Period*, 46–48.

36. Van Blarcom, *Getting Ready to Be a Mother*, 1.

37. Ibid., 1–2.

38. Ibid., 3. On being modern and "in the know," see Freidenfelds, *Modern Period*; Eisenberg, "Whole Nine Months."

39. Van Blarcom, *Getting Ready to Be a Mother*, 6.

40. Emily K. Abel, *The Inevitable Hour: A History of Caring for Dying Patients in America* (Baltimore: Johns Hopkins University Press, 2013), 54–56.

41. Harold J. Levis, "Salvarsan in Pregnancy," *Journal of the American Medical Association* 59, no. 8 (August 24, 1912).

42. Allan M. Brandt, *No Magic Bullet: A Social History of Venereal Disease in the United States since 1880* (New York: Oxford University Press, 1987), 149–150.

43. Van Blarcom, *Getting Ready to Be a Mother*, 76.

44. Wilcox, *Fertility and Pregnancy*, 264–265.

45. Van Blarcom, *Getting Ready to Be a Mother*, 47.

46. Ibid., 77.

47. *Obstetric Nursing*, 167.

48. Nicholson J. Eastman and Keith P. Russell, *Expectant Motherhood*, 5th ed. (Boston: Little, Brown, 1970), 114–115.

49. Leon Wilson, "Prenatal Care," *Journal of the National Medical Association* 20, no. 4 (1927): 181; also see Boston example in Eisenberg, "Whole Nine Months," 64, 82–83.

50. Loudon, "Maternal Mortality," 242S.

51. Ibid.

52. Klein, *A Population History of the United States*, 145–148. As historian Richard Meckel describes, the decline in infant mortality had many causes: in the late nineteenth century and early twentieth, it was most affected by declining fertility, a rising standard of living, and urban sanitary reforms and environmental improvements, including cleaning up the milk supply. Hygiene education efforts contributed too. After 1930 improved medical care substantially contributed as well (Richard A. Meckel, *Save the Babies: American Public Health Reform and the Prevention of Infant Mortality, 1850-1929* (Rochester, NY: University of Rochester Press, 1990), 6. Van Blarcom and others extrapolated these efforts and expected results to prenatal care.

53. Eisenberg, "Whole Nine Months," 8 and 50.

54. J. R. Torbert, "The Prenatal Care of Obstetric Cases," *The Canadian Medical Association Journal* (December 1914): 1087; Taylor, "Influence of Medical Work in Obstetrics."

55. Wilson, "Prenatal Care," 182.

56. William E. Hunter, "Prenatal Care," *California and Western Medicine* 26, no. 1 (January 1927): 46.

57. Ladd-Taylor, *Raising a Baby the Government Way*, 53; Adele Clarke, *Disciplining Reproduction: Modernity, American Life Sciences, and "the Problems of Sex"* (Berkeley: University of California Press, 1998), 45–46.

58. Freidenfelds, *Modern Period*, 123–127.

59. Eisenberg, "Whole Nine Months," 85–92.

60. Wendy Kline, *Building a Better Race: Gender, Sexuality, and Eugenics from the Turn of the Century to the Baby Boom* (Berkeley: University of California Press, 2001), 7–31.

61. Eisenberg, "Whole Nine Months," 24–31; Layne, *Motherhood Lost,* 67–74.

62. Van Blarcom, *Getting Ready to Be a Mother*, xi–xii.

63. See example in Eisenberg, "Whole Nine Months," 126–127.

64. Jean Aaberg, *ABCs for Mothers-to-Be* (Philadelphia: David McKay, 1944), 13.

65. Freidenfelds, *Modern Period*, 39.

66. Aaberg, *ABCs for Mothers-to-Be*, 13.

67. Anonymous, *Home Book of Health and Medicine* (Philadelphia: Key & Biddle, 1835), 84; on insect metaphors in nineteenth-century pregnancy advice literature, Withycombe, "Changing Bodies, Changing Behaviors".

68. For example, Edith Belle Lowry, *Herself: Talks with Women Concerning Themselves* (Chicago: Forbes & Company, 1911, reprinted 1920), 82; Nick Hopwood, "A Marble Embryo: Meanings of a Portrait from 1900," *History Workshop Journal* 73 (April 2012): 8.

69. Van Blarcom, *Getting Ready to Be a Mother*, 37, 39.

70. Anne A. Stevens and Margaret Ayer, *Maternity Handbook for Pregnant Mothers and Expectant Fathers* (New York G. P. Putnam's Sons, 1932), 25.

71. Rose Holz, "The Dickinson-Belskie Birth Series Sculptures: The Rise of Modern Visions of Pregnancy, the Roots of Modern Pro-Life Imagery, and Dr. Dickinson's Religious Case for Abortion," *Journal of Social History* 51, no. 4 (Summer 2018).

72. Ibid., 11–12.

73. Ibid., 13–14; Maternity Center Association, *A Baby Is Born: The Picture Story of a Baby from Conception through Birth* (New York: Grosset & Dunlap, 1957), 63 (republished in ten editions through 1977).

74. "Fetus, 18 Weeks," Time 100 Photos, http://100photos.time.com/photos/lennart-nilsson-fetus.

75. Solveig Julich, "The Making of a Best-Selling Book on Reproduction: Lennart Nillson's *a Child Is Born*," *Bulletin of the History of Medicine* 89, no. 3 (Fall 2015): 505–10; Barbara Duden, *Disembodying Women: Perspectives on Pregnancy and the Unborn* (Cambridge, MA: Harvard University Press, 1993), 11–24; Tatjana Buklijas and Nick Hopwood, "Making Visible Embryos," University of Cambridge, http://www.hps.cam.ac.uk/visibleembryos/ (http://www.sites.hps.cam.ac.uk/visibleembryos/s7_4.html#mydiv2). Nilsson continued to photograph embryos and fetuses and was increasingly able to do so in vivo: Nova Online, "Behind the Lens: An Interview with Lennart Nilsson," Thirteen, 1996, https://www.pbs.org/wgbh/nova/odyssey/nilsson.html.

76. "A Child Is Born: Photographs of the Foetus Developing in the Womb, by Lennart Nilsson," *The Telegraph*, http://www.telegraph.co.uk/news/health/pictures/6255474/A-Child-is-Born-Photographs-of-the-foetus-developing-in-the-womb-by-Lennart-Nilsson.html.

77. Anthropologist Emily Martin analyzed scientists' analogies in her much-reprinted paper, Emily Martin, "The Egg and the Sperm: How Science Has Constructed a Romance Based on Stereotypical Male-Female Roles," *Signs: Journal of Women in Culture and Society* 16, no. 3 (Spring 1991).

78. Nicholson J. Eastman, *Expectant Motherhood*, 1st ed. (Boston: Little, Brown, 1940), 25.

79. Ibid., 27–28.

80. This narrative is consistent in all editions of Eastman through the 1970s. For another dramatic tale of conception, with a similar shift in the drama starting at the moment of conception, see Niels H. Lauersen, *It's Your Pregnancy: An Obstetrician Answers Your Most Intimate Questions About Pregnancy and Childbirth* (New York: Simon & Schuster, 1987), 15–16.

81. Loudon, "Maternal Mortality," 243S.

82. Eisenberg, "Whole Nine Months," 225–237.

83. Leslie J. Reagan, *Dangerous Pregnancies: Mothers, Disabilities, and Abortion in Modern America* (Berkeley: University of California Press, 2010), 1.

84. Ibid., 55.

85. Ibid., 55–63.

86. Freidenfelds, "The History of Women in Biomedical Research"; Janet Golden, *Message in a Bottle: The Making of Fetal Alcohol Syndrome* (Cambridge, MA: Harvard University Press, 2006), 36-41; Randi Hutter Epstein, *Get Me Out: A History of Childbirth from the Garden of Eden to the Sperm Bank* (New York: W.W. Norton, 2010), 145-146.

87. Golden, *Message in a Bottle*, 96–97.

88. Victor Cohn, "FDA to Warn on Caffeine in Pregnancy," *The Washington Post*, September 4, 1980, https://www.washingtonpost.com/archive/politics/1980/09/04/fda-to-warn-on-caffeine-in-pregnancy/6d23546d-1fcc-46a6-83ab-bfc7f763a0ee/?utm_term=.687968dfb8ee.

89. This continues: Linsey Lanquist, "People Were Not Happy About Pink's Decision to Drink Coffee While Pregnant," *Self*, December 19, 2016, https://www.self.com/story/coffee-pregnancy.

90. Salim Al-Gailani, "Making Birth Defects 'Preventable': Pre-Conceptional Vitamin Supplements and the Politics of Risk Reduction," *Studies in History and Philosophy of Biological and Biomedical Sciences* 47 (September 2014): 286.

91. March of Dimes Archives, Medical Program Box 11 Series 13, Healthy Baby Week Radio Announcements.

92. Al-Gailani, "Making Birth Defects 'Preventable';" March of Dimes Archives, Senior VP for Education and Health Promotion Records Box 2 Series 1, Folic Acid Campaign Report 1999–2001.

93. Golden, *Message in a Bottle*, 66.

94. Eisenberg, Eisenberg Murkoff, and Eisenberg Hathaway, *What to Expect When You're Expecting*, 75–76.

95. Sue Mittenthal, "Viewpoint," *Glamour*, August 1984.

96. March of Dimes Archives, Senior VP for Education and Health Promotion Records Box 2 Series 1, Brand Identity Development report, 1997.

97. Babycenter was founded in 1997; Whattoexpect.com in 2005.

98. For example, Theodore R. Seidman, *Becoming a Mother*, 2nd ed. (Greenwich, CT: Fawcett Publications, 1963), 92, 1st edition 1956.

99. Jennifer Elias, "In 2016, Users Will Trust Health Apps More Than Their Doctors," *Forbes*, December 31, 2015, https://www.forbes.com/sites/jenniferelias/2015/12/31/in-2016-users-will-trust-health-apps-more-than-their-doctors/#6228e3ee7eb6. Nearly all women of childbearing age own smartphones: "Mobile Fact Sheet" (Pew Research Center, 2018).

100. Glow Nurture's umbrella company claimed four million users as of 2016: Jerry Beilinson, "Glow Pregnancy App Exposed Women to Privacy Threats, Consumer Reports Finds," *Consumer Reports*, July 28, 2016, https://www.consumerreports.org/mobile-security-software/glow-pregnancy-app-exposed-women-to-privacy-threats/. It is difficult to discern precise demographic details from Nurture's public logs, but they show evidence of ethnically and regionally diverse users, based on photos and descriptions. For example, Norelle, an African American woman, issued a "roll call!!!" "Where is everybody from? I'm from the Chicago area." Answers included: Washington, DC; Chicago; "A small town in Minnesota"; Southern Oregon; Chicago/Colorado; Southern California; Missouri, Victoria/WA Australia; "Cali!," Germany/expat from Oregon; Oakland, Iowa, Calfornia, Nebraska, Phoenix, DFW Texas, Rhode Island, Providence, Chicago area, Texas, Michigan, Georgia (and a "me too"), Lake Arrowhead, California, Hawaii, Central Oregon, North Carolina, Queensland Australia, Georgia, Colorado, Minnesota, Oklahoma, New York, Rhode Island.

101. I signed up as "Laura F." and logged responses through week nine of a simulated pregnancy. I modeled my logs on my first pregnancy (which miscarried), as best as I could recall, with a few deviations to be able to see how Nurture would respond to a variety of logged behaviors.

102. https://community.babycenter.com/post/a55329619/lol_the_glow_nurture_app_is_so_creepy accessed 12-06-17.

103. While Nurture has not publicly described its business model, Nurture's privacy policy is consistent with an intention to serve ads. Like other apps, its data-collection procedures have sparked privacy concerns (Natasha Felizi and Joana Varon, "Menstruapps—How to Turn Your Period into Money (for Others)," *Coding Rights*, https://chupadados.codingrights.org/en/menstruapps-como-transformar-sua-menstruacao-em-dinheiro-para-os-outros/).

CHAPTER 5

1. An identity I created for research purposes.

2. November 16, 2012 email from babycenter.com to lararesearch@gmail.com. Author's collection. BabyCenter's 2014 media kit claimed the website reaches

fifteen million American moms. http://www.babycentersolutions.com/docs/2014_BabyCenter_Media_Kit.pdf.

3. One example of the appearance of advertisers' influence on content: babycenter. com's content on cord blood banking reflects a major sponsor's promotional literature rather than the American Academy of Pediatrics' statement on cord blood banking, which definitively recommends against commercial, private banking.

4. Heidi Murkoff and Sharon Mazel, *What to Expect When You're Expecting* (New York: Workman Publishing Company, 2008).

5. http://www.babycentersolutions.com/marketing-solutions.html, accessed January 9, 2014.

6. babycenter, "Your Pregnancy: 5 Weeks," babycenter, https://www.babycenter. com/6_your-pregnancy-5-weeks_1094.bc.

7. "The Ultimate Pregnancy to-Do List: First Trimester" (2014), http://www. babycenter.com/0_the-ultimate-pregnancy-to-do-list-first-trimester_10341205. bc.

8. Lara Freidenfelds, "Buying for the Baby Too Soon? Marketing to Pregnant Women and Its Implications for Early Pregnancy Loss" (paper presented at the Hagley Museum Research Seminar, 2014). Historians have analyzed the development of children's role as consumers in the development of consumer culture much more deeply than they have attended to parents' role. The most relevant work on the history of parents in consumer culture includes Gary Cross's work, especially Gary S. Cross, *The Cute and the Cool: Wondrous Innocence and Modern American Children's Culture* (New York: Oxford University Press, 2004); Cheryl Lemus, "Save Your Baby, Save Ten Percent: National Baby Week, the Infants' Department, and the Modern Pregnant Woman, 1905-1925," *Journal of Women's History* 25, no. 3 (Fall 2013); Daniel Thomas Cook, *The Commodification of Childhood: The Children's Clothing Industry and the Rise of the Child Consumer* (Durham, NC: Duke University Press, 2004); Amy Bentley, *Inventing Baby Food: Taste, Health and the Industrialization of the American Diet* (Berkeley: University of California Press, 2014); Golden, *Babies Made Us Modern*; and Zelizer, *Pricing the Priceless Child*.

9. Phyllis Putnam, "Child-Bed Linen," Colonial Williamsburg Foundation, http://www.history.org/history/clothing/children/childbed.cfm. On the lack of specialized maternity clothes, Scholten, *Childbearing in American Society: 1650-1850*, 15.

10. Mark Jackson, "'Something More Than Blood': Conflicting Accounts of Pregnancy Loss in Eighteenth-Century England," in *The Anthropology of Pregnancy Loss: Comparative Studies in Miscarriage, Stillbirth and Neonatal Death*, ed. Rosanne Cecil (Oxford: Berg, 1996).

11. Betty Rollin, *Mothers Are Funnier Than Children* (New York: Doubleday, 1964).

12. Linda Baumgarten, *What Clothes Reveal: The Language of Clothing in Colonial and Federal America* (Williamsburg, VA: Colonial Williamsburg Foundation, 2002); Kevin M. Sweeney, "Furniture and the Domestic Environment in Wethersfield, Connecticut, 1639-1800," in *Material Life in America 1600-1860*, ed. Robert Blair St. George (Boston: Northeastern University Press, 1988); Richard Lyman Bushman, *The Refinement of America: Persons, Houses, Cities* (New York: Knopf, 1992); Mintz, *Huck's Raft*, 59.

13. Golden, *Babies Made Us Modern*, 74–75, 81–83.

14. Cross, *Cute and the Cool*, 70; T. J. Jackson Lears, *Fables of Abundance: A Cultural History of Advertising in America* (New York: Basic Books, 1994); Richard Tedlow, *New and Improved: The Story of Mass Marketing in America* (New York: Basic Books, 1990).

15. "Pushing the Sale of Infants' Wear," *New York Times*, July 3, 1921, cited in Lemus, "Save Your Baby, Save Ten Percent."
16. Ibid.
17. Sears, Roebuck and Company, *Catalog* (Chicago, IL, 1897), Hagley Museum & Library, Wilmington, DE, 19807.
18. Sears, Roebuck and Company, *The Baby Book* (Chicago, IL, 1907), ID #08078751, Hagley Museum & Library, Wilmington, DE, 19807.
19. *Woman's Home Companion* v. 37 (September 1910), 88.
20. Ibid.
21. *Printer's Ink* (November 7, 1912), 119.
22. Sears, Roebuck and Company, *The Baby Book* (Chicago, IL, 1907), 16, ID #08078751, Hagley Museum & Library, Wilmington, DE 19807.
23. Ibid., 18. Further, "These outfits are carefully selected in our Baby Department by women who are thoroughly versed in the proper clothing of the infant."
24. Sears, Roebuck and Company, *Catalog* (Chicago, IL, 1940), 253, Hagley Museum & Library, Wilmington, DE, 19807.
25. Sears, Roebuck and Company, *Catalog* (Chicago, IL, 1925), 156, 568, ID #08175781, Hagley Museum & Library, Wilmington, DE, 19807.
26. "Affairs of the Past Week in Local Society," *Los Angeles Times*, October 13, 1912, p. III3.
27. Marion Harland, "Marion Harland's Helping Hand: Colors for Babies," *Chicago Daily Tribune*, July 20, 1915, p. 14.
28. "Kirkwood Pre-School Age Circle Meets," *The Atlanta Constitution*, November 29, 1925, p. F4.
29. Advertising for baby goods increased during the baby boom, and so did lists of gifts parents recorded in baby books. Marketers worked with hospitals to send parents home with gift packages by the mid-1950s. Golden, *Babies Made Us Modern*, 186–187.
30. Ernest Dichter, *A Motivational Pilot Study of the Advertising and Product Factors Involved in the Sale of the Playtex Nurser* (Croton-on-Hudson, NY: Institute for Motivational Research, 1963), box 73 folder 1599D, Ernest Dichter papers (2407A), Hagley Museum & Library, Wilmington, DE, 19807.
31. Ernest Dichter, *A Motivational Research Study of the Sales and Advertising Problems of Clapp's Baby Foods* (Croton-on-Hudson, NY: Institute for Motivational Research, 1962), p. 2–3, box 68 folder 1484C, Ernest Dichter papers (2407A), Hagley Museum & Library, Wilmington, DE, 19807.
32. Dichter, *Playtex Nurser*, x.
33. Ibid., 84, 85, xxi.
34. Ibid., xvi, 40.
35. http://www.playtexbaby.com/Bottles/Dropins/Premium-Nurser, accessed January 26, 2014.
36. "American Baby," Echo Media, http://echo-media.com/medias/details/5117/american+baby+magazine; "Babytalk (Magazine)," in *Wikipedia* (2017). *American Baby* continues to be published; *Baby Talk* closed in 2013.
37. Greenwich Research Associates, *A Study of the Consumer Market for Infant Toys* (New York: American Baby, 1973), 3. Doing this kind of market research was not cheap, and at the time the results were almost certainly considered proprietary and kept private. Once they were out of date and useless as market data, these types of studies were generally thrown in the trash. This study found its way to the New York Public Library archives.

38. Erik Larson, *The Naked Consumer: How Our Private Lives Become Public Commodities* (New York: Henry Holt, 1992), 86–87.

39. *Your New Home: Plan Today for Tomorrow* (New York: The Parents' Institute, 1945), ID # 08142628, Hagley Museum & Library, Wilmington, DE, 19807.

40. Charles Duhigg, *The Power of Habit: Why We Do What We Do in Life and Business* (New York: Random House, 2012), 191–193.

41. Larson, *The Naked Consumer*, 86–87.

42. Other websites that solicit this information connected to their due date calculators include whattoexpect.com and webmd.com.

43. "Little Miracles Prenatal Mailing List," Mailing List Finder, https://lists.nextmark.com/market;jsessionid=E4B080570827B6C8F8B935C3D9FC0198?page=order/online/datacard&id=200311.

44. Duhigg, *The Power of Habit*, 192–197.

45. Cotton Delo, "Does Facebook Know You're Pregnant?", *Ad Age Digital*, September 10, 2012, https://adage.com/article/digital/facebook-pregnant/237073.

46. As of December 21, 2008, per comment date.

47. http://community.babycenter.com/post/a3508425/getting_baby_mail_still, accessed January 7, 2013.

CHAPTER 6

1. J. J. Keith, "My Miscarriages Made Me Question Being Pro-Choice," *Salon*, May 20, 2013, http://www.salon.com/2013/05/21/my_miscarriages_made_me_question_being_pro_choice/.

2. Lara Freidenfelds, "Without Choice or Life: The Impact of the Abortion Debates on Experiences of Early Pregnancy Loss since *Roe V. Wade*" (paper presented at the History of Science and Medicine Colloquia, Yale University, 2013).

3. Mohr, *Abortion in America*.

4. Ibid., 229.

5. Reagan, *When Abortion Was a Crime*, 19–22.

6. http://www.childbirthconnection.org/about/history/, accessed April 23, 2019.

7. In "Report of The First Year of Life. An Exhibit at the New York World's Fair. 1940," folder 7, box 39, Maternity Center Association Records, Archives & Special Collections, Health Sciences Library, Columbia University, New York City, NY.

8. Reagan, *When Abortion Was a Crime*, 160–181.

9. Ibid., 218–222.

10. Jeanie Kasindorf, "Abortion in New York," *New York*, September 18, 1989, 36.

11. Sarah Leavitt, "A Thin Blue Line: The History of the Pregnancy Test Kit," Stetten Museum, Office of NIH History, http://history.nih.gov/exhibits/thinblueline/index.html.

12. Katha Pollitt, "Children of Choice," *New York Times*, November 20, 1988, 28.

13. Medical abortion, which produces a miscarriage-like experience, has steadily increased in use since its introduction in the United States in 2000, and now accounts for almost a quarter of early abortions. It is also used to manage incomplete miscarriages detected via ultrasound. This may reduce this particular distinction between miscarriage and abortion. Tara C. Jatlaoui, et al., "Abortion Surveillance — United States, 2014," *Morbidity and Mortality Weekly Report* 66, no. 24 (2017).

14. Ibid.

15. For example, Susan Neiburg Terkel, *Abortion: Facing the Issues* (New York: Watts, 1988); Bonnie Szumski, *Abortion, Opposing Viewpoints* (St. Paul, MN: Greenhaven Press, 1986).

16. Cheryl McCall, "Denise's Decision," *Life*, March 1986, 74.
17. "The Fanatical Abortion Fight," *Time Magazine*, July 9, 1979, http://content.time.com/time/magazine/article/0,9171,920454,00.html.
18. "Choose Life License Plates," in *Wikipedia* (2017).
19. Storer, *Why Not?*, 28 and 31.
20. Jennifer L. Holland, "Abolishing Abortion: The History of the Pro-Life Movement in America," *The American Historian*, November (2016), http://tah.oah.org/november-2016/abolishing-abortion-the-history-of-the-pro-life-movement-in-america/.
21. For example http://www.heritagehouse76.com/default.aspx?GroupID=141 (accessed March 27, 2013). Celeste Condit, *Decoding Abortion Rhetoric: Communicating Social Change* (Chicago: University of Illinois Press, 1990), 88–89.
22. For example, http://www.labelledame.com/miscarriagejewelry/eternitycirclemiscarriagenecklace (accessed March 27, 2013); Reagan, "From Hazard to Blessing to Tragedy".
23. For example, Layne, "Designing a Woman-Centered Health Care Approach to Pregnancy Loss: Lessons from Feminist Models of Childbirth".
24. Ann Friedman, "What Should We Say Instead of 'Pro-Choice'?," *The Cut* (January 22, 2013), https://www.thecut.com/2013/01/what-should-we-say-instead-of-pro-choice.html.
25. Cristina Stanojevich, "Overlapping 'Pro-Choice' and 'Pro-Life' Identities," *Public Religion Research Institute* (January 28, 2013), https://www.prri.org/spotlight/graphic-of-the-week-overlapping-pro-choice-and-pro-life-identities/.
26. Jon A. Shields, "Almost Human: Ambivalence in the Pro-Choice and Pro-Life Movements," *Critical Review* 23, no. 4 (2011); Daniel K. Williams, "No Happy Medium: The Role of Americans' Ambivalent View of Fetal Rights in Political Conflict over Abortion Legalization," *Journal of Policy History* 25, no. 1 (January 2013).

CHAPTER 7

1. Sammie Mendez, "2 You Say?!?!?!," *thechroniclesofanonbellymama: Thoughts From The Other "Real" Mom* (June 15, 2014), https://thechroniclesofanonbellymama.wordpress.com/2014/06/15/2-you-say/.
2. Emily Malone, "The 20-Week Ultrasound," *Daily Garnish*, May 27, 2011, http://www.dailygarnish.com/2011/05/the-20-week-ultrasound.html.
3. Lara Freidenfelds, "New Losses: The Emergence of Very Early Miscarriage in the Twentieth Century" (paper presented at the Berkshires Conference on the History of Women, 2008).
4. Joseph Woo, "A Short History of the Development of Ultrasound in Obstetrics and Gynecology," http://www.ob-ultrasound.net/history1.html; H. P. Robinson, "Detection of Fetal Heart Movement in First Trimester of Pregnancy Using Pulsed Ultrasound," *British Medical Journal* 4, no. 838 (November 25, 1972); "Sonar Measurement of Fetal Crown-Rump Length as Means of Assessing Maturity in First Trimester of Pregnancy," *British Medical Journal* 4, no. 5883 (October 6, 1973); H. P. Robinson and J. E. Fleming, "A Critical Evaluation of Sonar 'Crown-Rump Length' Measurements," *British Journal of Obstetrics and Gynaecology* 82, no. 9 (September 1975).
5. Janelle S. Taylor, *The Public Life of the Fetal Sonogram: Technology, Consumption, and the Politics of Reproduction* (New Brunswick, NJ: Rutgers University Press, 2008), 177 n.2.

In Europe, in 1980 Germany led the way in guaranteeing women access to two routine scans; by 1996, scholars had documented the routinization of scanning in the United Kingdom, Iceland, Norway, Canada, and Greece. Gillian Harris et al., "'Seeing the Baby': Pleasures and Dilemmas of Ultrasound Technologies for Primiparous Australian Women," *Medical Anthropology Quarterly* 18, no. 1 (March 2004): 25. Doppler exams, in which the device produces an auditory representation of the fetal heartbeat, have become ubiquitous as well. Unlike ultrasound, they can be done by medical personnel without extensive specialized training and without expensive equipment.

6. Eugenia Georges, *Bodies of Knowledge: The Medicalization of Reproduction in Greece* (Nashville: Vanderbilt University Press, 2008); Tsipy Ivry, *Embodying Culture: Pregnancy in Japan and Israel* (New Brunswick, NJ: Rutgers University Press, 2009), 37–64, 216–222.

7. Taylor, *Public Life of the Fetal Sonogram*; Lisa M. Mitchell, *Baby's First Picture: Ultrasound and the Politics of Fetal Subjects* (Toronto, ON: University of Toronto Press, 2001). See Sanger, *About Abortion*, 131 for how mandatory pre-abortion ultrasounds "are meant to create a visual construction of loss for women awaiting an abortion." Also 120–122 on the ultrasound ritual.

8. Duden, *Disembodying Women*, 30–33.

9. Taylor, *Public Life of the Fetal Sonogram*, 1–5, 42–44, 107–111.

10. Ibid., 136–37.; Mitchell, *Baby's First Picture*, 1, 5, 139, 48–49.

11. http://209.157.64.200/focus/f-news/1406153/posts?q=1&&page=1, accessed May 20, 2015. Thank you to Gayle Kirshenbaum for sharing her archived copies of these posts.

12. Ryan Murphy, "Throwdown (Season 1, Episode 7)," in *Glee* (2009).

13. Gayle Kirshenbaum, "Caught in the Act of Becoming: 'Baby's First Picture' Is Now in Utero, but What If You Don't Feel Like a Mom?," *Newsweek*, May 23, 2005.

14. "FreeRepublic,"http://209.157.64.200/focus/f-news/1406153/posts?q=1&&page=1, accessed May 20, 2015.

15. Albert Mohler, "The Ultrasound and the Fetus–a Scary Article in *Newsweek*," May 17, 2005, https://albertmohler.com/2005/05/17/the-ultrasound-and-the-fetus-a-scary-article-in-newsweek/.

16. This is the scan Kirshenbaum describes. The purpose of this exam is to conduct a nuchal translucency screening, an ultrasound measurement that can detect the possibility of Down syndrome. We might expect this to be an uneasy translation, since this earlier test is much more clearly for the purpose of detecting a problem that would likely prompt a therapeutic abortion. However, I have found only occasional evidence of resistance to this translation from pregnant women or their health care providers.

17. H. P. Robinson, "The Diagnosis of Early Pregnancy Failure by Sonar," *British Journal of Obstetrics and Gynaecology* 82, no. 11 (November 1975).

18. Christine Morton, personal communication, e-mail January 31, 2010.

19. http://www.youtube.com/watch?v=7J8ys7WgC_A&NR=1, accessed November 9, 2009.

20. Layne, *Motherhood Lost*, 87–93.

21. http://www.youtube.com/watch?v=HNE5e5buP2I&NR=1, accessed November 9, 2009.

22. http://www.youtube.com/watch?v=XFVsX6y2OZE&NR=1, accessed November 9, 2009.

23. Here I use the term "bonding" as my sources use it, not in a technical sense as it may be used in psychology research.

24. Mitchell, *Baby's First Picture*, 132–133.
25. A Doppler exam, in which a transducer is used to detect a fetal heartbeat and project an auditory representation of it, can have a similar effect, at ten to twelve weeks' gestation. The obstetrician or midwife might suggest "listening to the baby," rather than looking at it, but it is also a test that is understood to be for both monitoring the health of the pregnancy and "showing the baby." It is somewhat less technologically spectacular and does not engage the sense of sight, which some scholars have suggested is an important part of the impact of ultrasound. But it nonetheless sits at the center of an important and emotional ritual that, like ultrasound, women often experience as making the pregnancy "real," or showing that "there really is a baby in there." Doppler monitors are so inexpensive and easy to use that they are now marketed as rentals for home use, though there are serious questions about the safety of frequent use, especially during the first trimester. (http://www.pregnancy. org/article/fetal-doppler-rental, accessed November 9, 2009.)
26. Even when a woman has been diagnosed with repeated pregnancy loss, the chances of the pregnancy going to term are still 82 percent, according to this small (three hundred women with repeated pregnancy loss and three hundred matching women without repeated pregnancy loss) prospective study. J. S. Hyer, S. Fong, and W. H. Kutteh, "Predictive Value of the Presence of an Embryonic Heartbeat for Live Birth: Comparison of Women with and without Recurrent Pregnancy Loss," *Fertility and Sterility* 82, no. 5 (November 2004).
27. J. West, "Mail Call: Understanding Motherhood," *Newsweek* (June 6, 2005).
28. See also Leslie Reagan's story, which opens her article: Reagan, "From Hazard to Blessing to Tragedy".
29. Half of first-trimester miscarriages are anembryonic pregnancies (blighted ovum): "Blighted Ovum," WebMD, https://www.webmd.com/baby/blighted-ovum#1.

CHAPTER 8

1. Lorie Parch, "Pregnancy Testing: 1000 Women's Trials and Triumphs," BabyCenter. com, http://www.babycenter.com/0_pregnancy-testing-1-000-womens-trials-and-triumphs_10315799.bc.
2. See Jesse Olszynko-Gryn, "Pregnancy Testing in Britain, C.1900-1967: Laboratories, Animals, and Demand from Doctors, Patients, and Consumers" (PhD diss., University of Cambridge, 2014), 23, for an example of a doctor's statement on the embarrassment of misdiagnosing pregnancy.
3. Duden, *The Woman Beneath the Skin*.
4. Charles D. Meigs, *Obstetrics: The Science and the Art*. 3rd ed. (Philadelphia: Blanchard and Lea, 1856), 280.
5. Ibid.
6. Ibid., 280–281.
7. Ibid., 281.
8. American doctor James Read Chadwick had not actually described the phenomenon from his own research, but it was named for him after he read a paper to the American Gynecological Society in 1886 calling attention to French physician Étienne Joseph Jacquemin's earlier observations. James E. Gleichert, "Etienne Joseph Jacquemin, Discoverer of 'Chadwick's Sign'," *Journal of the History of Medicine and Allied Sciences* 26, no. 1 (January 1971): 75.
9. These pregnancy signs remain standard today: https://learningext.com/students/student_resources/f/22/t/2677.

10. Van Blarcom, *Getting Ready to Be a Mother,* 11–12.
11. Gladys Denny Shultz, *Better Homes & Gardens' Baby Book* (Des Moines: Meredith, 1943), 18.
12. Deborah Brunton, "The Rise of Laboratory Medicine," in *Medicine Transformed: Health, Disease and Society in Europe 1800-1930,* ed. Deborah Brunton (Manchester, UK: Manchester University Press, 2004).
13. Olszynko-Gryn, "Pregnancy Testing in Britain," 37.
14. Nelly Oudshoorn, *Beyond the Natural Body: An Archaeology of Sex Hormones* (New York: Routledge, 1994), 15–16.
15. Olszynko-Gryn, "Pregnancy Testing in Britain," 51–52; Sarah Leavitt, "'A Private Little Revolution': The Home Pregnancy Test in American Culture," *Bulletin of the History of Medicine* 80, no. 2 (Summer 2006): 322.
16. "Prenatal Care," ed., United States Department of Labor Children's Bureau (Washington, DC: United States Government Printing Office, 1930), 3–4.
17. Aaberg, *ABCs for Mothers-to-Be,* 24–25.
18. Eastman, *Expectant Motherhood,* 1st ed. (Boston: Little, Brown, 1940), 15–16. These recommendations remained consistent in the fourth edition, 1964 (p. 16). The fifth edition (1970) contained minor editing in the form of a paragraph acknowledging accurate immunological test at seven weeks' gestation, and yet maintained the assertions that a doctor cannot really tell and that a woman should remain patient (pp. 15–16).
19. "Prenatal Care," ed. Social Security Administration Children's Bureau (Washington, DC: US Government Printing Office, 1949), 5. See also example in Leavitt, "Private Little Revolution," 326.
20. "A Thin Blue Line: The History of the Pregnancy Test Kit," Stetten Museum, Office of NIH History, http://history.nih.gov/exhibits/thinblueline/index.html.
21. Predictor ad in McCall's, July 1979, reprinted in http://pictorial.jezebel.com/selling-american-women-on-the-first-at-home-pregnancy-t-1722665070; Andrea Tone, "Medicalizing Reproduction: The Pill and Home Pregnancy Tests," *Journal of Sex Research* 49, no. 4 (2012): 324.
22. For the connection between pregnancy testing, abortion, and feminism in Great Britain's women's health movement, see Jesse Olszynko-Gryn, "The Feminist Appropriation of Pregnancy Testing in 1970s Britain," *Women's History Review* (2017).
23. Kelly Faircloth, "Selling American Women on the First At-Home Pregnancy Tests," *Jezebel.com,* August 17, 2015, http://pictorial.jezebel.com/selling-american-women-on-the-first-at-home-pregnancy-t-1722665070.
24. These oral histories are collected on a multifaceted interpretive historical website called The Thin Blue Line, which Leavitt created for the National Institutes of Health's Office of NIH History to document the history of home pregnancy testing and the NIH's role in the science that made it possible. Leavitt, "Thin Blue Line."
25. Faircloth, "Selling American Women on the First At-Home Pregnancy Tests," http://pictorial.jezebel.com/selling-american-women-on-the-first-at-home-pregnancy-t-1722665070
26. Leavitt, "Private Little Revolution," 327–329; Layne, "The Home PregnancyTest".
27. Faircloth, "Selling American Women on the First at-Home Pregnancy Tests," http://pictorial.jezebel.com/selling-american-women-on-the-first-at-home-pregnancy-t-1722665070.
28. Leavitt, "Private Little Revolution," 332.

29. Faircloth, "Selling American Women on the First at-Home Pregnancy Tests," http://pictorial.jezebel.com/selling-american-women-on-the-first-at-home-pregnancy-t-1722665070.

30. Susan Lapinksi and Michael deCourcy Hinds, "Are We Ready for a Baby? Will We Ever Be?," *Glamour*, January 1983, 60.

31. Leavitt, "Thin Blue Line."

32. https://www.youtube.com/watch?v=A1_CWNatOMA, accessed May 17, 2017); "Private Little Revolution," 331.

33. "Thin Blue Line."

34. Faircloth, "Selling American Women on the First at-Home Pregnancy Tests," http://pictorial.jezebel.com/selling-american-women-on-the-first-at-home-pregnancy-t-1722665070; "Bringing Medicine Home: Self-Test Kits Monitor Your Health," *Consumer Reports*, October 1996.

35. L. L. Jeng et al., "How Frequently Are Home Pregnancy Tests Used? Results From the 1988 National Maternal and Infant Health Survey," *Birth* 18, no. 1 (March 1991).

36. See also marketing info in Leavitt, "Private Little Revolution," 330.

37. Pagan Kennedy, "Who Made That Home Pregnancy Test?," *New York Times Magazine*, July 27, 2012, http://www.nytimes.com/2012/07/29/magazine/who-made-that-home-pregnancy-test.html?_r=0.

38. Freidenfelds, "New Losses."

39. Leavitt, "Thin Blue Line."

40. A typical example is Jenny Silverstone, "25 of the Most Memorable Pregnancy Announcement Ideas Ever," (2018), https://momlovesbest.com/pregnancy/pregnancy-announcement-ideas.

41. Anna Prushinskaya, "The Quantified Baby," *The Atlantic*, April 10, 2015, https://www.theatlantic.com/health/archive/2015/04/the-quantified-baby/389009/.

42. Leavitt, "Thin Blue Line."

43. Ibid.

44. http://www.mothering.com/forum/178-trying-conceive/1166726-faint-line-hpt.html accessed 07-29-16.

45. Rosalind Pollack Petchesky, "Fetal Images: The Power of Visual Culture in the Politics of Reproduction," *Feminist Studies* 13, no. 2 (Summer 1987); Lara Freidenfelds, "Making Miscarriage: Technologies of Early Pregnancy Loss" (paper presented at the Gender and Science Program, University of California at Berkeley, 2010).

46. March 1978 E.P.T. ad, http://clickamericana.com/eras/1970s/early-home-pregnancy-tests-1978-1985, accessed December 1, 2017.

47. August 1982 ad, http://clickamericana.com/eras/1970s/early-home-pregnancy-tests-1978-1985.

48. November 1985 ad, http://clickamericana.com/eras/1970s/early-home-pregnancy-tests-1978-1985.

49. David N. Danforth, et al., *Danforth's Obstetrics and Gynecology*, 8th ed. (New York: Lippincott Williams & Wilkins, 1999), 67–68.

50. Andrew Adam Newman, "Maker of Pregnancy Test Finds Opportunity in Personal Stories," *New York Times*, May 2, 2010.

51. http://www.mothering.com/forum/178-trying-conceive/1166726-faint-line-hpt.html accessed July 29, 2016.

52. Prushinskaya, "The Quantified Baby," https://www.theatlantic.com/health/archive/2015/04/the-quantified-baby/389009/.

53. Melissa Byers, "The Secret World of Pregnancy Test Tweaking, Demystified," *babycenter blog* (2015), https://blogs.babycenter.com/mom_stories/03272015-do-you-know-how-to-properly-tweak-a-pregnancy-test/; Kaitlin Stanford, "So Pregnancy Test 'Tweaking' Is a Thing That's Happening. Why?!," *Bustle* (2015), https://www.bustle.com/articles/95462-so-pregnancy-test-tweaking-is-a-thing-thats-happening-why; https://itunes.apple.com/us/app/pregnancy-test-checker-free/id854689871?mt=8 ad for tweaking app, accessed May 26, 2017.

54. http://www.fertilethoughts.com/forums/ivf-high-tech/703219-february-cycle-buddy-group-last-thread-2011-a.html, accessed April 2, 2011.

55. Leavitt, "Thin Blue Line."

56. To arrive at these figures, researchers conducted laboratory hCG tests much more sensitive than home pregnancy tests, and each study defined slightly different thresholds for defining an hCG surge as indicative of a pregnancy. Most researchers measured in terms of nanograms of hCG, rather than International Units of hCG, which makes their thresholds difficult to compare with the sensitivities claimed by home pregnancy test manufacturers, which are always in terms of International Units. The comparison is not straightforward because IUs are defined by effect in the body, and are not directly translatable into grams of hCG, since samples of hCG differ in their purity and therefore in IUs per gram. One study, however, did include an estimate of hCG peaks for "occult" (pre-clinical) pregnancy losses at 1 to 2 nanograms per mililiter and 13 to 26 microIUs per mililiter (M. J. Zinaman et al., "Estimates of Human Fertility and Pregnancy Loss," *Fertility and Sterility* 65, no. 3 (March 1996)). Most home pregnancy tests claim sensitivity in the range of 30–50 mIU/mL, but First Response Early Result has been demonstrated to be sensitive to 12.5 mIU/mL (http://www.peeonastick.com/hpts.html).

57. J. H. E. Promislow et al., "Bleeding Following Pregnancy Loss before 6 Weeks' Gestation," *Human Reproduction* 22, no. 3 (March 2007). Leavitt argues that home pregnancy tests can be seen as oppressive rather than liberating when they reveal miscarriages a woman might otherwise have not known about (see Leavitt, "Private Little Revolution," 320, 38–39).

58. http://www.babycenter.com/400_after-having-a-miscarriage-how-early-can-you-start-trying-ag_810197_402.bc?startIndex=10 accessed December 1, 2017.

59. Leavitt, "Thin Blue Line."

60. Sallie Han, "The Chemical Pregnancy: Technology, Mothering and the Making of a Reproductive Experience," *Journal of the Motherhood Initiative* 5, no. 2 (2014): 50–51. Han also describes the intolerance for ambiguity and ambivalence around pregnancy more generally.

61. Krissi Danielsson, "What Is a Chemical Pregnancy? A Type of Early Miscarriage That Usually Goes Unnoticed," https://www.verywell.com/chemical-pregnancy-a-very-early-miscarriage-2371493.

62. Fan Xiao-Guang and Zheng Zhen-Qun, "A Study of Early Pregnancy Factor Activity in Preimplantation," *American Journal of Reproductive Immunology* 37 (May 1997).

63. "Early Pregnancy Factor (Epf)," *Fertility Smarts*, https://www.fertilitysmarts.com/definition/1150/early-pregnancy-factor-epf, accessed May 1, 2017.

CONCLUSION

1. Emily Malone, "New Beginnings," *Daily Garnish*, October 30, 2017, http://www.dailygarnish.com/2017/10/new-beginnings.html.

2. "Baby Talk," *Daily Garnish*, November 13, 2017, http://www.dailygarnish.com/2017/11/baby-talk.html.

3. Ibid.

4. Promislow et al., "Bleeding Following Pregnancy Loss before 6 Weeks' Gestation".

5. This approach would also mesh well with the goal of providing pre-conception care to all women. Many interventions, such as folic acid supplementation, are most effective in the first weeks of pregnancy, before most women know they are pregnant. For a related discussion of parenting, and the role of parents as "gardeners" (i.e., responsive nurturers) rather than "carpenters" (i.e., controlling creators), see Alison Gopnik, *The Gardener and the Carpenter: What the New Science of Child Development Tells Us About the Relationship Between Parents and Children* (New York: Farrar, Straus and Giroux, 2016).

6. Malone, "Baby Talk," http://www.dailygarnish.com/2017/11/baby-talk.html.

7. Charles J. Lockwood, "Prediction of Pregnancy Loss," *The Lancet*, no. 9212 (April 15, 2000).

8. Tracy Wilson Peters and Laurel Wilson, *The Attachment Pregnancy: The Ultimate Guide to Bonding with Your Baby* (New York: Adams Media, 2014).

9. Layne, "The Home Pregnancy Test" notes the profit motive, and argues against using the tests at all.

10. Thanks to Conevery Valencius, Kara Swanson, and John Freidenfelds for these ideas.

11. Lara Freidenfelds, "Enforcing Death Rituals After Miscarriage Is Just Plain Cruel," *Nursing Clio* (2016), https://nursingclio.org/2016/04/13/enforcing-death-rituals-after-miscarriage-is-just-plain-cruel/.

12. Drs. Yvonne Bohn, Allison Hill, and Alane Park provide an excellent model for addressing miscarriage in their guide for pregnant women: Yvonne Bohn, Allison Hill, and Alane Park, *The Mommy Docs' Ultimate Guide to Pregnancy and Birth* (New York: Da Capo Lifelong Books, 2011).

13. I disagree with Linda Layne and Janet Bronstein on this point (Layne, "Designing a Woman-Centered Health Care Approach to Pregnancy Loss", and Janet M. Bronstein, *Preterm Birth in the United States: A Sociocultural Approach* (New York: Springer, 2016). Layne advocates teaching about stillbirth in prenatal preparation classes, and Bronstein would like to see more education about pre-term birth in pregnancy guides. I suggest that it is important to distinguish between likely and unlikely bad outcomes, so as to limit our concern to outcomes we are actually likely to need to address.

14. Some examples of the many articles that urge readers to be careful about minimizing someone's miscarriage include Devan McGuinness, "8 Things Not to Say to Someone Who's Had a Miscarriage," *Parents*, http://www.parents.com/pregnancy/complications/miscarriage/things-not-to-say-to-someone-whos-had-a-miscarriage/, accessed September 13, 2017; Rachel Paula Abrahamson, "Five Things You Should Never Say to a Woman Who Has Had a Miscarriage," *Us Weekly*, July 15, 2016, http://www.usmagazine.com/celebrity-moms/news/what-not-to-say-to-a-woman-who-has-had-a-miscarriage-w429449; Christine O'Brien, "10 Things You Should Never Say to a Woman Who's Had a Miscarriage," *WhatToExpect.com*, September 16, 2014, https://www.whattoexpect.com/wom/pregnancy/10-things-you-should-never-say-to-a-woman-who-s-had-a-miscarriage.aspx; Becky Hoh, "9 Things Not to Say to a Woman Who Has Had a Miscarriage," *Cosmopolitan*, January 26, 2016, http://www.cosmopolitan.com/uk/body/health/news/a40850/not-to-say-woman-miscarriage/; among many others.

15. Murkoff and Mazel, *What to Expect When You're Expecting*, 539.

16. Murkoff and Mazel, *What to Expect When You're Expecting*, 5th ed. (New York: Workman, 2016), 592.

17. Layne, *Motherhood Lost*.

18. Others may appreciate the social support from sharing the news: Lara Freidenfelds, "Yes, We Should Tell About Our Miscarriages on Facebook," *Nursing Clio* (2015), http://nursingclio.org/2015/08/18/yes-we-should-tell-about-our-miscarriages-on-facebook/.

19. Malone, "New Beginnings," http://www.dailygarnish.com/2017/10/new-beginnings.html.

20. As historian of childhood Paula Fass describes it, "The sense of control becomes the defining illusion of our time." Fass, *The End of American Childhood*, 225.

21. Senior, *All Joy and No Fun*. It also may set up some of the parenting issues that have been the focus of attention lately (helicopter parenting, a lack of "grit" or "resilience," and so on): Wendy Mogel, *The Blessing of a Skinned Knee: Using Timeless Teachings to Raise Self-Reliant Children* (New York: Scribner, 2001); Julie Lythcott-Haims, *How to Raise an Adult: Break Free of the Overparenting Trap and Prepare Your Kid for Success* (New York: Henry Holt, 2015); Caren Baruch-Feldman and Thomas R. Hoerr, *The Grit Guide for Teens: A Workbook to Help You Build Perseverance, Self-Control, and a Growth Mindset* (Oakland, CA: Instant Help, 2017). This post on freerangekids.com links pregnancy perfectionism to parenting perfectionism: http://www.freerangekids.com/driven-crazy-by-pregnancy-perfectionists-especially-on-the-web/, accessed December 2, 2017.

22. The impact of blaming parents for events beyond their control falls especially hard on economically disadvantaged families. On disadvantaged parents sharing child-rearing values with middle-class parents and faulting themselves for falling short, see Knight, *Addicted.Pregnant.Poor*, 157–158. On blaming parents for children's accidents rather than sympathizing with them, see Melissa Fenton, "Stop Blaming Parents for Accidents. Please," *4 Boys Mother*, June 16, 2016, https://4boysmother.com/stop-blaming-parents-for-accidents-please/.

INDEX

Note: For the benefit of digital users, indexed terms that span two pages (e.g., 52–53) may, on occasion, appear on only one of those pages.

Figures are indicated by an italic *f* following the page/paragraph number.

social sciences. A true ratio scale has a meaningful zero point, so that zero means "nothingness." This mean that if we could devise a legitimate ratio testing instrument for measuring the achievement of nursing students in biochemistry, students scoring 0 would have absolutely no knowledge of the biochemistry objectives tested. This is not possible in educational measurement, obviously, since even the least capable student will have some minimal knowledge. (True ratio scales are often found in the physical sciences, but not in the social sciences.)

The main point of this discussion of number-types is that most of the assessment data we obtain in health professions education is considered or assumed to be interval data, so that we can perform nearly all types of statistical analyses on the results. For instance, data from a multiple-choice achievement test in pharmacology is always assumed to be interval data, so that we can compute summary statistics for the distribution of scores (means, standard deviations), correlations between scores on this test and other similar tests or subtests, and may even perform a paired t-test of mean pre-post differences in scores. If these data were ordinal, we would have some limitations on the statistical analyses available, such as using only the Spearman rank-order correlation coefficient. All psychometric models of data used in assessment, such as the various methods used to estimate the reproducibility or reliability of scores or ratings, are derived with the underlying assumption that the data are interval in nature.

Fidelity to the Criterion

Another familiar concept in assessment for the health professions is that of "fidelity." The full term, as used by most educational measurement professionals, is "fidelity to the criterion," implying some validity-type relationship between scores or ratings on the assessment and the ultimate "criterion" variable in real life. "Fidelity to the criterion" is often shortened to "fidelity." What does this actually mean? Think of a dichotomy between a high fidelity and a low fidelity assessment. A simulation of an actual clinical problem, presented to pharmacy students by highly trained actors, is thought to be "high fidelity," because the test appears to be much like an authentic, real-life situation that the future pharmacists may encounter with a real patient. On the other hand, a multiple-choice test of basic knowledge in chemistry might be considered a very low-fidelity simulation of a real-life situation for the same students. High-fidelity assessments are said to be "more proximate to the criterion," meaning that the assessment itself appears to be fairly lifelike and authentic, while low-fidelity assessments appear to be far removed from the criterion or are less proximate to the criterion (Haladyna, 1999). Most highly structured performance exams, complex simulations, and less well structured observational methods of assessment are of higher fidelity than written exams, and are all intended to measure different facets of learning.

The concept of fidelity is important only as a superficial trait or characteristic of assessments. Fidelity may have little or nothing to do with true scientific validity evidence and may, in fact, actually interfere with objectivity of measurement, which tends to decrease validity evidence (Downing, 2003); this topic will be explored in some depth in Chapter 2. Students and their faculty, however, often prefer (or think they prefer) more high-fidelity assessments, simply because they look more like real-life situations. One fact is certain: the higher the fidelity of the assessment, the higher the cost and the more complex are the measurement issues of the assessment.

Formative and Summative Assessment

The concepts of formative and summative assessment are pervasive in the assessment literature and date to the middle of the last century; these concepts originated in the program evaluation literature, but have come to be used in all areas of assessment (Scriven, 1967). These useful concepts are straightforward in meaning. The primary purpose of formative testing is to provide useful feedback on student strengths and weaknesses with respect to the learning objectives. Classic formative assessment takes place *during* the course of study, such that student learners have the opportunity to understand what content they have already mastered and what content needs more study (or for the instructor, needs more teaching). Examples of formative assessments include weekly short quizzes during a microbiology course, shorter written tests given at frequent intervals during a two semester-long course in pharmacology, and so on.

Summative assessment "sums up" the achievement in a course of study and typically takes place at or near the end of a formal course of study, such as an end of semester examination in anatomy which covers the entire cumulative course. Summative assessments emphasize the final measurement of achievement and usually count heavily in the grading scheme. Feedback to students may be one aspect of the summative assessment, but the primary purpose of the summative assessment is to measure what students have learned during the course of instruction. The ultimate example of a summative assessment is a test given at the conclusion of long, complex courses of study, such as a licensure test in nursing which must be taken and passed at the very end of the educational sequence and before the newly graduated nurse can begin professional work.

Norm- and Criterion-Referenced Measurement

The basic concept of norm- and criterion-referenced measurement or assessment is also fairly simple and straightforward. Norm-referenced test scores are interpreted relative to some well-defined normative group, such as all students who took the test. The key word is *relative*; norm-referenced scores or ratings tell us a lot about how well students score or are rated relative to some group of other students, but may tell us less about what exact content they actually know or can do. Criterion-referenced scores or ratings, on the other hand, tell us how much of some specific content students actually know or can do. Criterion-referenced testing has been popular in North America since the 1970s (Popham & Husek, 1969). This type of assessment is most closely associated with competency or content-based teaching and testing. Other terms used somewhat interchangeably with criterion-referenced testing are "domain-referenced," "objectives-referenced," "content-referenced," and "construct-referenced." There are some subtle differences in the usage of these terms by various authors and researchers, but all have in common the strong interest in the content actually learned or mastered by the student and the lack of interest in rank-ordering students by test scores.

Mastery testing is a special type of criterion-referenced testing, in that the assessments are constructed to be completed nearly perfectly by almost all students. For mastery tests, the expected score is 100 percent-correct. Mastery teaching strategies and testing methods imply that all students can learn up to some criterion of "mastery," and the only difference may be in the time needed to complete the mastery learning and testing. Some special theories and methods of assessment are required for true mastery testing, since almost all of testing theory is based on norm-referenced testing. Many norm-referenced testing statistics are inappropriate for true mastery tests.

A final note on this important topic. Any assessment score or rating can be interpreted in either a norm-referenced or criterion-referenced manner. The test, the methods used to construct the test, and the overarching philosophy of the instructor about testing and student learning and achievement determine the basic classification of the test as either norm- or criterion-referenced. It is perfectly possible, for example, to interpret an inherently normative score, like a percentile or a z-score, in some absolute or criterion-referenced manner. Conversely, some criterion-referenced tests may report only percent-correct scores or raw scores but interpret these scores relative to the distribution of scores (i.e., in a normative or relative fashion).

The concepts of norm- and criterion-referenced testing will be revisited often in this book, especially in our treatment of topics like standard setting or establishing effective and defensible passing scores. For the most part, the orientation of this book is criterion-referenced. We are most interested in assessing what our students have learned and achieved and about their competency in our health professions disciplines rather than ranking them in a normative distribution.

High-stakes and Low-stakes Assessments

Other terms often used to describe assessments are high- and low-stakes assessments. These terms are descriptive of the consequences of testing. If the results of a test can have a serious impact on an examinee, such as gaining or loosing a professional job, the stakes associated with the test are clearly high. High-stakes tests require a much higher burden, in that every facet of such tests must be of extremely high quality, with solid research-based evidence to support validity of interpretations. There may even be a need to defend such high-stakes tests legally, if the test is perceived to cause some individuals or groups harm. Examinations used to admit students to professional schools and tests used to certify or license graduates in the health professions are good examples of very high-stakes tests. Assessments used to determine final grades in important classes required for graduation or final summative exams that must be passed in order to graduate are also high stakes for our students.

A low- to moderate-stakes test carries somewhat lower consequences. Many of the formative-type assessments typically used in health professions education are low to moderate stakes. If the consequences of failing the test are minor or if the remediation (test retake) is not too difficult or costly, the exam stakes might be thought of as low or moderate.

Very high-stakes tests are usually professionally produced by testing experts and large testing agencies using major resources to ensure the defensibility of the resulting test scores and pass-fail decisions. Lower stakes tests and assessments, such as those used by many health professions educators in their local school settings, require fewer resources and less validity evidence, since legal challenges to the test outcomes are rare. Since this book focuses on assessments developed at the local (or classroom) level by highly specialized content experts, the assessments of interest are low to moderate stakes. Nevertheless, even lower stakes assessments should meet the basic minimum standards of quality, since important decisions are ultimately being made about our students from our cumulative assessments over time.

Large-scale and Local or Small-scale Assessments

Another reference point for this book and its orientation toward assessment in the health professions is the distinction between large- and small-scale assessments. Large-scale assessments refer to standardized testing programs, often national or international in scope, which are generally designed by testing professionals and administered to large numbers of examinees. Large-scale tests such as the Pharmacy College Admissions Test (PCAT) and the Medical College Admissions Test (MCAT) are utilized to help selected students for pharmacy and medical schools. Tests such as the National Council Licensure Examination (NCLEX®) for Registered Nurses is another example of a large-scale test, which is used for licensure of registered nurses by jurisdictions in the United States.

Small-scale or locally developed assessments—the main focus of this book—are developed, administered, and scored by "classroom" instructors, clinical teaching faculty, or other educators at the local school, college, or university level. Too frequently, health professions educators "go it alone" when assessing their students, with little or no formal educational background in assessment and with little or no support from their institutions for the critically important work of assessment. This book aims to provide local instructors and other health professions educators with sound principles, effective tools, and defensible methods to assist in the important work of student assessment.

Summary

This introduction provided the general context and overview for this book. Most of the concepts introduced in this chapter are expanded and detailed in later chapters. We hope that this introductory chapter provides even the most novice assessment learner with the basic vocabulary and some of the most essential concepts and principles needed to comprehend some of the more technical aspects of following chapters.

Christine McGuire, a major contributor to assessment theory and practice in medical education, once said: "Evaluation is probably the most logical field in the world and if you use a little bit of logic, it just fits together and jumps at you. . . . It's very common sense." (Harris & Simpson, 2005, p. 68). We agree with Dr. McGuire's statement. While there is much technical nuance and much statistical elaboration to assessment topics in health professions education, we should never lose sight of the mostly commonsense nature of the enterprise. On the other hand, Voltaire noted that "Common sense is very rare" (Voltaire, 1962, p. 467), so the goal of this book is to bring state-of-the art assessment theory and practice to health professions educators, so that their students will benefit from quality assessments that become "common" in their curricula.

References

Accreditation Council for Graduate Medical Education. (2000). ACGME Outcome Project. Retrieved December 2, 2005, from http://www.acgme.org/outcome/assess/assHome.asp/

Accreditation Council for Graduate Medical Education & American Board of Medical Specialties. (2000). Toolbox of assessment methods. Retrieved December 2, 2005, from http://www.acgme.org/outcome/assess/toolbox.asp/

American Educational Research Association, American Psychological Association, & National Council on Measurement in Education. (1999). *Standards for educational and psychological testing.* Washington DC: American Educational Research Association.

Anderson, M.B., & Kassebaum, D.G. (Eds.). (1993). Proceedings of the AAMC's consensus conference on the use of standardized patients in the teaching and evaluation of clinical skills. *Academic Medicine, 68,* 437–483.

Barrows, H.S., & Abrahamson, S. (1964). The programmed patient: A technique for appraising student performance in clinical neurology. *Journal of Medical Education, 39,* 802–805.

Bloom, B.S., Engelhart, M.D., Furst, E.J., Hill, W.H., & Krathwohl, D.R. (1956). *Taxonomy of educational objectives.* New York: Longmans Green.

Downing, S.M. (2002). Assessment of knowledge with written test forms. In G.R. Norman, C.P.M. Van der Vleuten, & D.I. Newble (Eds.), *International handbook for research in medical education* (pp. 647–672). Dordrecht, The Netherlands: Kluwer Academic Publishers.

Downing, S.M. (2003). Validity: On the meaningful interpretation of assessment data. *Medical Education, 37,* 830–837.

Gordon, M.S. (1999). Developments in the use of simulators and multimedia computer systems in medical education. *Medical Teacher, 21*(1), 32–36.

Haladyna, T.M. (1999, April). When should we use a multiple-choice format? A paper presented at the annual meeting of the American Educational Research Association, Montreal, Canada.

Harden, R., Stevenson, M., Downie, W., & Wilson, M. (1975). Assessment of clinical competence using objective structured examinations. *British Medical Journal, 1,* 447–451.

Harris, I.B., & Simpson, D. (2005). Christine McGuire: At the heart of the maverick measurement maven. *Advances in Health Sciences Education*, 10, 65–80.

Howell, D.C. (2002). *Statistical methods for psychology* (5th ed.). Pacific Grove, CA: Duxbury-Wadsworth Group.

Miller, G. (1990). The assessment of clinical skills/competence/performance. *Academic Medicine*, 65, S63–S67.

National Board of Medical Examiners. (2006). USMLE Bulletin of Information. Federation of State Medical Boards and National Board of Medical Examiners. Retrieved December 2, 2005, from http://www.usmle.org/bulletin/2006/2006bulletin.pdf/

Popham, W.J., & Husek, T.R. (1969). Implications of criterion-referenced measurement. *Journal of Educational Measurement*, 7, 367–375.

Scriven, M. (1967). The methodology of evaluation. In R. Tyler, R. Gagne, & M. Scriven (Eds.), *Perspectives of curriculum evaluation* (pp. 39–83). Chicago: Rand McNally.

Sireci, S.G., & Zenisky, A.L. (2006). Innovative item formats in computer-based testing: In pursuit of improved construct representation. In S.M. Downing & T.M. Haladyna (Eds.), *Handbook of test development* (pp. 329–348). Mahwah, NJ: Lawrence Erlbaum Associates.

Voltaire. (1962). *Philosophical dictionary* (P. Gay, Trans.). New York: Basic Books, Inc.

Wallace, P. (1997). Following the threads of an innovation: The history of standardized patients in medical education. *CADUCEUS*, 13 (2), 5–28.

Welch, C. (2006). Item and prompt development in performance testing. In S.M. Downing & T.M. Haladyna (Eds.), *Handbook of test development* (pp. 303–328). Mahwah, NJ: Lawrence Erlbaum Associates.

William, R.G., Klaman, D.A., & McGaghie, W.C. (2003). Cognitive, social, and environmental sources of bias in clinical performance ratings. *Teaching and Learning in Medicine*, 15(4), 270–292.

2

VALIDITY AND ITS THREATS

STEVEN M. DOWNING AND
THOMAS M. HALADYNA

Validity is the *sine qua non* of all assessment data, without which assessment data has little or no meaning. All assessments require validity evidence and nearly all topics in assessment involve validity in some way. Thus, validity gets to the heart or essence of all assessment and is the single most important topic in testing.

Many books on assessment place a chapter on validity toward the end of the text. The placement of this validity chapter early in the book emphasizes a major point: Validity is the single most important characteristic of assessment data. If you understand validity at some deep level, you will know most of what is important concerning assessments and their application in health professions educational settings.

The purpose of this chapter is to present an overview of contemporary validity theory, illustrated by specific examples from health professions education together with concrete examples of the various types of scientific data required as validity evidence. Threats to validity will also be discussed in some detail, since such threats abound.

In the absence of solid scientific evidence of validity, most assessment data has little or no meaning. For instance, if you are given a distribution of numbers, ranging from 3 to 100, for a class of pharmacy students, what do you know about these students? Obviously, very little without much more information. Unless you know what the numbers are supposed to represent, it's very difficult to assign a valid or meaningful interpretation to the numbers. You would need to know, for example: Do these numbers represent a count of the questions answered correctly on a multiple-choice test? Or, are these numbers some type of percent-correct score, on either a selected-response, constructed-response test or a performance test or on some observational rating scale? If the numbers represent a number-correct or percent-correct score, what content is measured by the written or performance test? How was this content sampled? How representative is the sampled content to the entire domain or universe of content? How scientifically sound was the measurement? Are the numbers/scores scientifically reproducible? And so on and on with inquiry of this type, posing and answering essential questions about the assessment, the answers to which help provide meaning to the numbers. This scientific inquiry aimed at establishing a certain meaning or interpretation for assessment data is the essence of validity.

What is Validity?

Validity refers to the evidence presented to support or to refute the meaning or interpretation assigned to assessment data or results (Messick, 1989). Kane discusses validity and validation thus: "To validate a proposed interpretation or use of test scores is to evaluate the claims being based on the test scores. The specific mix of evidence needed for validation depends on the inferences being drawn and the assumptions being made." (Kane, 2006a, p. 131) In common parlance, it is said that validity has to do with a test measuring what it is supposed to measure. This is a generally true statement, but a statement in need of considerable elaboration, which is the intended purpose of this chapter.

Validation as Scientific Research

Contemporary validity theory is primarily concerned with a process of scientific inquiry, based on sound theory and focused on hypotheses, which guides the gathering of scientific evidence from multiple sources, to either support or refute specific interpretations or meanings associated with assessment data, used for a specific purpose. Validity evidence is associated with scores or data resulting from tests or assessments, not the assessment forms or instruments which produce the data. Validity evidence is case and time specific; the data presented to support or refute a specific score interpretation or the arguments for a given score meaning are not good for all time, but rather only for the specific uses specified by the assessment user and the purpose of the assessment. Validity evidence used for one test administration does not necessarily apply to a different test administration; the argument for generalizing validity evidence must be made on a case-by-case basis.

Validity is the application of the scientific method to assessment data, for the purpose of establishing reasonable interpretations or legitimate meanings to data. In this conceptualization, assessment data are more or less valid for some very specific purpose, meaning or interpretation, at a specific point in time and only for some well defined population. The assessment itself is never said to be *valid* or *invalid*; rather one speaks of the scientifically sound evidence presented to either support or refute the specific proposed interpretation of assessment scores, at a particular time period in which the validity evidence was collected from some specific population.

Validity theory, like many theories in education and psychology, has evolved over time. The formal theory and practice of educational measurement is only about 100 years old, dating back to the early twentieth century in the United States with the introduction of the U. S. Army Alpha test, used to test large numbers of recruits for World War I (Ebel, 1972). The history of the evolution of validity theory in assessment is summarized succinctly by a review of successive editions of a document currently titled *Standards of Educational and Psychological Testing* (AERA, APA, & NCME, 1999). This *Standards* document represents the best consensus thinking about acceptable testing practice by the three North American organizations which are most involved with testing: the American Educational Research Association (AERA), the American Psychological Association (APA), and the National Council on Measurement in Education (NCME). The *Standards* are updated periodically, with the last update published in 1999. Previous editions of the *Standards* were published in 1955, 1966, 1974, and 1985; a careful reading of the *Standards*, over various editions, gives an historical overview of an evolving view of validity (Linn, 2006).

A complete overview of the evolution of validity theory is beyond the scope of this chapter, but it is important to understand that the theory, definitions, and methods of validity and validation research have changed considerably over the past fifty years or so. In earlier editions of the *Standards* (e.g., 1955 and 1966), validity was discussed as the trinitarian or three-level model of validity: content, criterion-related, and construct validity. Criterion-related validity was often thought of as either "concurrent" or "predictive," depending on the timing of data collection for the criterion variable (Cureton, 1951). Such a trinitarian view of validity is dated and is generally no longer used in educational measurement research and writing, given the evolution of validity theory in the late twentieth century.

Contemporary Validity Theory

In its contemporary conceptualization, validity is a unitary concept, which requires multiple sources of scientific evidence to support or refute the meaning associated with assessment data (e.g., AERA, APA, & NCME, 1999; Cronbach, 1988, 1989; Kane, 1992, 1994, 2006 a, b; Messick, 1989, 1995). These evidentiary sources are logically suggested by the desired types of interpretation or meaning associated with measures, firmly rooted in theory and the scientific method. All validity is construct validity in this framework, described most philosophically and eloquently by Messick (1989) and Kane (2006b) and embodied in the *Standards* (AERA, APA, & NCME, 1999).

Constructs

Why is construct validity now considered the sole type of validity? The complex answer is found in the philosophy of science from which, it is posited, there are many complex webs of inter-related inference associated with sampling content in order to make meaningful and reasonable inferences from a sample to a domain or larger population of interest. The more straightforward answer is: Nearly all assessments in the social sciences deal with *constructs*— intangible collections of abstract concepts and principles, which are inferred from behavior and explained by educational or psychological theory.

Cronbach and Meehl (1955) set the course for development of contemporary views of test validity as early as the mid-1950s, defining a construct as a hypothesized attribute assumed to be tested by the assessment. Note that their definition of a construct is fairly circular, but it captures the essence of the scientific point we attempt to establish with our work in validation.

Educational achievement is a construct, usually inferred from performance on assessments such as written tests over some well-defined domain of knowledge, oral examinations over specific problems or cases, or highly structured performance examinations such as standardized-patient examinations of history taking, communication or physical examination skills. The educational achievement construct is the primary assessment focus of this book. While constructs such as *ability* or *aptitude*, or *intelligence* are important in some educational settings, they are not the primary focus of this book.

Because constructs are necessarily intangible, validation of our assessment data requires an evidentiary chain which clearly links the interpretation of the assessment scores or data to an inter-related, complex network of theory, hypotheses and logic, which are presented to support or refute the reasonableness of some specific desired interpretations. Validity is an ongoing process of hypothesis generation, data collection and testing, critical evaluation, and logical inference.

The validity argument relates theory, predicted relationships, and empirical evidence in ways to suggest which particular interpretative meanings are reasonable and which are not reasonable for a specific assessment use or application (Kane, 1992, 1994, 2006 a, b). The notion of validity as argument is now prominent since the publication of the fourth edition of *Educational Measurement* in which Michael Kane's chapter discusses the validity model as a process of building logical, scientific and empirical arguments to support or refute very specific intended interpretations of assessment scores (Kane, 2006b). Kane's validity argument requires an overt linking of inferences, with all the interconnections and intermediate steps, which trace the specific content tested by items or performance prompts back to the content domain—or the population of knowledge, skills, or ability to which one wishes to make inferences or to generalize.

The Negative Case—Refuting the Intended Interpretation of Test Scores

Too often in validation research and in our thinking about validity theory, we forget or ignore the negative case for validity (Haladyna, 2006). We have discussed validity and validation research in terms of hypothesis driven research in search of hard scientific evidence to either support or refute specific interpretations or meanings associated with assessment data. The "negative case" refers to serious attempts to refute or falsify the hypothesis or overturn our expectations or beliefs about the interpretative meaning. "A proposition deserves some degree of trust only when it has survived serious attempts to falsify it." (Cronbach, 1980, p. 103.) Again, this sounds much like solid scientific research. Using experimental research methods, we set out to objectively test hypotheses. When research is conducted in a sound scientific manner, controlling for all important nuisance variables that could spoil the study, the researcher must always be open to negative findings. This is the essence of all scientific research; this is the major point of validation research. An alternate meaning or interpretation of assessment data may always be found, thus falsifying our hypotheses or our beliefs about the meaning or proper interpretation of our assessment data.

Meaningful Interpretation of Scores

In order to meaningfully interpret scores, some assessments, such as achievement tests of cognitive knowledge, may require only fairly straightforward content-related evidence of the adequacy of the content tested (in relationship to instructional objectives), statistical evidence of score reproducibility and item statistical quality and evidence to support the defensibility of passing scores or grades. Other types of assessments, such as complex performance examinations, may require both evidence related to content and considerable empirical data demonstrating the statistical relationship between the performance examination and other measures of ability or achievement, the generalizability of the sampled cases to the population of skills, the reproducibility of the score scales, the adequacy of the standardized patient training, and so on. There can never be too much validity evidence, but there is often too little evidence to satisfy the skeptic. Validation research for high-stakes tests is an on-going task, with data collected routinely over time to address specific validity questions (e.g., Haladyna, 2006).

The higher the stakes associated with assessments, the greater the requirement for validity evidence, from multiple sources, which are collected on an on-going basis and continually re-evaluated (Linn, 2002). The on-going documentation of validity evidence for a high-stakes testing program, such as a licensure or certification examination in any of the health professions, may require the allocation of many resources and the contributions of many different professionals with a variety of skills—content specialists, psychometricians and statisticians, test editors and administrators (Haladyna, 2006). For low-to-medium stakes assessment programs, such as formative classroom tests in the basic sciences, less validity evidence is required.

Five Sources of Validity Evidence

According to the *Standards*: "Validity refers to the degree to which evidence and theory support the interpretations of test scores entailed by proposed uses of tests" (AERA, APA, & NCME, 1999, p. 9). The *Standards* closely parallel Messick's seminal chapter in *Educational Measurement* (Messick, 1989), which considers all validity to be construct validity. Kane (1992, 1994, 2006 a, b) discusses validity as an investigative process through which constructs are carefully defined, data and evidence are gathered and assembled to form an argument, which either supports or refutes some very specific interpretation of assessment scores.

In this context, the validity hypothesis is tested as a series of propositions—usually interrelated—concerning the sufficiency of the evidence supporting or refuting a specific score interpretation.

The *Standards*

The *Standards* discuss five distinct sources or types of validity evidence, which are summarized in Table 2.1: Content, Responses, Internal structure, Relationship to other variables, and Consequences. Each source of validity evidence is associated with some examples of the types of data that might be collected to support or refute specific assessment interpretations (validity). Some assessment formats or types demand a stronger emphasis on one or more sources of evidence as opposed to other sources and not all sources of data or evidence are required for all assessments. For example, a written, objectively scored test covering several weeks of instruction in microbiology, might emphasize content-related evidence, together with some evidence of response quality, internal structure, and consequences, but very likely would not seek much or any evidence concerning relationship to other variables. On the other hand, a high-stakes summative Objective Structured Clinical Examination (OSCE), using standardized patients to portray and rate student performance on a examination that must be passed in order to proceed in the curriculum, might require all of these sources of evidence and many of the data examples noted in Table 2.2, to support or refute the proposed interpretation of the scores.

The construct validity model, using five major sources or aspects of validity evidence, is now being used in the health professions education settings. For example, several recent publications used this model to examine multiple sources of validity evidence for clinical teaching (Beckman & Cook, 2005), assessments of all types in internal medicine (Cook & Beckman, 2006), and for an integrated assessment system in an undergraduate clinical teaching setting (Auewarakul, Downing, Jaturatumrong, & Praditsuwan, 2005).

Examples: Sources of Validity Evidence

Each of the five sources of validity evidence are considered, in the context of a written assessment of cognitive knowledge or achievement and a performance examination in health professions education.

Table 2.1 Five Major Sources of Test Validity: Evidence Based on Messick (1989) and AERA, APA, & NCME (1999)

1. **Content**—relationship between test content and the construct of interest; theory; hypothesis about content; independent assessment of match between content sampled and domain of interest; solid, scientific, quantitative evidence.

2. **Response Process**—analysis of individual responses to stimuli; debriefing of examinees; process studies aimed at understanding what is measured and the soundness of intended score interpretations; quality assurance and quality control of assessment data

3. **Internal Structure**—data internal to assessments such as: reliability or reproducibility of scores; inter-item correlations; statistical characteristics of items; statistical analysis of item option function; factor studies of dimensionality; Differential Item Functioning (DIF) studies

4. **Relations to Other Variables**—data external to assessments such as: correlations of assessment variable(s) to external, independent measures; hypothesis and theory driven investigations; correlational research based on previous studies, literature

    a. Convergent and discriminant evidence: relationships between similar and different measures

    b. Test-criterion evidence: relationships between test and criterion measure(s)

    c. Validity generalization: can the validity evidence be generalized?
    Evidence that the validity studies may generalize to other settings.

5. **Evidence Based on Consequences of Testing**—intended and unintended consequences of test use; differential consequences of test use; impact of assessment on students, instructors, schools, society; impact of assessments on curriculum; cost/benefit analysis with respect to tradeoff between instructional time and assessment time.

Both example assessments are high-stakes, in that the consequences of passing or failing are very important to students, faculty, and ultimately the patients or clients of the health professions' provider.

The example written assessment is a summative comprehensive examination in the basic sciences—a test consisting of 250 multiple-choice questions (MCQs) covering all the pre-clinical instruction in the basic sciences—and a test that must be passed in order to proceed into clinical training. The performance examination example is a standardized patient (SP) examination, administered to students toward the end of their clinical training, after having completed all of their required clerkship rotations. The purpose of the SP examination is to comprehensively assess graduating students' ability to take a history and do a focused physical examination in an ambulatory primary-care setting. The SP examination consists of ten twenty-minute SP cases, presented by a lay, trained standardized patient who simulates the patient's presenting problem and rates the student's

Table 2.2 Some Sources of Validity Evidence for Proposed Score Interpretations and Examples of Some Types of Evidence

Source of Evidence	Content	Response Process	Internal Structure	Relationship to Other Variables	Consequences

Examples of Evidence	• Examination blueprint
	• Representativeness of test blueprint to achievement domain
	• Test specifications
	• Match of item content to test specifications
	• Representativeness of items to domain
	• Logical/empirical relationship of content tested to achievement domain
	• Quality of test questions
	• Item writer qualifications
	• Sensitivity review
		• Student format familiarity
		• Quality control of electronic scanning/scoring
		• Key validation of preliminary scores
		• Accuracy in combining different item format scores
		• Quality control/accuracy of final scores/marks/grades
		• Accuracy of applying pass–fail decision rules to scores
		• Quality control of score reporting to students/faculty
		• Understandable/accurate descriptions/interpretations of scores for students
			• Item analysis data
			• Item difficulty/discrimination
			• Item/test characteristic curves (ICCs/TCCs)
			• Inter-item correlations
			• Item-total correlations
			• Score scale reliability
			• Standard errors of measurement (SEM)
			• Subscore/subscale analyses
			• Generalizability
			• Dimensionality
			• Item factor analysis
			• Differential Item Functioning (DIF)
			• Psychometric model
				• Correlation with other relevant variables
				• Convergent correlations—internal/external
				  • Similar tests
				• Divergent correlations—internal/external
				  • Dissimilar measures
				• Test-criterion correlations
				• Generalizability of evidence
					• Impact of test scores/results on students/society
					• Consequences on learners/future learning
					• Positive consequences outweigh unintended negative consequences?
					• Reasonableness of method of establishing pass–fail (cut) score
					• Pass/fail consequences
					• P/F Decision reliability—Classification accuracy
					• Conditional standard error of measurement at pass score (CSEM)
					• False positives/negatives
					• Instructional/learner consequences

performance at the conclusion of the examination. The SP examination must be passed in order to graduate. (These examples from medical education generalize easily to all types of health professions education which have a classroom-type component and a practical or clinical teaching/learning component.)

Documentation of these five sources of validity evidence consists of the systematic collection and presentation of information and data to present a convincing argument that it is reasonable and defensible to interpret the assessment scores in accordance with the purpose of the measurement. The scores have little or no intrinsic meaning; thus the evidence presented must convince the skeptic that the assessment scores can reasonably be interpreted in the proposed manner.

Content Evidence

For our written assessment example, documentation of validity evidence related to the content tested is the most essential. The outline and plan for the test, described by a detailed test blueprint and test specifications (Downing, 2006b), clearly relates the content tested by the 250 MCQs to the domain of the basic sciences as described by the course learning objectives. This type of blueprinting and its documentation form the logical basis for the essential validity argument (Kane, 2006b).

Test Blueprint

The process of defining the content to sample on an assessment can be an exacting and complex process. The scientific methods used to study and define test content—especially for credentialing examinations—can be elaborate and entail complex research designs using specialized data analysis methods, all of which are beyond the scope of this book (e.g., Raymond & Neustel, 2006). As the test stakes increase, so must the scientific evidence linking the content on the assessment to the domain or population of interest. This is an essential validity requirement. Since all assessments are samples of knowledge or behavior, the unbiased methods used to sample content form an essential basis for content-related validity evidence. A test blueprint defines and precisely outlines the proportion of test questions or performance prompts allocated to each major and minor content area and the proportion of these stimuli designed to test which specific cognitive knowledge levels or performance skill levels (Linn, 2006).

Test specifications and the specific test blueprints arising from these detailed specifications form an exact sampling plan for the content domain to be tested. These documents and their rationales form a solid foundation for all systematic test development activities and for the content-related validity evidence needed to support score inferences to the domain of knowledge or performance and the meaningful interpretation of test scores with respect to the construct of interest.

The test blueprint should be sufficiently detailed to describe subcategories and subclassifications of content and specifies precisely the proportion of test questions in each category and the cognitive level of those questions. At minimum, the blueprint documentation must show a direct linkage of the stimuli on the test to the instructional objectives and should clearly document the rationale for specific content selected. Independent content experts should evaluate the reasonableness of the test blueprint with respect to the course objectives and the cognitive levels tested. In our current example, the logical relationship between the content tested by the 250 MCQs and the major instructional objectives and teaching/learning activities of the course should be obvious and demonstrable, especially with respect to the proportionate weighting of test content to the actual emphasis of the basic science courses taught. Further, if most learning objectives were at the application or problem-solving level, most test questions should also be directed to these cognitive levels.

Test Item Quality

The quality of the test items is a source of content-related validity evidence. Do the MCQs adhere to the best-evidence-based principles of effective item writing (Haladyna, Downing, & Rodriguez, 2002)? Are the item writers qualified as content experts in the disciplines? Are there sufficient numbers of questions to adequately sample the large content domain? Have the test questions been edited for clarity, removing all ambiguities and other common item flaws? Have the test questions been reviewed for cultural sensitivity? (Zieky, 2006).

For the SP performance examination, some of the same content issues must be documented and presented as validity evidence. For example, each of the ten SP cases fits into a detailed content blueprint of ambulatory primary-care history and physical examination skills. There is evidence of faculty content-expert agreement that these specific ten cases are representative of primary-care ambulatory cases. Ideally, the content of the ten clinical cases is related to population demographic data and population data on disease incidence in primary-care ambulatory settings. Evidence is documented that expert clinical faculty have created, reviewed, and revised the SP cases together with the checklists and ratings scales used by the SPs, while other expert clinicians have reviewed and critically critiqued the SP cases. Exacting specifications detail all the essential clinical information to be portrayed by the SP. Evidence that SP cases have been competently edited and that detailed SP training guidelines and criteria have been prepared, reviewed by faculty experts, and implemented by experienced SP trainers are all important sources of content-related validity evidence.

There is documentation that during the time of SP administration, the SP portrayals are monitored closely to ensure that all students experience nearly the same case. Data is presented to show that a different SP, trained on the same case, rates student case performance in about the same manner, thus assuring the equivalence of the content tested. Many basic quality-control issues concerning performance examinations contribute to the content-related validity evidence for the assessment (Boulet, McKinley, Whelan, & Hambleton, 2003).

Response Process

As a source of validity evidence, *response process* may seem a bit strange or inappropriate. *Response process* is defined here as evidence of data integrity such that all sources of error associated with the test administration are controlled or eliminated to the maximum extent possible.

Response process has to do with aspects of assessment such as ensuring the accuracy of all responses to assessment prompts, the quality control of all data flowing from assessments, the appropriateness of the methods used to combine various types of assessment scores into one composite score, and the usefulness and the accuracy of the score reports provided to examinees. (Assessment data quality-control issues could also be discussed as content evidence.)

For evidence of *response process* for the written comprehensive examination, documentation of all practice materials and written information about the test and instructions to students is important. Documentation of all quality-control procedures used to ensure the absolute accuracy of test scores is also an important source of evidence: the final *key validation* after a preliminary scoring—to ensure the accuracy of the scoring key and eliminate from final scoring any poorly performing test items; a rationale for any combining rules, such as the combining into one final composite score of MCQ, multiple-true-false, and short-essay question scores.

Other sources of evidence may include documentation and the rationale for the type of scores reported, the method chosen to report scores, and the explanations and interpretive materials provided to fully explain the score report and its meaning, together with any materials discussing the proper use and any common misuses of the assessment score data.

For the SP performance examination, many of the same response process sources may be presented as validity evidence. For a performance examination, documentation demonstrating the accuracy of the SP rating is needed and the results of an SP accuracy study is a particularly important source of response-process evidence. Basic quality control of the large amounts of data from an SP performance examination is important to document, together with information on score calculation and reporting methods, their rationale, and, particularly, the explanatory materials discussing an appropriate interpretation of the performance-assessment scores (and their limitations).

Documentation of the rationale for using global versus checklist rating scores, for example, may be an important source of response evidence for the SP examination. Or, the empirical evidence and

logical rationale for combining a global rating-scale score with checklist item scores to form a composite score may be one very important
source of *response process evidence.*

Internal Structure

Internal structure, as a source of validity evidence, relates to the statistical or psychometric characteristics of the examination questions
or performance prompts, the scale properties—such as reproducibility
and generalizability, and the psychometric model used to score and
scale the assessment. For instance, scores on test items or sets of
items intended to measure the same variable, construct, or content
area should be more highly correlated than scores on items intended
to measure a different variable, construct, or content area.

Many of the statistical analyses needed to support or refute evidence of the test's internal structure are often carried out as routine
quality-control procedures. Analyses such as statistical item analyses
—which computes the difficulty (or easiness) of each test question
(or performance prompt), the discrimination of each question (a
statistical index indicating how well the question separates the high
scoring from the low scoring examinees), and a detailed count of the
number or proportion of examinees who responded to each option of
the test question—are completed. Summary statistics are usually
computed, showing the overall difficulty (or easiness) of the total test
scale, the average discrimination, and the internal-consistency reliability of the test.

Reliability is one very important aspect or facet of validity evidence
for all assessment data. Reliability refers to the reproducibility of the
data or scores on the assessment; high score reliability indicates that if
the test were to be repeated over time, examinees would receive about
the same scores on retesting as they received the first time. Unless
assessment scores are reliable and reproducible (as in an experiment) it
is nearly impossible to interpret the meaning of those scores—thus,
validity evidence is lacking (Axelson & Kreiter, Chapter 3, this volume).

There are many different types of reliability, appropriate to various
uses of assessment scores. In both example assessments described

above, in which the stakes are high and a passing score has been established, the reproducibility of the pass–fail decision is a very important source of validity evidence. That is, analogous to score reliability, if the ultimate outcome of the assessment (passing or failing) cannot be reproduced at some high level of certainty, the meaningful interpretation of the test scores is questionable and validity evidence is compromised.

For performance examinations, such as the SP example, a specialized type of reliability, derived from Generalizability Theory (GT) is an essential component of the internal structure aspect of validity evidence (Brennan, 2001; Crossley, Davies, Humphris, & Jolly, 2002; Kreiter, Chapter 4, this volume). GT is concerned with how well the specific samples of behavior (in this example, SP cases) can be generalized to the population or universe of behaviors. GT is also a useful tool for estimating the various sources of contributed error in the SP exam, such as error due to the SP raters, error due to the cases (case specificity), and error associated with examinees. Since rater error and case specificity are major threats to meaningful interpretation of SP scores, GT analyses are important sources of validity evidence for most performance assessments such as OSCEs, SP exams, and clinical performance examinations.

The measurement model itself can serve as evidence of the internal structure aspect of construct validity. For example, Item Response Theory (IRT) measurement models (e.g., Downing, 2003b; Embretson & Reise, 2000; van der Linden & Hambleton, 1997), might be used to calibrate and score our example comprehensive examination, in which case the factor structure, item-intercorrelation structure, and other internal statistical characteristics of the examination can all contribute to validity evidence.

Issues of bias and fairness also pertain to internal test structure and are important sources of validity evidence. All assessments, presented to heterogeneous groups of examinees, have the potential of validity threats from statistical bias. Bias analyses, such as Differential Item Functioning (DIF) analyses (e.g., Holland & Wainer, 1993; Penfield & Lam, 2000) and the sensitivity review of item and performance prompts are sources of internal structure validity evidence

(Baranowski, 2006; Zieky, 2006). Documentation of the absence of statistical test bias permits the desired score interpretation and therefore adds to the validity evidence of the assessment.

Relationship to Other Variables

This familiar source of validity evidence is statistical and correlational. The correlation or relationship of assessment scores to a criterion measure's scores is a typical design for a validity study, in which some newer (or simpler or shorter) measure is validated against an existing, older measure with well known characteristics.

This source of validity evidence embodies all the richness and complexity of the contemporary theory of validity in that the *relationship to other variables* aspect seeks both confirmatory and counter-confirmatory evidence. For example, it may be important to collect correlational validity evidence which shows a strong positive correlation with some other measure of the same achievement or ability *and* evidence indicating no correlation (or a negative correlation) with some other assessment that is hypothesized to be a measure of some completely different achievement or ability.

The concept of convergence or divergence of validity evidence (or discriminant validity evidence) is best exemplified in the classic research design first described by Campbell and Fiske (1959). In this multitrait-multimethod design, multiple measures of the same trait (achievement, ability, performance) are correlated with each other and with different measures of the same trait. The resulting pattern of correlation coefficients show the convergence and divergence of the different assessment methods on measures of the same and different abilities or proficiencies, thus triangulating appropriate interpretations of scores on measures.

In the written comprehensive examination example discussed here, it may be important to document the correlation of total and subscale scores with achievement examinations administered during the basic science courses. One could hypothesize that a subscale score for biochemistry on the comprehensive examination would correlate more highly with biochemistry course test scores than with behavioral science course scores. Additionally, the correlation of the written examination scores with the SP final examination may show a low (or no) correlation, indicating that these assessment methods measure some unique achievement, while the correlation of the SP scores with other performance examination scores during the students' clinical training may be high and positive.

As with all research, issues of the generalizability of the results of these studies and the limitations of data interpretation pertain. Interpretation of correlation coefficients, as validity coefficients, may be limited due to the design of the study, systematic bias introduced by missing data from either the test or the criterion or both, and statistical issues such as restriction of the range of scores (lack of variance).

Consequences

This aspect of validity evidence may be the most controversial, although it is solidly embodied in the 1999 *Standards*. The consequential aspect of validity refers to the impact on examinees from the assessment scores, decisions, and outcomes and the impact of assessments on teaching and learning. The consequences of assessments on examinees, faculty, patients, and society can be great and these consequences can be positive or negative, intended or unintended.

High-stakes examinations abound in North America, especially in health professions education. Extremely high-stakes assessments are often mandated as the final, summative hurdle in professional education. As one excellent example, the United States Medical Licensure Examination (USMLE) sequence, sponsored by the National Board of Medical Examiners (NBME), currently consists of three separate examinations (Steps 1, 2, and 3) which must be passed in order to be licensed by the state or jurisdiction as a physician. The consequences of failing any of these examinations is enormous, in that medical education is interrupted in a costly manner or the examinee is not permitted to enter graduate medical education or practice medicine. Likewise, most medical specialty boards in the United States mandate passing a high-stakes certification examination in the specialty or subspecialty, after meeting all eligibility requirements of post-graduate training.

The consequences of passing or failing these types of examinations are great, since false positives (passing candidates who should fail) may do harm to patients through the lack of a physician's specialized knowledge or skill and false negatives (failing candidates who should pass) may unjustly harm individual candidates who have invested a great deal of time and resources in graduate medical education.

Thus, consequential validity is one very important aspect of the construct validity argument. Evidence related to consequences of testing and its outcomes is presented to suggest that no harm comes directly from the assessment or, at the very least, more good than harm arises from the assessment. Much of this evidence is more judgmental, qualitative or subjective than other aspects of validity.

In both of our example assessments, sources of consequential validity may relate to issues such as passing rates (the proportion who pass), the subjectively judged appropriateness of these passing rates, data comparing the passing rates of each of these examinations to other comprehensive examinations such as the USMLE Step 1, and so on. Evaluations of false positive and false negative outcomes relate to the consequences of these two high-stakes examinations.

The passing score (or grade levels) and the process used to determine the cut scores, the statistical properties of the passing scores, and so on all relate to the consequential aspects of validity (Cizek, 2006; Norcini, 2003; Yudkowsky, Downing, & Tekian, Chapter 6, this volume). Documentation of the method used to establish a pass–fail score is key consequential evidence, as is the rationale for the selection of a particular passing score method. The psychometric characteristics of the passing score judgments and the qualification and number of expert judges—all may be important to document and present as evidence of consequential validity.

Other psychometric quality indicators concerning the passing score and its consequences—for both example assessments—include a formal, statistical estimation of the pass–fail decision reliability or classification accuracy (e.g., Subkoviak, 1988). and some estimation of the standard error of measurement at the cut score (Angoff, 1971)

Equally important consequences of assessment methods on instruction and learning have been discussed by Newble and Jaeger (1983).

The methods and strategies selected to evaluate students can have a profound impact on what is taught, how and exactly what students learn, how this learning is used and retained (or not) and how students view and value the educational process.

These five sources or facets of validity evidence provide a systematic and concrete structure for validity studies and validation research. At least two different categories of validity evidence are required for most measures, with more evidence needed for higher-stakes test and assessment data. As Haladyna notes: "Without research, a testing program will have difficulty generating sufficient evidence to validate its intended test score interpretations and uses" (Haladyna, 2006, p. 739). For on-going high-stakes testing programs, validation research is a fairly open-ended loop in that too much validity evidence can never be presented, but often too little data is offered to support the particular score interpretations desired.

Threats to Validity

There are many threats to validity; in fact, there may be many more threats to validity than there are sources of validity evidence. Any factors that interfere with the meaningful interpretation of assessment data are a threat to validity. Messick (1989) noted two major sources of validity threats: construct underrepresentation (CU) and construct-irrelevant variance (CIV). CU refers to the undersampling or biased sampling of the content domain by the assessment instrument. CIV is systematic error (rather than random error) introduced into the assessment data by variables unrelated to the construct being measured. Both CU and CIV reduce the ability to interpret the assessment results in the proposed manner and thus decrease evidence for validity.

Table 2.3 lists examples of some typical threats to validity for written assessments, performance examinations, such as Objective Structured Clinical Examinations (OSCEs) or standardized patient (SP) examinations, and clinical performance ratings. These threats to validity are organized by CU and CIV, following Mesick's model.

Table 2.3 Threats to Validity of Assessments

	Written Test	Performance Examination	Ratings of Clinical Performance
Construct Underrepresentation (CU)	Too few items to sample domain adequately	Too few cases/OSCEs for generalizability	Too few observations of clinical behavior
	Biased/unrepresentative sample of domain	Unstandardized patient raters	Too few independent raters
	Mismatch of sample to domain	Unrepresentative cases	Incomplete observations
	Low score reliability	Low reliability of ratings	Low reliability of ratings/Low generalizability
Construct-irrelevant Variance (CIV)	Flawed item formats	Flawed cases/checklists/rating scales	Inappropriate rating items
	Biased items (DIF)	DIF for SP cases/rater bias	Rater bias
	Reading level of items inappropriate	SP use of inappropriate jargon	Systematic rater error: Halo, Severity, Leniency, Central tendency
	Items too easy/too hard/non-discriminating	Case difficulty inappropriate (too easy/too hard)	Inadequate sample of student behaviors
	Cheating/Insecure items	Bluffing of SPs	Bluffing of raters
	Indefensible passing score methods	Indefensible passing score methods	Indefensible passing score methods
	Teaching to the test	Poorly trained SPs	Poorly trained raters

Written Examinations

In a written examination, such as an objective test in a basic science course, CU is exemplified in an examination that is too short to adequately sample the domain being tested. Other examples of CU are: test item content that does not match the examination specifications well, so that some content areas are oversampled while others are undersampled; use of many items that test only low level cognitive behavior, such as recall or recognition of facts, while the instructional objectives required higher level cognitive behavior, such as application or problem solving; and, use of items which test trivial content that is unrelated to future learning (Downing, 2002b).

The remedies for the CU threats to validity are straightforward, although not always easily achieved. For any test taker, an achievement test should be a representative sample of items from the domain. That is, the domain may have subdomains, and these subdomains must be adequately sampled on any test. The length of the test should be adequate for the use of the test. For example, for a high-stakes pass–fail test, several hundred items are desired. For a test where assessment of learning is made, approximately 40 items might be minimally sufficient. One dimension of all achievement testing is the cognitive demand required. Does the test taker have to remember, understand or apply information? The proportion of items on such tests should be clearly specified and items should be written to test higher cognitive levels, if the instructional objectives require higher-order learning. Items should test important information, not trivia.

CIV may be introduced into written examination scores from many sources (Haladyna & Downing, 2004). CIV represents systematic "noise" in the measurement data, often associated with the scores of some but not all examinees. CIV is a type of nuisance variable and comprises the unintended measurement of some construct that is off-target, not associated with the primary construct of interest, and therefore interferes with the validity evidence for assessment data. For instance, flawed or poorly crafted item formats, which make it more difficult for some students to give a correct answer, introduce CIV into the measurement (Downing, 2002a, 2005), as does the use of many test items that are too difficult or too easy for student achievement levels and items that do not discriminate high-achieving from low-achieving students. CIV is also introduced by including statistically biased items on which some subgroup of students under- or over-performs compared to their expected performance or by including test items which offend some students by their use of culturally insensitive language. If some students have prior access to test items and other students do not have such access, this type of test security breach represents CIV and makes score interpretation difficult or impossible by seriously reducing the validity evidence for the assessment data. Likewise, other types of test irregularities, such as cheating, introduce CIV and compromise the ability to interpret scores meaningfully. A related CIV issue is "teaching to the test," such that the instructor uses actual test items for teaching, thus creating misleading or incorrect inferences about the meaning of scores (if the construct of interest is student achievement and not simply the ability to memorize answers to test items).

If the reading level of achievement test items is inappropriate for students, reading ability becomes a CIV variable which is unrelated or only minimally related to the construct intended to be measured, thereby introducing CIV (Abedi, 2006). Reading level issues may be particularly important for students taking tests written in their non-native language. By using complex sentence structures, challenging vocabulary, and idiosyncratic jargon, we run the risk of underestimating the achievement of any student whose first language is not English. While guessing is generally not a major issue on long tests, composed of well-crafted multiple-choice test items with at least three options (Haladyna & Downing, 1993; Rodriguez, 2005), random guessing of correct answers on multiple-choice items can introduce CIV, because the student's propensity to guess is a personality factor which is not directly related to the achievement construct intended to be measured (Downing, 2003a). Poorly crafted items, which violate one or more of the standard principles of effective item writing, may introduce CIV (Downing, 2005) by providing clues to the correct answer for some students who do not know the correct answer or by leading other students to answer incorrectly in spite of the fact that they actually know the correct answer.

If one accepts the consequential aspects of validity as a major source of validity evidence, then anything that interferes with the accurate determination of pass–fail status for some students on an assessment, may be considered CIV, since it adds non-random error to the measurement outcomes. All passing score determination methods, whether relative or absolute, are arbitrary. However, these methods and their results should not be capricious nor random (Norcini, 2003). If passing scores or grade-levels are determined in a manner such that they lack reproducibility, are statistically biased for some groups or subgroups, or produce cut scores that are so unrealistic that unacceptably high (or low) numbers of students fail, this introduces systematic CIV error into the final outcome of the assessment.

What are the solutions for these types of CIV problems? On written achievement tests, items should be well crafted and follow the basic evidence-based principles of effective item writing (Case & Swanson, 1998; Haladyna, Downing, & Rodriguez, 2002). The item format itself should not be an impediment to student assessment. The reading ability of students should not be a major factor in the assessment of the achievement construct. Most items should be targeted in difficulty to student achievement levels. All items that are empirically shown to be biased or use language that offends some cultural, racial, or ethnic group should be eliminated from the test. Test items must be maintained securely and tests should be administered in proctored, controlled environments so that any potential cheating is minimized or eliminated. Instructors should not teach directly to the content of the test. Instead, teaching should be to the content domain of which the test is a small sample. And, finally, passing scores (or grading standards) should be established in a systematic and defensible manner, which is unbiased and fair to all students.

Performance Examinations

OSCEs or SP examinations increase the fidelity of the assessment and are intended to measure performance, rather than knowledge or skills (Miller, 1990; Yudkowsky, Chapter 9, this volume). Performance assessments are closer in proximity to the actual criterion performance of interest, but these types of assessment also involve constructs, because they sample performance behavior in a standardized or simulated context. Such tests approximate the real world, but are not the real world. The performance of students, rated by trained SPs in a simulated and controlled environment on a finite number of selected cases requiring maximum performance, is not *actual* performance in the real world; rather, inferences must be made from performance ratings to the domain of performance, with a specific interpretation or meaning attributed to the checklist or the rating-scale data. Validity evidence must be documented to support or refute the proposed meanings associated with these performance-type constructs.

There are many potential CU and CIV threats to validity for performance assessments. In Table 2.3, some examples of validity threats are presented. Many threats are the same as noted for written tests. One major CU threat arises from using too few performance cases to adequately sample or generalize to the domain. The case specificity of performance cases is well documented (e.g., Elstein, Shulman, & Sprafka, 1978; Norman, Tugwell, Feightner, Muzzin, & Jacoby, 1985). Approximately 10 to 12 SP encounters, lasting up to 20 or 25 minutes each, may be required to achieve even minimal generalizability in order to support inferences to the domain (van der Vleuten & Swanson, 1990). Lack of sufficient generalizability is a CU threat to validity. If performance cases are unrepresentative of the performance domain of interest, CU threatens validity by misrepresenting or biasing the inferences to the domain. For example, in an SP examination of patient communication skills, if the medical content of the cases is atypical and unrepresentative of the domain, it may be impossible for students to demonstrate their patient communication skills adequately.

Many SP examinations use trained lay simulated patients to portray actual patient medical problems and to rate student performance, after the encounter, using standardized checklists or rating scales. The quality of the SP portrayal is extremely important, as is the quality of the SPs training in the appropriate use of checklists and rating scales. If the SPs are not well trained to consistently portray the patient in a standardized manner, different students effectively encounter different patients and slightly different patient problems. The construct of interest is, therefore, misrepresented, because all students do not encounter the same patient problem or stimulus.

Remedies for CU in SP examinations include the use of large numbers of representative cases, using well-trained SP raters. SP monitoring, during multi-day performance examinations, is critical, such that any slippage in the standard portrayal can be corrected during the time of the examination.

For a performance examination, such as an OSCE or SP

examination, there are many potential CIV threats. CIV on a SP examination concerns issues such as systematic rater error which is uncorrected statistically, such that student scores are systematically higher or lower than they should be. SP cases that are flawed or of inappropriate difficulty for students and checklist or rating scale items that are ambiguous may introduce CIV. Statistical bias for one or more subgroups of students, which is undetected and uncorrected, may systematically raise or lower SP scores, unfairly advantaging some students and penalizing others. Racial or ethnic rater bias on the part of the SP rater creates CIV and makes the score interpretation difficult or impossible. Also, all the classic rater errors, such as severity/leniency, halo, central tendency, restriction of the range and many other idiosyncratic types of rater error add CIV, since this type of error is systematic rather than random (e.g., Engelhard, 2002).

It is possible for students to bluff SPs, particularly on non-medical aspects of SP cases, making ratings higher for some students than they actually should be. Establishing passing scores for SP examinations is challenging; if these cut scores are indefensibly established, the consequential aspect of validity will be reduced and CIV will be introduced to the assessment, making the evaluation of student performance difficult or impossible.

The remedies for CU in performance examinations are obvious, but may be difficult and costly to implement. Low reliability is a major threat to validity (Messick, 1989), thus using sufficient numbers of reliable and representative cases to adequately generalize to the proposed domain is critical. Generalizability must be estimated for most performance-type examinations, using Generalizability Theory (Brennan, 2001). For high-stakes performance examinations, Generalizability coefficients should be at least 0.80; the phi-coefficient is the appropriate estimate of generalizability for criterion-referenced performance examinations, which have absolute, rather than relative passing scores (van der Vlueten & Swanson, 1990). SPs should be well trained in their patient roles and their portrayals monitored throughout the time period of the examination to ensure standardization. To control or eliminate CIV in performance examinations, checklists and rating scales must be well developed, critiqued, edited, and tried-out and must be sufficiently accurate to provide reproducible data, when completed by the SPs who are well trained in their use. Methods to detect statistical bias in performance-examination ratings should be implemented for high-stakes examinations (De Champlain & Floreck, 2002). Performance cases should be pretested with a representative group of students prior to their final use, testing the appropriateness of case difficulty and all other aspects of the case presentation. SP training is critical, in order to eliminate sources of CIV introduced by variables such as SP-rater bias and student success at bluffing the SP. If passing scores or grades are assigned to the performance examination results, these scores must be established in a defensible, systematic, reproducible, and fair manner.

Ratings of Clinical Performance

In health professions education, ratings of student clinical performance in clerkships or preceptorships are often a major assessment modality. This method depends primarily on faculty observations of student clinical performance behavior in a naturalistic setting (McGaghie, Butter, & Kaye, Chapter 8, this volume). Clinical performance ratings are unstandardized, often unsystematic, and are frequently completed by faculty who are not well trained in their use. Thus, there are many threats to validity of clinical performance ratings by the very nature of the manner in which they are typically obtained.

The CU threat is exemplified by too few observations of the target or rated behavior by the faculty raters (Table 2.3). Williams, Klamen, and McGaghie (2003) suggest that 7 to 11 independent ratings of clinical performance are required to produce sufficiently generalizable data to be useful and interpretable. The use of too few independent observations and ratings of clinical performance is a major CU threat to validity.

CIV is introduced into clinical ratings in many ways. The major CIV threat is due to systematic rater error. Raters are the major source of measurement error for these types of observational assessments, but CIV is associated with systematic rater error, such as rater severity or leniency errors, central tendency error (rating in the center of the rating scale) and restriction of range (failure to use all the points on the rating scale). The halo rater effect occurs when the rater ignores the traits to be rated and treats all traits as if they were one. Thus, ratings tend to be repetitious and inflate estimates of reliability.

Although better training may help to reduce some undesirable rater effects, another way to combat rater severity or leniency error is to estimate the extent of severity (or leniency) and adjust the final ratings to eliminate the unfairness that results from harsh or lenient raters. Computer software is available to estimate these rater-error effects and adjust final ratings accordingly. While this is one potentially effective method to reduce or eliminate CIV due to rater severity or leniency, other rater-error effects, such as central tendency errors, restriction in the use of the rating scale, and idiosyncratic rater error remain difficult to detect and correct (Haladyna & Downing, 2004).

Rating scales are frequently used for clinical performance ratings. If the items are inappropriately written, such that raters are confused by the wording or misled to rate a different student characteristic from that which was intended, CIV may be introduced. Unless raters are well trained in the proper use of the observational rating scale and trained to use highly similar standards, CIV may be introduced into the data, making the proposed interpretation of ratings difficult and less meaningful. Students may also attempt to bluff the raters and intentionally try to mislead the observer into one or more of the systematic CIV rater errors noted.

As with other types of assessment, the methods used to establish passing scores or grades may be a source of CIV. Additionally, methods of combining clinical performance observational data with other types of assessment data, such as written test scores and SP performance examination scores may be a CIV source. If the procedures used to combine different types of assessment data into one composite score are inappropriate, CIV may be introduced such that the proposed interpretation of the final score is incorrect or diminished in meaning (Norcini & Guille, 2002).

Remedies for the CU and CIV threats to validity of clinical performance data are suggested by the specific issues noted. For CU, many independent ratings of behavior are needed, by well trained raters who are qualified to make the required evaluative judgments and are motivated to fulfill these responsibilities. The mean rating, over several independent raters, may tend to reduce the CIV due to systematic rater error, but will not entirely eliminate it, as in the case of a student who luckily draws two or more lenient raters or is unlucky in being rated by two or more harsh raters.

Passing score determination may be more difficult for observational clinical performance examinations, but is an essential component of the assessment and a potential source of CIV error. The method and procedures used to establish defensible, reproducible, and fair passing scores or grades for clinical performance examinations are as important as for other assessment methods and similar procedures may be used (Downing, Tekian, & Yudkowsky, 2006; Norcini & Shea, 1997).

What about Face Validity?

The term *face validity*, despite its popularity in some health professions educator's usage and vocabulary, has been derided by educational measurement professionals since at least the 1940s. *Face validity* can have many different meanings. The most pernicious meaning, according to Mosier, is: "the validity of the test is best determined by using common sense in discovering that the test measures component abilities which exist both in the test situation and on the job" (Mosier, 1947, p. 194). This type of face validity represents a belief and has no place in the science of validation research (Downing, 2006a). Clearly, this meaning of *face validity* has no place in the literature or vocabulary of health professions educators. Further, reliance on this type of face validity as a major source of validity evidence for assessments is a major threat to validity and a potential source of harm to our students and society.

Face validity, in the meaning above, is not endorsed by any contemporary educational measurement researchers (Downing, 1996). Face validity is not any type of legitimate source of validity evidence and can never substitute for any of the many evidentiary sources of validity discussed in this chapter (Messick, 1989; Kane, 2006b).

Can face validity have any legitimate meaning in health professions education? If by *face validity* one means that the assessment has superficial qualities that make it appear to measure the intended construct (e.g., the SP case looks like it assesses history taking skills or communications skills), this may be an important characteristic of the assessment, but it is not validity. Such an SP characteristic has to do with acceptance of the assessment by students and faculty or is important for administrators and even the public, but it is not validity. But, the avoidance of this type of *face invalidity* was endorsed by Messick (1989). The appearance of validity is not validity; appearance is not scientific evidence, derived from hypothesis and theory, supported or unsupported, more or less, by empirical data and formed into logical arguments.

Alternate terms for *face validity* might be considered. For example, if an objective test looks like it measures the achievement construct of interest, one might consider this some type of value-added and important trait of the assessment that may be required for the overall success of the assessment program, its acceptance and its utility, but this clearly is not sufficient scientific evidence of validity. The appearance of validity may be necessary, but it is not sufficient evidence of validity. The congruence between the superficial look and feel of the assessment and solid validity evidence might be referred to as *congruent* or *social-political meaningfulness*, but it is clearly not a primary type of validity evidence and can not, in any way, substitute for any of the five suggested primary sources of validity evidence (AERA, APA, & NCME, 1999).

Summary

This chapter has reviewed the contemporary meaning of validity, a unitary concept with multiple facets, which considers construct validity as the whole of validity. Validity evidence refers to the data and information collected in order to assign meaningful interpretation to assessment scores or outcomes, which were designed for a specific purpose and at one specific point in time. Validity always refers to score interpretations or the desired meanings associated with score data and never to the assessment itself. The process of validation is closely aligned with the scientific method of theory development, hypothesis generation, data collection for the purpose of hypothesis testing, and forming conclusions concerning the accuracy of the desired score interpretations. Validity refers to the impartial, scientific collection of data, from multiple sources, to provide more or less support for the validity hypothesis and relates to logical arguments, based on theory and data, which are formed to assign meaningful interpretations to assessment data.

The chapter discussed five typical sources of validity evidence—Content, Response process, Internal structure, Relationship to other variables, and Consequences—as described by validity theorists such as Messick and Kane and embodied in the 1999 *Standards*.

This chapter also summarized two broad general threats to validity in the context of the contemporary meaning of validity. These threats are construct underrepresentation (CU) and construct-irrelevant variance (CIV). CU threats relate primarily to undersampling or biased sampling of the content domain or the selection or creation of assessment items or performance prompts that do not match the appropriate construct definition and thus fail to sample the proper domain. CIV adds "noise" to the assessment data and introduces systematic, rather than random, measurement error, which reduces our ability to interpret assessment outcomes in the proposed manner. Face validity was rejected as any type of legitimate source of validity evidence. Sole reliance on this pernicious type of validity is a threat to validity.

References

Abedi, J. (2006). Language issues in item development. In S.M. Downing & T.M. Haladyna (Eds.), *Handbook of test development* (pp. 377–398). Mahwah, NJ: Lawrence Erlbaum Associates.

American Educational Research Association, American Psychological Association, & National Council on Measurement in Education. (1999). *Standards for educational and psychological testing*. Washington, DC: American Educational Research Association.

Angoff, W.H. (1971). Scales, norms, and equivalent scores. In R.L. Thorndike (Ed.), *Educational measurement* (2d ed., pp. 508–600). Washington: American Council on Education.

Auewarakul, C., Downing, S.M., Jaturatumrong, U., & Praditsuwan, R. (2005). Sources of validity evidence for an internal medicine student evaluation system: An evaluative study of assessment methods. *Medical Education*, 39, 276–283.

Baranowski, R. (2006). Item editing and editorial review. In S.M. Downing & T.M. Haladyna (Eds.), *Handbook of test development* (pp. 349–357). Mahwah, NJ: Lawrence Erlbaum Associates.

Beckman, T.J., & Cook, D.A. (2005). What is the validity evidence for assessments of clinical teaching? *Journal of General Internal Medicine*, 20, 1159–1164.

Boulet, J.R., McKinley, D.W., Whelan, G.P., & Hambleton, R.K. (2003). Quality assurance methods for performance-based assessments. *Advances in Health Sciences Education*, 8, 27–47.

Brennan, R.L. (2001). *Generalizability theory*. New York: Springer-Verlag.

Campbell, D.T., & Fiske D.W. (1959). Convergent and discriminant validation by the multitrait-multimethod matrix. *Psychological Bulletin*, 56, 81–105.

Case, S.M., & Swanson, D.B. (1998). *Constructing written test questions for the basic and clinical sciences* (2nd ed.). Philadelphia, PA: National Board of Medical Examiners.

Cizek, G.J. (2006). Standard setting. In S.M. Downing & T.M. Haladyna (Eds.), *Handbook of test development* (pp. 225–258). Mahwah, NJ: Lawrence Erlbaum Associates.

Cook, D.A., & Beckman, T.J. (2006). Current concepts in validity and reliability for psychometric instruments: Theory and application. *American Journal of Medicine*, 119(2), e7–16.

Cronbach, L.J. (1980). Validity on parole: How can we go straight? New directions for testing and measurement: Measuring achievement over a decade. *Proceedings of the 1979 ETS Invitational Conference* (pp. 99–108). San Francisco: Jossey-Bass.

Cronbach, L.J. (1988). Five perspectives on validity argument. In H. Wainer & H. Braun (Eds.), *Test validity* (pp. 3–17). Hillsdale, NJ: Lawrence Erlbaum.

Cronbach, L.J. (1989). Construct validation after thirty years. In R.E. Linn (Ed.), *Intelligence: Measurement, theory, and public policy* (pp. 147–171). Urbana, IL: University of Illinois Press.

Cronbach, L.J., & Meehl, P.E. (1955). Construct validity in psychological tests. *Psychological Bulletin*, 52, 281–302.

Crossley, J., Davies, H., Humphris, G., & Jolly, B. (2002). Generalisability; a key to unlock professional assessment. *Medical Education*, 36, 972–978.

Cureton, E.E. (1951). Validity. In E.F. Lingquist (Ed.), *Educational measurement* (pp. 621–694). Washington: American Council on Education.

De Champlain, A.F., & Floreck, L.M. (2002, April). Assessing potential bias in a large-scale standardized patient examination: An application of common DIF methods for polytomous items. Paper presented at the Annual Meeting of the American Educational Research Association, New Orleans, LA.

Downing S.M. (1996). Test validity evidence: What about face validity? *CLEAR Exam Review*, Sum, 31–33.

Downing S.M. (2002a). Construct-irrelevant variance and flawed test questions: Do multiple-choice item writing principles make any difference? *Academic Medicine*, 77, S103–S104.

Downing, S.M. (2002b). Threats to the validity of locally developed multiple-choice tests in medical education: Construct-irrelevant variance and construct underrepresentation. *Advances in Health Sciences Education*, 7, 235–241.

Downing, S.M. (2003a). Guessing on selected-response examinations. *Medical Education*, 37, 670–671.

Downing, S.M. (2003b). Item response theory: Applications in modern test theory in medical education. *Medical Education*, 37, 1–7.

Downing, S.M. (2005). The effects of violating standard item writing principles on tests and students: The consequences of using flawed test items on achievement examinations in medical education. *Advances in Health Sciences Education*, 10, 133–143.

Downing, S.M. (2006a). Face validity of assessments: Faith-based interpretations or evidence-based science? *Medical Education*, 40, 7–8.

Downing, S.M. (2006b). Twelve steps for effective test development. In S.M. Downing & T.M. Haladyna (Eds.), *Handbook of test development* (pp. 3–25). Mahwah, NJ: Lawrence Erlbaum Associates.

Downing, S.M., Tekian, A., & Yudkowsky, R. (2006). Procedures for establishing defensible absolute passing scores on performance examinations in health professions education. *Teaching & Learning in Medicine*, 18(1), 50–57.

Ebel, R.L. (1972). *Essentials of educational measurement* (2nd ed.). Englewood Cliffs, NJ: Prentice-Hall.

Elstein, A.S, Shulman, L.S, & Sprafka, S.A. (1978). *Medical problem solving: An analysis of clinical reasoning*. Cambridge, MA: Harvard University Press.

Embretson, S.E., & Reise, S.P. (2000). *Item response theory for psychologists*. Mahwah, NJ: Lawrence Erlbaum Associates.

Engelhard, G. Jr. (2002). Monitoring raters in performance assessments. In G. Tindal & T.M. Haladyna (Eds.), *Large-scale assessment programs for all students: Validity, technical adequacy, and implementation* (pp. 261–288). Mahwah, NJ: Lawrence Erlbaum Associates.

Haladyna, T.M. (2006). Roles and importance of validity studies in test development. In S.M. Downing & T.M. Haladyna (Eds.), *Handbook of test development* (pp. 739–755). Mahwah, NJ: Lawrence Erlbaum Associates.

Haladyna, T.M., & Downing, S.M. (1993). How many options is enough for a multiple-choice test item? *Education and Psychological Measurement*, 53, 999–1010.

Haladyna, T.M, & Downing, S.M. (2004). Construct-irrelevant variance in high-stakes testing. *Educational Measurement: Issues and Practice*, 23(1), 17–27.

Haladyna, T.M., Downing, S.M., & Rodriguez, M.C. (2002). A review of multiple-choice item-writing guidelines for classroom assessment. *Applied Measurement in Education*, 15(3), 309–334.

Holland, P.W., & Wainer, H. (Eds.). (1993). *Differential item functioning*. Mahwah, NJ: Lawrence Erlbaum.

Kane, M.T. (1992). An argument-based approach to validation. *Psychological Bulletin*, 112, 527–535.

Kane, M.T. (1994). Validating interpretive arguments for licensure and certification examinations. *Evaluation and the Health Professions*, 17, 133–159.

Kane, M. (2006a). Content-related validity evidence in test development. In S.M. Downing & T.M. Haladyna (Eds.), *Handbook of test development* (pp. 131–153). Mahwah, NJ: Lawrence Erlbaum Associates.

Kane, M. (2006b) Validation. In R.L. Brennan (Ed.), *Educational measurement* (4th ed., pp. 17–64). New York: American Council on Education and Greenwood.

Linn, R.L. (2002). Validation of the uses and interpretations of results of state assessment and accountability systems. In G. Tindal & T. Haladyna (Eds.), *Large-scale assessment programs for all students: Development, implementation, and analysis* (pp. 27–48). Mahwah, NJ: Lawrence Erlbaum Associates.

Linn, R.L. (2006). The standards for educational and psychological testing: Guidance in test development. In S.M. Downing & T.M. Haladyna (Eds.), *Handbook of test development* (pp. 27–38). Mahwah, NJ: Lawrence Erlbaum Associates.

Messick, S. (1989). Validity. In R.L. Linn (Ed.), *Educational measurement* (3rd ed., pp. 13–104). New York: American Council on Education and Macmillan.

Messick, S. (1995). Validity of psychological assessment: Validation of inferences from persons' responses and performances as scientific inquiry into score meaning. *American Psychologist*, 50, 741–749.

Miller, G.E. (1990). The assessment of clinical skills/competence/performance. *Academic Medicine*, 65, s63–67.

Mosier, C.I. (1947). A critical examination of the concepts of face validity. *Educational and Psychological Measurement*, 7, 191–205.

Newble, D.I., & Jaeger, K. (1983). The effects of assessment and examinations on the learning of medical students. *Medical Education*, 17, 165–171.

Norcini, J.J. (2003). Setting standards on educational tests. *Medical Education*, 37, 464–469.

Norcini, J., & Guille, R. (2002). Combining tests and setting standards. In G.R. Norman, C.P.M. van der Vleuten, & D.I. Newble (Eds.),

International handbook of research in medical education (pp. 811–834). Dordrecht, The Netherlands: Kluwer Academic Publishers.

Norcini, J.J., & Shea, J.A. (1997). The credibility and comparability of standards. *Applied Measurement in Education*, 10, 39–59.

Norman, G.R., Tugwell, P., Feightner, J.W., Muzzin, L.J., & Jacoby, L.L. (1985). Knowledge and problem-solving. *Medical Education*, 19, 344–356.

Penfield, R.D., & Lam, R.C.M. (2000). Assessing differential item functioning in performance assessment: Review and recommendations. *Educational Measurement: Issues and Practice*, 19, 5–15.

Raymond, M., & Neustel, S. (2006). Determining the content of credentialing examinations. In S.M. Downing & T.M. Haladyna (Eds.), *Handbook of test development* (pp. 181–223). Mahwah, NJ: Lawrence Erlbaum Associates.

Rodriguez, M.C. (2005). Three options are optimal for multiple-choice items: A meta-analysis of 80 years of research. *Educational Measurement: Issues and Practice*, Summer, 3–13.

Subkoviak, M.J. (1988). A practitioner's guide to computation and interpretation of reliability indices for mastery tests. *Journal of Educational Measurement*, 25, 47–55.

Van der Linden, W.J., & Hambleton, R.K. (1997). Item response theory: Brief history, common models, and extensions. In W.J. van der Linden & R.K. Hambleton (Eds.), *Handbook of modern item response theory* (pp. 1–28). New York: Springer-Verlag.

van der Vleuten, C.P.M., & Swanson, D.B. (1990). Assessment of clinical skills with standardized patients: State of the art. *Teaching and Learning in Medicine*, 2, 58–76.

Williams, R.G., Klamen, D.A., & McGaghie, W.C. (2003). Cognitive, social and environmental sources of bias in clinical competence ratings. *Teaching and Learning in Medicine*, 15, 270–292.

Zieky, M. (2006). Fairness review in assessment. In S.M. Downing & T.M. Haladyna (Eds.), *Handbook of test development* (pp. 359–376). Mahwah, NJ: Lawrence Erlbaum Associates.

3

RELIABILITY

RICK D. AXELSON AND CLARENCE D. KREITER

Introduction

Reliability plays a central role in educational measurement and social science research. It provides a set of concepts and indices for assessing the proportionate amount of random error contained in data. While all educational measurements contain some level of measurement error, the particular types of assessments used in the social sciences are especially vulnerable to measurement error.

To illustrate the concept of error, consider the following situation. You and a friend are having a conversation over lunch in a busy restaurant. There are also a number of other sounds—conversations at other tables, rattling of dishes, traffic noises from outside, and air whooshing through the heating vent. This makes it difficult to hear the message of interest. The types of sounds that you hear at lunch could be classified either as distracting background noise (random sounds) or your friend's words (meaningful sound or information). The proportion of your friend's remarks that you heard and could interpret could range from 0 (background noise completely drowned out the conversation) to 1.0 (clearly understood every word he said). The closer you are to 1.0 on this scale, the more likely it would be that you could give a trustworthy and reliable account of the conversation. Similarly, one could look at research and assessment data in this same way; it contains two sources of variation—random error or noise and systematic information. The reliability of assessment data increases as it contains less random error.

Reliable data are fundamental to effective assessment practices and comprise an essential element of validity. Reliable data provide the foundation of trustworthy evidence needed to inform and enhance effective practices. Although reliability and validity are often treated as distinct and separate aspects or indicators of data quality, they are in fact inextricably linked. Perhaps the most succinct description of this relationship is conveyed by the observation that reliability is a necessary but not sufficient condition for validity. It is obvious that if a score is totally unreliable it will also be invalid and meaningless for any particular use or interpretation. This is true because measures with reliability of zero are totally composed of random error and hence cannot be measuring any meaningful aspect of an individual. But, on the other hand, it is possible to imagine scores that are perfectly reliable but totally invalid for certain purposes or interpretations. For example, although a measure of adult height would likely produce highly reliable and consistent values, it would not be valid to use these values as a measure of individuals' general intelligence.

In this chapter, we will explore the concept of reliability in greater detail, show how it can be assessed and enhanced in different assessment contexts, and how it can help determine the adequacy and validity of assessment data for particular uses. We begin with a conceptual discussion of reliability and its relationship to variance, and then move toward a more precise formulation of reliability through a discussion of its role in classical test theory (CTT), which is also often referred to as classical measurement theory (CMT). Each concept is also demonstrated with an applied example from within the context of health science education. The goal is to provide the reader with meaningful ways of understanding, assessing, and applying information about reliability.

The Conceptual Foundation of Reliability in Classical Test Theory

The concept and estimation of reliability assumes a central role in educational assessment. While all measurements are prone to some level of error, individual educational assessment measures often contain high levels of error. For example, consider a single global rating of a nursing or medical student's performance within a clinical setting.

Measurement studies have suggested that such ratings are not primarily dependent on a student's clinical ability, but rather a reflection of the particular circumstances (e.g. the medical case, rater, and so forth) in which the rating took place (e.g., Carline, Wenrich, & Ramsey, 1989; Kreiter, Gordon, Elliott, & Callaway, 1998). When considering the high level of error in such ratings, one might be tempted to reject their usefulness as an educational assessment. Fortunately, however, an understanding of reliability theory and the statistical quantification of error allows educators to generate valid and reliable judgments even when the individual measures employed are quite error prone. In this section we will discuss procedures for understanding and quantifying the measurement error affecting reliability. While simply calculating reliability will not improve measurement precision, we will demonstrate how utilizing reliability related concepts can improve the accuracy of the judgments, grades, and other summary scores employed in health science education.

Statistical Definition of Reliability

Test or assessment data are reliable to the degree to which they can be replicated or reproduced. For instance, imagine the repeated measurement of some characteristic of a single person, for example their height. The dispersion, variation, scatter, or variance of these repeated measures around that person's mean score (height) is referred to as *error variance* (σ^2_{error}), and is an indication of the imprecision of measurement. An individual's mean score across an infinite number of repeated measurements will cancel out all of the random error or "noise" in the measurement and is considered that person's "*true score.*" Note that the *observed* score (the score we record from the test or assessment) is comprised of the true score plus error.

Given the true score distribution across a group of persons, commonly summarized as *true score variance* (σ^2_{true}), and the distribution of repeated measures within examinees (σ^2_{error}), it is possible to represent *reliability* as the ratio of true score variance divided by the sum of true score variance plus error score variance.

$$\text{Reliability} = \frac{\text{True score variance}}{\text{True score variance} + \text{error variance}}$$

$$= \frac{\sigma^2_{\text{true}}}{\sigma^2_{\text{true}} + \sigma^2_{\text{error}}} = \frac{\sigma^2_{\text{true}}}{\sigma^2_{\text{observed}}} \tag{3.1}$$

Using the noisy room metaphor we began with, we can think of reliability as the proportion of data available that is useful information or "signal":

$$\text{Reliability} = \frac{\text{signal}}{\text{signal} + \text{noise}} \tag{3.2}$$

Note that in CTT, systematic variation is solely attributable to variation in true scores. However, in practice, there are other sources of systematic variation, such as rater or measurement bias. For example, a scale that consistently registers 10 pounds heavier than the object's true weight produces a systematic rather than a random source of error. Systematic measurement error will not be detected in reliability analyses, but it will negatively impact the interpretability of the measure and, hence, its validity. Chapter 2 (Downing & Haladyna, this volume) provides a discussion of systematic error, also called Construct-irrelevant Variance, which is a general threat to test score validity. Chapters 7 to 12 provide recommendations for decreasing systematic error in various types of testing formats.

The Theory: Statistical Foundations of Reliability

In thinking about the statistical estimation of reliability, it is important again to remember its close association with the concept of replication. Conceptually and statistically, when considering how closely two separate measurements or replications agree, we usually think in terms of correlation. Indeed, a correlation coefficient can be used to estimate reliability.

Reliability and Randomly Parallel Tests

As an example, let's suppose that test x and test x' are two "randomly parallel" tests. In this case, the term "randomly parallel" implies that each test is generated by randomly sampling items from the same item bank. If each test were composed of 50 unique biochemistry items sampled at random from a large common item bank, the tests would be quite similar except for the slight variations resulting from sampling error. If both of these tests were administered to a single sample of examinees, the correlation between the two randomly parallel tests could serve as an estimate of the reliability of scores generated by test x.

Although this is a valid methodology for estimating reliability, in practice, instructors seldom have the time or resources to generate and administer randomly parallel tests. Nonetheless, the practice of correlating parallel test scores to derive an estimate of reliability underlies the logic for deriving reliability estimates based on the correlated scores from random halves of a single test (such as internal consistency reliability estimates). Because estimating reliability using split-half methods is efficient and generally reflects the overall replicability or internal test consistency, it is by far the most common technique used in health science assessments. A discussion of procedures for estimating reliability from a single administration of a test is provided in the next section.

The Practice: Practical Methods for Estimating Reliability

In considering a practical method for estimating reliability in a real assessment context, such as a multiple-choice (MC) test, how can we separate random score variation (i.e., measurement error) from systematic variation (i.e., true score)?

Test–Retest Reliability

One way would be to have individuals take the same test multiple times. Then, under classical test theory assumptions, a person's true score (systematic score component) is equal to his/her average score over a very large number of tests, and the differences between a person's average score and each of his/her separate test scores would be error. A major difficulty with using such a test–retest approach to estimate reliability is the impracticality of arranging repeated testing sessions for individuals. Additionally, obtaining accurate estimates with this approach rests upon the dubious assumption that examinees do not remember information from earlier testing sessions. The test–retest method of estimating reliability is of only theoretical and conceptual interest now, since far more efficient techniques—such as the internal consistency methods—are now available.

Single Test Reliability: Internal Consistency

Consequently, rather than replicating testing sessions to estimate reliability, practitioners generally opt for an internal-consistency method. Using an internal-consistency method, only one testing session is needed and it is the consistency among the subparts of the test that becomes the basis for estimating reliability. One early way of doing this was to split the test into two random halves and calculate the correlation between respondents' scores on the two sets of items. This correlation provided an estimate of the agreement between test replications.

The difficulty with the split-half method described above occurs when separating the items into two groups. There are multiple ways of splitting the items. Even in a relatively simple case of separating six items into two groups of three, there are ten possible ways to do this. Each of the ten splits will likely yield different estimates of the coefficient of reliability. Since the selection of any one configuration is arbitrary, what estimate of reliability should be used? One way out of this conundrum is to calculate the average correlation across all splits. This is effectively what coefficient alpha does.

Coefficient alpha, often referred to as Cronbach's alpha, is a widely used measure of internal-consistency reliability. Like other measures of reliability, it represents the proportion of systematic or true score variance in the total test score variance. Consider each item in the test as an attempt to measure an underlying ability or construct such as "knowledge of biochemistry." Then coefficient alpha reflects how strongly the responses to the different items on the test all depend on examinee ability in biochemistry. Greater shared variance or correlations among the items results in higher coefficient alpha values; this indicates closer alignment around the common underlying construct "knowledge of biochemistry."

As an example consider the scores obtained on a five-item biochemistry quiz. Ten examinees who took the quiz had the patterns of correct = 1 and incorrect = 0 responses displayed in Table 3.1.

Using commonly available statistical software applications, we find that coefficient alpha for these five items equals 0.538. An alpha of 0.538 indicates that just over half of the observed variation in total scores is due to variation in examinee ability (true score). Or, conversely, just under half of the observed score variation $(0.462 = 1 - 0.538)$ is due to random error rather than examinee ability. The large random error component is due to the fact that any given item is an imperfect measure of the underlying construct of "knowledge of biochemistry."

Reliability coefficients of less than 0.50 are not uncommon for very short tests and quizzes. Whether this alpha indicates a sufficient level of reliability depends upon how the test will be used. Downing (2004) notes that educational measurement professionals generally suggest the following interpretative guidance for alpha:

Table 3.1 Hypothetical Five-Item MC Quiz Results for 10 Students

Student ID	Item 1	Item 2	Item 3	Item 4	Item 5	Students' Total Correct
A	0	0	1	0	0	1
B	0	1	1	0	1	3
C	0	1	1	0	0	2
D	1	0	0	0	0	1
E	0	0	0	1	1	2
F	1	1	1	0	1	4
G	1	0	0	1	1	3
H	0	0	0	0	0	0
I	0	0	0	0	0	0
J	1	1	1	0	1	4

Notes: Mean score for the class = 2   Standard Deviation (SD) = 1.49

- 0.90 or higher is needed for very high stakes tests (e.g., licensure, certification exams)
- 0.80–0.89 is acceptable for moderate stakes tests (e.g., end-of-year summative exams in medical school, end-of-course exams)
- 0.70–0.79 would be acceptable for lower stakes assessments (e.g., formative or summative classroom-type assessments created and administered by local faculty.

Although many in-course or classroom-type educational assessments have reliabilities below 0.70, there may still be a sound rationale for using test score information with relatively low levels of reliability. For example, test scores with a reliability coefficient below 0.70 might be useful as one component of an overall composite score.

As we will discuss later, adding additional items to a test, or adding total scores from multiple tests, often times yields an enhanced total score reliability.

Standard Error of Measurement (SEM)

To gain a clearer sense of the instrument's reliability, one can also calculate the standard error of measurement (SEM) and form confidence intervals for an obtained score (Downing, 2004; Downing, Chapter 5, this volume). For example, an instructor can interpret a 90% confidence interval as the score range around an obtained score that includes an examinee's true score 90% of the time. Equation 3.3 displays a method for deriving the SEM from a reliability coefficient.

$$\text{SEM} = \text{standard deviation} * \sqrt{(1 - \text{Reliability})} \tag{3.3}$$

For our example quiz, the SEM = $1.49 * \sqrt{(1 - 0.538)}$
= $1.49 * 0.6797 = 1.01$.

Multiplying the SEM by 1.65 will provide the needed value to construct a 90% confidence interval around an obtained score. The value 1.65 is appropriate for a 90% confidence interval because for any distribution, the scores that fall within 1.65 standard deviations of the mean will include 90% of all the scores in the distribution.

90% CI = predicted value ± (1.65 * 1.01) = predicted value ± 1.67

So, for examinees who score at the test average of 2.0, 90% of them will have true scores in the interval ranging from 0.33 to 3.67 (2.0 ± 1.67). Given that possible test scores range only from 0 to 5, this 90% confidence interval is very large and is a reflection of the low reliability of this five-item test.

If the reliability of this quiz is too low for the given purpose, there are some options for increasing alpha. One approach is to increase the number of test items. The Spearman-Brown formula can be used to estimate the likely impact on reliability of a lengthened test (see also Downing, Chapter 5, this volume). The formula, shown in Equation 3.4 below, assumes that the items added to the test will have internal consistency, difficulty, and discrimination levels similar to those items already on the test.

$$r_{predicted} = f * r_{current} / (1 + (f - 1) * r_{current}), \tag{3.4}$$

where $r_{predicted}$ = the predicted reliability of the lengthened test; f is the factor by which the test will be lengthened; $r_{current}$ = the reliability coefficient for the current test.

For the 5-item quiz with a reliability of 0.538, what would the likely reliability be for a test of 10 items, i.e., increasing the length of the test by a factor of 2? Using the Spearman-Brown formula,

$$r_{predicted} = 2 * 0.538 / (1 + (2 - 1) * 0.538)$$

$$= 2 * 0.538 / 1.538$$

$$= 0.70$$

Using the Spearman-Brown formula, we find that the reliability of the new lengthened test is likely to be approximately 0.70.

How to Increase Reliability

If this level of reliability is still too low for the given purpose, what else could be done to improve it? Some options are:

a. Adding even more test items;

b. Conducting an item analysis and removing, revising, or replacing items that are not working well (see Downing, Chapter 5, this volume); and

c. Combining the current test with other types of measures to produce a composite score that may be more reliable than some of the tests or measures individually (see composite scores, below).

Assessing and Improving the Reliability of Rater Data

Up to this point, our focus has been on assessment instruments producing data that can be objectively scored as correct (1) or incorrect (0). However, many educational assessments within the health sciences are conducted through structured observation and the rating of performance (see Yudkowsky, Chapter 9, this volume). Methods for assessing and improving the reliability of such data are discussed next.

Rater data are generated, for example, when observers assign scores to examinees' performances or products. Since scoring a performance or test is typically a labor-intensive process, scoring duties are often distributed across multiple judges. For rating data to be reliable, each rater must be scoring performances consistently and in a manner comparable to the other raters. To enhance the replicability of the scores awarded by judges, an explicit set of scoring guidelines, often referred to as a scoring rubric, should be used to guide their work. In addition, after the judges have assigned scores, it is important to check on the extent to which the scoring rules have been consistently applied by examining inter-rater reliability.

In discussing the wide array of statistics to assess inter-rater reliability, Stemler (2004) identifies three ways of conceptualizing and estimating them:

1. **consensus estimates**—based on exact agreement among raters (*statistics: percent agreement, Cohen's kappa*);

2. **consistency estimates**—based on raters' similar ordering of performances (*statistics: Pearson's r, Spearman's rho, Cronbach's alpha*); and

3. **measurement estimates**—based on using all information from

judges' ratings in a model and providing statistics related to the various facets of the ratings (*models: generalizability theory, principal components, many-facets Rasch model*).

Each of these approaches is discussed below.

Consensus Estimates of Inter-rater Reliability

Consensus estimates are perhaps the most straightforward approach to assessing inter-rater reliability. They examine the percentage of items that are scored the same way by the raters. To illustrate, consider the data in Table 3.2 showing two judges' cross-classified ratings of a student's communication skills (0 = unsatisfactory, 1 = satisfactory, 2 = exemplary). The cases where the judges awarded the same score are found in the diagonal cells of the table. The percent-agreement statistic is calculated by adding the diagonal elements (40 + 60 + 35 = 135) and dividing this sum by the total number of cases (200). Percent agreement = 135/200 * 100 = 67.5%.

The interpretation of this statistic, however, is not as clear-cut as it would first appear. Just by chance alone, there will be some cases of apparent agreement even when there is no relationship between the judges' ratings. To disentangle the systematic agreement from those attributable to chance Cohen developed the kappa statistic, calculated by subtracting the expected value of random occurrences of agreement from the total observed instances of agreement. As a guide for interpreting the level of agreement indicated by kappa values, Landis and Koch (1977) note that values above 0.60 are considered substantial

Table 3.2 Hypothetical Communication Skills Ratings for 200 Students by Two Judges

		Judge 2:			
	Scores:	0	1	2	Total
Judge 1:	0	40	10	20	70
	1	5	60	5	70
	2	15	10	35	60
	Total	60	80	60	200

levels of agreement and values of 0.41 to 0.60 are considered moderate.

For the data displayed in Table 3.2 kappa can be obtained from statistical programs and is found to be 0.511. The programs will also provide statistics to test the null hypothesis that the judges' ratings are independent; or, in other words, that there is no more agreement among the judges ratings than would be expected by chance.

In reflecting on the information obtained from kappa, note that it is based on dividing data into classes—agreement and disagreement. When there are only two rating categories, kappa's mapping of responses into agreement and disagreement is unproblematic. Raters either picked the same category (agree) or they did not (disagree). But, what happens, as in the preceding example, if there are three or more rating categories? In such cases, one has to decide which ratings should be classified as "agreement" and "disagreement." In our numerical example, cases that received the same score were defined as "agreement" and the two types of non-identical responses were lumped together in the "disagreement" category. Note, that by lumping the two cases of disagreement together we effectively discard information about the types of disagreements. In our example, it is likely that we would want to consider the disagreements where judges' ratings were two levels apart (0, 2) as more serious than those that only differed by one level (e.g., (0,1) or (1,2)). Thus, when judges are rating performance on an ordinal or interval scale with three or more categories, kappa does not take full advantage of the available information about distances between data categories. For such situations, one could either use a weighted kappa statistic that adjusts for different levels of disagreement; or one of the available consistency- or measurement-based estimates of inter-rater reliability discussed below.

Consistency Estimates of Inter-rater Reliability

Consistency estimates focus on the correspondence among raters' ordering of observed performances. In our example the overall clinical performance of ten pharmacy students is rated by preceptors on a

5-point scale with "4" indicating outstanding performance and "0" indicating unsatisfactory performance; see Table 3.3.

To examine the level of agreement in preceptors' ratings of students, a correlation coefficient such as Pearson's r could be calculated among all possible pairs of preceptors. However, Pearson's r assumes that the raters' scores are based on an at least interval scale of measurement, which like integers on a number line, requires equal distances between each of the adjacent scores. This may not be true, if, for example, raters are only giving failing scores of 0 in the most extreme cases. Such a practice could result in the distance between a 0 and 1 score being much larger than the distance between any of the other adjacent categories (e.g., (1,2), (2,3), and (3,4)). When such a situation is of concern, Spearman's rho should be used since it is based on the rank ordering of the data and does not require an interval scale of measurement. Table 3.4 provides the Spearman's rho correlations obtained from a statistical program:

These coefficients are interpreted in the same way as Pearson's correlation coefficients. Possible values range from −1 to +1, with values closer to −1 or +1 indicating stronger linear relationships between the variables. Note that Rater #4's scores for students do not correspond very well ($r < .30$) with the scores given by Raters #1, #2, and #3. Also, there is a low correspondence between the scores given by Rater #3 and Rater #5 ($r = 0.218$). To improve inter-rater reliability, the sources

Table 3.3 Hypothetical Clinical Performance Ratings of 10 Students by 5 Judges/Raters

Student ID	Rater #1	Rater #2	Rater #3	Rater #4	Rater #5	Student Totals
A	1	1	4	1	0	7
B	2	4	4	2	4	16
C	3	4	4	2	3	16
D	4	0	2	2	3	11
E	0	0	1	4	4	9
F	4	4	4	2	4	18
G	4	3	2	4	4	17
H	1	0	1	1	3	6
I	0	1	0	0	2	3
J	4	4	4	1	4	17
Rater Totals	23	21	26	19	31	

Table 3.4 Spearman Rho Correlations of Rater Agreement

	RATER 1	RATER 2	RATER 3	RATER 4	RATER 5
RATER 1	1.00				
RATER 2	.475	1.0			
RATER 3	.541	.765	1.0		
RATER 4	.297	.023	.079	1.0	
RATER 5	.436	.399	.218	.639	1.0

of the disagreement among these raters could be investigated, identified, and used to improve rating procedures (see Yudkowsky, Chapter 9, this volume).

The above correlation coefficients limited our analysis to pairwise comparisons between raters. To assess the average correlation across all raters Cronbach's alpha could be calculated. The alpha is 0.744, indicating that the shared (true score) variance in the judges ratings accounts for nearly three-quarters of the variance in students' overall clinical performance rating.

Measurement Estimates of Inter-rater Reliability

Judges' ratings are often utilized to assess performance in more complex context than that described above. For example, several judges might rate a student's performance on one task and another set of judges might rate performance on another task. If we wanted to estimate the reliability of a student's obtained score, a comprehensive measure of score reliability would need to take into account the overall judges agreement and the number and variability of tasks presented to the examinee. We might want to ask how replicable a score might be if a different set of judges and tasks were selected and the entire measurement process were repeated. In more complex assessment environments where there are two or more sources of systematic variation simultaneously impacting an assessment score, more sophisticated approaches are needed to estimate reliability. Such instances require partitioning of error sources according to the different facets (e.g., judges, tasks). Generalizability theory, discussed by Kreiter, (Chapter 4, this volume), is more appropriate in these situations.

Reliability of Composites

Health science instructors often need to generate a summary score based on multiple diverse measures. For example, a course grade might be derived by summing written test scores assessing knowledge achievement and ratings of clinical performance. Given that the final grade is usually the most important and consequential score awarded for a course, it may be important to accurately assess its reliability.

Composite score reliability is a special topic, which requires some unique assumptions, formulas, and software to estimate properly. Wainer and Thissen (2001) provide a thorough treatment of composite score reliability. The key points are that in order to accurately estimate the reliability of composite scores, any differential weighting of the input test or assessment scores must be included in the estimation process. And, composite scores are almost always more reliable than the sum of their respective parts, as alluded to earlier in this chapter.

Nominal and Effective Weights: Standard Scores

In calculating a grade or composite score and its reliability, it is important to first transform each component of the summary score to a standard score (see Downing, Chapter 5, this volume). If an instructor simply applies weights to each component score without first standardizing them to a common scale, the nominal weights applied will often be quite different than the effective weights. For example, when simply summing unstandardized score components (i.e. applying nominal weights of 1.0 to each component), those component scores with larger observed standard deviations will contribute more to the composite score. To eliminate the disparity between nominal and effective weights, it is good practice to standardize all component scores to a common mean and standard deviation before weighting and summing. This will allow the applied weights to equal the effective weights.

Depending on the correlation between scores, it is often observed that a composite score can exhibit higher reliability than any of the component scores individually. The composite reliability will depend on the reliability of the components, the weights chosen, and the correlation between component scores (Kreiter, Gordon, Elliott, & Calloway, 2004).

Summary

In a fashion similar to the noisy restaurant example at the beginning of the chapter, assessment scores usually contain error or noise that hampers our ability to accurately measure an examinee's ability or achievement. Reliability analysis allows educators to quantify error and facilitates the correct interpretation and use of scores containing error.

To provide a conceptual framework for reliability analyses, CTT was introduced as a method for partitioning total test score variance into two components: 1) true score; and 2) error. It was emphasized that the notion of replications provides the necessary framework for representing reliability.

Methods for estimating reliability were discussed and illustrated with numerical examples. For MC exams, the internal consistency of item responses can be used to estimate reliability using Cronbach's alpha or KR-20. Guidelines for interpreting alpha were provided and it was suggested that item analysis, lengthening the test, and creating composite scores are possible approaches for improving reliability.

Procedures for estimating the reliability of rater data were discussed next. Such data are produced when two or more judges rate a student product or performance. Cohen's kappa, Pearson's r, and Spearman's rho assess the correspondence of ratings between pairs of judges. These measures can be used to identify instances of poor agreement among particular judges and to monitor the effectiveness of scoring rubrics and rater training. Cronbach's alpha was mentioned as a measure of the overall inter-rater reliability among judges.

Just as lengthening a test can increase its reliability, creating a composite score by combining tests and other measures can also provide increased reliability over the individual measures.

References

Carline, J.D., Wenrich, M.D., & Ramsey, P.G. (1989). Characteristics of ratings of physician competence by professional associates. *Evaluation and the Health Professions*, 12, 409–23.

Cohen, J. (1960). A coefficient for agreement for nominal scales. *Educational and Psychological Measurement*, 20, 37–46.

Downing, S. M. (2004). Reliability: On the reproducibility of assessment data. *Medical Education*, 38, 1006–1012.

Kreiter, C.D., Ferguson, K., Lee, W.C., Brennan, R.L., & Densen, P. (1998). A generalizability study of a new standardized rating form used to evaluate students' clinical clerkship performance. *Academic Medicine*, 73, 1294–1298.

Kreiter, C.D., Gordon, J.A., Elliott, S., & Callaway, M. (2004). Recommendations for assigning weights to derive an overall course grade. *Teaching and Learning in Medicine*, 16(2), 133–138.

Landis, J.R., & Koch, G.G. (1977). The measurement of observer agreement for categorical data. *Biometrics*, 33, 159–174.

Pedhazur, E.J., & Schmelkin, L.P. (1991). *Measurement, design, and analysis: An integrated approach*. Hillsdale, NJ: Lawrence Erlbaum Associates.

Schmitt, N. (1996). Uses and abuses of coefficient alpha. *Psychological Assessment*, 8(4), 350–353.

Stemler, S.E. (2004). A comparison of consensus, consistency, and measurement approaches to estimating inter-rater reliability. *Practical Assessment, Research & Evaluation*, 9(4), available online from http://PAREonline.net/getvn.asp?v=9&n=4

Wainer, H., & Thissen, D. (2001). True score theory: The traditional method. In D. Thissen & H. Wainer (Eds.), *Test scoring*. Mahwah, NJ: Lawrence Erlbaum Associates, Inc.

4

GENERALIZABILITY THEORY

CLARENCE D. KREITER

Introductory Comments

Since this treatment of generalizability theory (G theory) is limited to a single chapter, it necessarily provides only a brief introduction to many important aspects of the theory. Despite the brevity, the reader is provided with an overview of all the basic concepts and procedures used in G theory. The primary objective of the chapter is to provide the learner with the background to comprehend common health science education applications of the theory in practice and in research. To achieve this goal, generalizability concepts are presented within the context of a hypothetical performance assessment measurement problem. Computational methods and equations are presented only when they promote the reader's conceptual understanding of the theory. To assist those interested in delving deeper into the technical aspects of the theory, notation and terminology is largely consistent with Brennan's authoritative text: *Generalizability Theory* (Brennan, 2001). Although some research, validity, and reliability applications become apparent only with a more in-depth treatment, this chapter will allow the reader to apply and interpret most of the commonly encountered generalizability designs.

The two appendices at the end of this chapter provide a brief description of the ANOVA-based statistical methods used in generalizability analyses. Understanding the material covered in this chapter does not require familiarity with ANOVA, hence, the two statistical appendices can be regarded optional reading.

Background and Overview

As discussed in Chapter 2, in classical test theory (CTT) there is an assumption that an observed score is composed of two components, a "true" score and random error. A shorthand way of representing this concept is:

$$Observed\ Score = True\ Score + Error, \tag{4.1}$$

and the CTT expression for reliability as:

$$Reliability = True\ Score\ /\ True\ Score + Error. \tag{4.2}$$

Similar to CTT, G theory also assumes that the variance of an observed score is partitioned between true score variance and error variance. However, G theory differs from CTT in allowing the examination of multiple sources of error, and hence expands on the CTT equation as:

$$Observed\ Score = True\ Score + Error_1 + Error_2 + Error_3 \ldots, \tag{4.3}$$

and the expression for reliability as:

$$Reliability = True\ Score\ /\ True\ Score + Error_1 + Error_2 \\ + Error_3. \ldots \tag{4.4}$$

In conceptualizing score variance to fall into two broad categories (true score and error), G theory shares a common theoretical framework with CTT. However, G theory differs dramatically from CTT in the details related to estimating the variances associated with both the true score and error, and in its use of these variance estimates to calculate multiple reliability-like coefficients that are appropriate to specific applications.[1] In Chapter 3 it was noted that in CTT, when a measurement process has more than one dimension or *facet* over which measures are averaged, different reliability coefficients can characterize the score. For example, if a measurement process uses raters to rate tasks on a multiple-item form, CTT methods could calculate an inter-rater reliability coefficient, an "inter-task" reliability coefficient, or an internal consistency (split-half) alpha statistic. However, it would be difficult to meaningfully integrate these different CTT measures and globally assess reliability. On the other hand,

G theory can characterize how accurately an obtained score estimates a hypothetical score derived by averaging across many replications of a multi-faceted measurement process. In G theory, this average score, or *universe score*, similar to a "true" score in CTT, is carefully defined in relation to all identified *facets* of the measurement process, and provides a more comprehensive assessment of reliability. In G theory, the *facets* of a measurement problem specify the *conditions of measurement*. In explaining the concepts associated with the *facets* and the *conditions of measurement*, it is useful at this point to introduce a hypothetical performance assessment problem that will be used throughout this chapter to demonstrate the concepts and procedures used in G theory. This problem, designed for instructional purposes, employs a small synthetic data set to demonstrate generalizability study (G study) procedures and to allow the reader to confirm reported statistical findings with simple hand calculations.

The Instructional Problem

A medical education researcher is asked to report on the reliability of test scores from a piloted version of an Objective Structured Clinical Examination (OSCE), and to make recommendations for structuring a larger operational version of the test. The researcher has been provided with global ratings of ten examinees' videotaped performances on a 5-station OSCE exam. The hypothetical ratings, displayed in Table 4.1, represent ratings by two expert physician raters independently rating the ten examinees' performances on a 10-point scale. CTT methods could be used to calculate an inter-rater reliability coefficient or an inter-task reliability coefficient, but it would be difficult to simultaneously represent the multiple sources of error and to meaningfully integrate the CTT coefficients. Therefore, the researcher decides to use G theory to address the measurement problem.

Defining the G Study Model

Before analyzing the information presented in Table 4.1, the researcher must first define the G study measurement model. Reflecting on the

Table 4.1 Data for the Example OSCE Measurement Problem: Ratings from a Piloted Version of the OSCE Examination

| | STA 1 | | STA 2 | | STA 3 | | STA 4 | | STA 5 | |
	R1	R2	R1	R2	R1	R2	R1	R2	R1	R2
Ex1	5	5	5	5	4	5	5	5	4	5
Ex2	4	7	4	4	4	7	8	9	5	4
Ex3	6	6	8	8	8	7	6	6	5	5
Ex4	0	5	5	5	4	5	5	4	1	1
Ex5	4	4	3	5	5	6	6	4	4	4
Ex6	3	6	5	8	6	4	7	7	4	3
Ex7	2	2	6	5	7	5	5	5	1	2
Ex8	4	5	8	7	8	7	6	6	5	4
Ex9	2	2	7	6	6	7	5	5	3	3
Ex10	3	7	4	7	4	6	4	4	2	3

Notes: STA = Station R = Rater Ex = Examinee

conditions of measurement, or how the data was collected, the researcher observes that the same two expert raters rated all examinees on each of the five stations, and that the exam was designed to assess students' clinical skills. With this information, the researcher can define some important aspects of the G study model. First, since the exam was designed as a measure of examinee performance, as opposed to rater or station performance, the researcher can conclude that the examinee is the *object of measurement.* Once the *object of measurement* has been identified, the researcher can further assume that the remaining conditions of measurement, raters and stations, represent *facets* in the G study measurement model. In this example, there are two *facets,* raters and stations. It should be noted that there may be other important measurement *facets* or influences related to the measures obtained in Table 4.1, however, the researcher does not have information characterizing these other influences.

The researcher is now ready to formally specify a G study model that will represent how the measures within the OSCE exam were collected. In doing so, it is important to first provide some formal definitions along with the notational conventions used in model specifications. First, we must define what we mean by an *object of measurement.* The *object of measurement* is defined as the member of the sample or population that the examination is designed to assess. In most testing applications, the *object of measurement* is the examinee, commonly referred to as the person (p). The notational convention in the majority of G studies is to represent persons, the *object of measurement*, with the small letter "p". After identifying the *object of measurement*, the *facets* within a G study are identified by default as the other main sources of variation in the G study model. A *facet* represents a dimension or source of variation across which the researcher wishes to generalize. In our example problem, we have two *facets*, raters (r) and stations (s), with the first letter of their spelled name representing the *facet*. Hence, in this problem "r" and "s" will represent raters and stations respectively.

Again, considering our example problem, every person (p) experiences every station (s) and is rated by the same two raters (r) on each station. The shorthand way of expressing this concept in generalizability terminology is to say all conditions of measurement are completely *crossed*. The notation for the *crossed* concept is the symbol "x". So, with these simple notational conventions, we can write a symbolic expression that summarizes the G study model as: [p x s x r]. Hence, our G study model is a persons *crossed* with stations *crossed* with raters design. Not all G study models are completely *crossed*. For example, it would be possible to conduct an OSCE exam, similar to the one described in the example problem, using a different pair of raters for each station. In generalizability terminology, this is called a *nested* design and is represented by the symbol ":". For instance, had the ratings been collected using two different raters for each station, we would have represented the G study design as: [p x (r : s)]. In G theory terminology, this would be a persons *crossed* with raters *nested* within stations model design. There will be additional discussions of design variations throughout this chapter.

All G study models must define whether the facets are *random* or *fixed*. A facet is considered *random* when observed values of the facet within the G study are regarded as a sample from a larger population. In our example problem, both raters and stations are considered *random* variables. Hence, in G theory terminology, we would define our G study model from the example problem as being a *random model*.

The reason we consider stations as *random* is that our interest is not focused solely on the five stations observed. Rather, the goal of the measurement process is to generalize from performance on the five stations to performance on a universe of similar stations from which the five stations are a sample. In the example problem, the same argument applies to raters. The two expert physician raters employed in the pilot exam are considered a sample from a population of potential expert physician raters we might use or consider acceptable to rate performance. For example, if no special rater training of the physician raters was provided, the population of acceptable raters might reasonably be defined as: academic physicians at U.S. medical schools. However, if the two academic physician raters in the study received special rater training, we would need to modify our definition of the rater universe as academic physicians who received the special rater training. A facet is regarded as *fixed* when all levels of a facet are observed in the G study. An example of a fixed facet will be presented later in the chapter.

Obtaining G Study Results

Now that the basic G study model has been presented, the next step in the G study is to obtain G study results. *Variance components* (VCs) represent the primary output of a G study analysis. VCs are estimates of the magnitude of variability of each effect in the G study model. The model in the example problem has three main effects: the object of measurement, persons (p), and the two facets, stations (s) and raters (r). In addition, as in analysis of variance (ANOVA), there are also interactions. So, in addition to p, s and r, there are four interaction effects; ps, pr, sr and psr. Therefore, in the example problem, the G study will estimate a total of seven VCs (p, s, r, ps, pr, sr, psr). A description of these effects and how to interpret them is presented shortly. The statistical procedures for the estimation of the VCs are presented in Appendix 4.1.

Table 4.2 displays the G study output for the data displayed in Table 4.1. The VCs in Table 4.2 can be calculated using GENOVA® software (Crick & Brennan, 1982), which is specially designed for

Table 4.2 G Study Results for Example Problem [p x s x r]

Effect	DF	Variance Component (VC)	Standard Error (SE)	Percent Variance
p	9	0.5706	0.3745	16
s	4	1.0156	0.7003	29
r	1	0.0361	0.0851	1
ps	36	0.6694	0.2823	19
pr	9	0.1139	0.1355	3
sr	4	0.1528	0.1439	4
psr	36	0.9372	0.2150	27

conducting G study and decision study (D study) analyses and automatically outputs VCs and other statistical information important in the G study analysis. These same results can also be derived with SAS's VARCOMP procedure or with BMDP's V8 statistical software.

Interpreting G Study Results

The first column of Table 4.2 lists each of the effects estimated in the G study, the *main* effects (p, s, r) and the *interaction* effects (ps, pr, sr, psr). The second column displays the degrees of freedom. The third column of Table 4.2 displays the VC values for each of the seven effects estimated. The fourth column of Table 4.2 lists the standard error (SE) for each VC estimate. The fifth column provides the percentage of the total variance represented by each VC.

In the first row of Table 4.2 we observe that 16% of the variance is attributable to systematic differences between examinees (p). This is object of measurement variance and is similar to "true" score variance in CTT. The ratio definition of reliability provided in Equation 4.4 suggests that the larger the percentage of variance accounted for by p, the higher will be the obtained reliability. The second row of Table 4.2 displays the systematic variance attributable to station, and it reflects the degree to which the stations have different means. The station effect, accounting for the largest percentage of variance (29%) in the model, implies that there were considerable differences in the level of difficulty between stations in our sample. The third row shows the variance associated with the systematic effects of rater, and it reflects the difference in raters' overall mean scores across stations and persons. In the example problem, the small proportion of variance related to raters (1%) suggests that the mean difference between raters is small, or stated another way, that the two raters were approximately equal in their overall level of stringency.

The fourth row in Table 4.2 displays the person by station (ps) interaction. This indicates the degree to which stations tended to rank-order persons (examinees) differently. The relatively large amount of variance (19%) attributed to this interaction (ps) suggests that examinee rank orders would change considerably depending on which station(s) were sampled. The person by rater (pr) interaction is relatively small at just 3%, and suggests that raters tended to agree on the ratings assigned to an examinee at a given station, or that rank orders would not change dramatically based upon which single rater's ratings were used. The station by rater (sr) interaction was also small (4%), indicating that the level of station difficulty changed little depending on which rater assigned the ratings. The psr VC accounted for 27% of the total variance and is a confounded measure of the triple interaction of person, station, and rater, and influences not modeled in the [p x s x r] design.

The standard errors (SE) in the fourth column of Table 4.2 convey the level of precision with which we were able to estimate the population VCs. The SE can be interpreted as an estimated standard deviation of a VC estimate upon multiple estimations from multiple replications using the same sample sizes. It should be observed that the SE estimates in Table 4.2 are rather large relative to the size of the VC estimates. This can be attributed to the small sample sizes employed within the G study and suggest that the estimates are likely to display large variability between replications employing these sample sizes.

Conducting the D Study

In the description of our example problem, it was noted that the researcher was asked not only to characterize the reliability of the scores from the pilot test, but also to make recommendations for how an operational version of the test might best be structured. A *decision study* (D study) can provide reliability estimates both for the scores collected in the G study and also for tests employing different designs and sample sizes. Hence, a D study can address questions related to how best to optimize test design. The structure of the G study determines what designs a D study can address. Completely crossed designs allow for the maximum number of addressable designs. A D study uses VCs from the G study to calculate estimated reliability coefficients given variations in the conditions of measurement. In this instance, the researcher using a D study could estimate not only the reliability of the test with the observed conditions of measurement (a completely crossed random model with two raters crossed with five stations), but could also estimate the reliability of a test using any number of raters or stations administered using either the same crossed OSCE test design or a different design (e.g., a nested design). Using a series of D studies to examine various test structure options can help the researcher determine how best to structure an operational version of the test.

Before proceeding further, it is useful here to discuss D study notation. In the G study model of the example problem, we employed small letter notation to represent the facets. The small letter notation is a way of indicating that in the G study analysis, estimated effects are for one rating on a single station by one rater. However, in a D study we are interested in representing average ratings across a sample of conditions, and capital letters are used to indicate this. For this reason, our notational system for the D study model employs capital letters to express the D study model design. For instance, a D study model for the design in our example measurement problem is represented as: [p x S x R].

The D study can generate two types of reliability-like coefficients: a generalizability coefficient (G or $E\rho^2$) and a measure of dependability (Phi or Φ). The G coefficient is sensitive to relative error and is useful for expressing the reproducibility of examinee rankings. The dependability measure, commonly referred to as Phi, expresses the absolute reproducibility of a score and reflects the degree to which an obtained score is likely to change upon replication of the measurement process.

Hence, if one imagines a complete replication of the OSCE measurement procedure as documented in our example problem (i.e., a sample of five different stations and two different raters), a Phi will reflect how closely a replication is likely to reproduce an examinee's final score. The G coefficient estimates how consistently a replication will rank examinees. Because of this distinction, the Phi coefficient is useful for answering questions related to criterion-referenced testing, while a G coefficient is most informative for norm-referenced testing applications. A tangible impact of the difference between the G and the Phi coefficients in our example problem is that the large variation in station difficulty (29% of the total variance) lowers Phi substantially; however this variability in station difficulty does not impact the G coefficient. This difference is best understood by considering the outcome of a replication of a [p x S x R] design. Within each replication, all examinees will experience the same stations. Hence, variation in station difficulty will not change the rank ordering of examinees across replications, and therefore will not affect the G coefficient. However, variations in station difficulty will obviously produce variation in the magnitude of the obtained mean scores across replications, and hence will lower Phi. Building on the very general definition of reliability provided in Equation 4.4, we can now write the symbolic expression for these two reliability-like coefficients as:

$$G = E\rho^2 = \frac{\sigma^2(p)}{\sigma^2(p) + \sigma^2(\delta)} \tag{4.5}$$

and

$$Phi = \Phi = \frac{\sigma^2(p)}{\sigma^2(p) + \sigma^2(\Delta)} \tag{4.6}$$

where:

$\sigma^2(p)$ = the variance associated with person,
$\sigma^2(\delta)$ = the sum of relative error variances, and
$\sigma^2(\Delta)$ = the sum of absolute error variances.

Absolute error variance (Δ) includes all sources of error. Relative error (δ) includes only those sources of error variance that will impact examinee rank ordering. This implies that for all D study designs, absolute error will always be greater than or equal to relative error. Hence, Phi (Φ) will always be less than or equal to G ($E\rho^2$). Appendix 4.2 provides additional detail regarding what VCs, or sources of error, are included as part of absolute and relative error calculations. Colliver et al. (Colliver, Verhulst, Williams, & Norcini, 1989) provide an excellent in-depth treatment of how various reliability-like measures can be computed and interpreted within a performance assessment context. As part of the D study in our example problem, Phi (Φ) and G ($E\rho^2$) results were calculated, using Equations 4.12 and 4.13 from Appendix 4.2, and displayed in Table 4.3.

Interpreting the D Study

In interpreting a D study, it is often helpful to graphically display the results as shown in Figure 4.1. When the G coefficients from Table 4.3 are graphed across levels of the two facets, several important outcomes become apparent. First, small gains in reliability are observed by using more than one rater, and increasing the number of raters beyond two yields negligible improvements. On the other hand, utilizing multiple stations substantially increases reliability. For example, increasing the number of stations from one to five increases G by as much as 0.35. In addition, this D study also suggests that the addition

Table 4.3 D Study Results for Example Problem [p x S x R]

Number of Raters	Number of Stations	G ($E\rho^2$)	Phi (Φ)
1	1	0.25	0.16
1	5	0.56	0.45
1	10	0.67	0.57
2	1	0.32	0.20
2	5	0.67*	0.52*
2	10	0.77	0.66
3	1	0.36	0.21
3	5	0.71	0.55
3	10	0.81	0.69

Note: * G and Phi for the mean scores obtained in the G study.

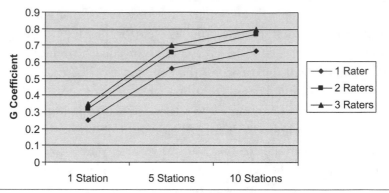

Figure 4.1 G Coefficient for Various Numbers of Raters and Stations.

of stations after the fifth continues to produce appreciable gains in the estimated reliability. To obtain a summary of how the number of raters and stations impacts the dependability of scores, the Phi values in the last column of Table 4.3 could also be plotted in a similar fashion to aid in interpretability. Although the pattern is much the same for Phi and G in our example problem, because stations tended to exhibit considerable variability in difficulty, Phi values are smaller compared to the G coefficients for a given number of stations and raters.

There is a broad G study literature on SP assessments. Van der Vlueten and Swanson (van der Vlueten & Swanson, 1990) provide a useful summary of major findings. For example, they note that in most SP studies the primary source of measurement error is due to variation in examinee performance from station to station (ps variance—sometimes referred to as content specificity variance). This implies that in most instances adding stations is considerably more effective in increasing reliability than adding raters. This finding is particularly true for SP exams employing checklists where inter-rater agreement is generally high.

G and D Study Model Variations

As previously discussed, specialized software is capable of handling many of the technical aspects in G and D study analyses. However, to successfully utilize G study software it is essential that the researcher accurately specify G and D study models. This section briefly discusses two additional measurement examples and considers commonly encountered G and D study model variations.

Our example OSCE problem presented a two-faceted [p x s x r] random model design. However, many commonly encountered G study models use only one facet. For example, a typical standardized multiple-choice test can be modeled as a simple persons (p) crossed (x) with items (i) one-faceted random model design [p x i]. A [p x i] G study design yields estimates for three effects: p, i and pi, and the G coefficient for this design would be:

$$G = E\rho^2 = \frac{\sigma^2(p)}{\sigma^2(p) + \sigma^2(pi) / n_i} \qquad (4.7)$$

and is equivalent to Cronbach's coefficient alpha. The Phi for the multiple-choice test example is:

$$Phi = \Phi = \frac{\sigma^2(p)}{\sigma^2(p) + \sigma^2(i) / n_i + \sigma^2(pi) / n_i} \qquad (4.8)$$

To demonstrate a *fixed* facet within a G study, imagine a written test employing two formats (f), multiple-choice (MC) and true–false (TF). Since it is logically impossible for an item to be in both formats, the reader should recognize first that a test employing both formats (MC & TF) implies that items must be nested within format (i : f). Second, since the two formats do not represent a sample from a population of many possible formats, the MC and TF formats are quite likely the only two formats of interest in the study. Given that the two observed levels of format are not a sample from a larger population of formats, and that the two formats represent the only two formats of interest, format (f) is regarded as a *fixed* rather than a random facet. This further implies that the model is *mixed* since it contains both a random facet (items) and a fixed facet (format). Hence, the G study design would be a persons (p) crossed (x) with items (i) nested (:) within format (f) mixed model design [p x (i : f)].

This chapter has briefly discussed modeling concepts of just four G study designs ([p x i], [p x (i : f)], [p x s x r] and [p x (r : s)]).

Even though variants of G study models grow rapidly with the addition of facets, nesting, and mixed model conditions, these four models provide the reader with the building blocks and core concepts to model most commonly encountered designs. As it is beyond the scope of this chapter to provide the reader with an exhaustive list of models, the reader is encouraged to reference texts offering a wider presentation on model detail and design (Brennan, 2001; Shavelson & Webb, 1991; Norman, 2003).

Final Considerations

G theory provides a powerful method for examining a wide array of both simple and complex measures. A thorough consideration of G and D study results can provide a better understanding of the measurement process and how to improve it. Through the facilitation of insights regarding validity and reliability, G theory methods provide social scientists with a powerful research tool. The reader is encouraged to explore more advanced demonstrations of the theory to gain an appreciation of G theory's many applications to health science education.

APPENDIX 4.1: STATISTICAL FOUNDATIONS OF A GENERALIZABILITY STUDY

To understand the derivation of the VC, it is necessary to briefly review methods employed in ANOVA. In ANOVA, *sums of squares* (SS) characterize the distribution of scores around a mean. For example, the total SS in our example problem can be computed as:

$$\sum_p \sum_s \sum_r (X_{psr} - \overline{X})^2 \tag{4.9}$$

where:

$\sum$ is the summation operator,
X_{psr} is a rating for a single person on one station by a single rater,
$\overline{X}$ is the grand mean across all raters, stations and persons.

Hence, the total SS in our example problem is simply the sum of the squared difference of each rating subtracted from the overall mean. The three summation operators (Σ) in Equation 4.9 simply indicate this sum is performed across all persons (p), stations (s) and raters (r). To continue with this example, the SS for stations (s) can be calculated using Equation 4.10. This equation contains just one summation operator, indicating the sum is across just stations. Hence, Equation 4.10 indicates that the SS for stations equals the sum of the squared differences between each stations mean and the grand mean, multiplied by the number of persons (n_p) and raters (n_r). A derivation for the SS for each SS follows similar notation and techniques. It is beyond the scope of this chapter to provide the complete derivation of all SS, however, an in-depth treatment of ANOVA estimation methods is provided in Kirk's *Experimental Design* (Kirk, 1982).

$$SS_{(s)} = n_p \, n_r \, \Sigma_s \, (\overline{X}_s - \overline{X})^2 \tag{4.10}$$

Table 4.4 displays the ANOVA results from the data set in Table 4.1. In the first column is the source of the variance, and the second column displays the degrees of freedom (df) for that source of variance. Dividing the SS (column 3) by the degrees of freedom yields the mean squares (MS) displayed in the fourth column of Table 4.4.

The fifth column of Table 4.4 expresses the expected mean squares (EMS) in terms of variance components (σ^2), and the number of raters (n_r), stations (n_s), and persons (n_p) sampled. The EMSs describes the composition of the MSs, or what elements of variance comprise a MS

Table 4.4 ANOVA Table [p x s x r]

Effect	DF	Sum-of-Squares (SS)	Mean Square (MS)	Expected Mean Square (EMS)
p	9	76.96	8.55	$\sigma^2(psr) + n_s \, \sigma^2(pr) + n_r \, \sigma^2(ps) + n_s \, n_r \, \sigma^2(p)$
s	4	96.46	24.12	$\sigma^2(psr) + n_p \, \sigma^2(sr) + n_r \, \sigma^2(ps) + n_p \, n_r \, \sigma^2(s)$
r	1	4.84	4.84	$\sigma^2(psr) + n_p \, \sigma^2(sr) + n_s \, \sigma^2(pr) + n_p \, n_s \, \sigma^2(r)$
ps	36	81.94	2.28	$\sigma^2(psr) + n_r \, \sigma^2(ps)$
pr	9	13.56	1.51	$\sigma^2(psr) + n_s \, \sigma^2(pr)$
sr	4	9.86	2.47	$\sigma^2(psr) + n_p \, \sigma^2(sr)$
psr	36	33.74	0.94	$\sigma^2(psr)$

obtained from a sample. The MS values in Table 4.4 are for the sample data in Table 4.1. It is important to note that because the MSs are calculated on a sample, only in the case of the psr interaction will the sample MS act as an estimator of the population VC ($\hat{\sigma}^2$) (the "^" symbol over the σ^2 indicates that it is an estimate of the population variance). As shown in the fifth column of Table 4.4, for MS values calculated from a sample, the MS includes both the effect of interest and also other interactions. An estimate of a population VC is derived algebraically, solving in reverse for each VC using observed sample MSs. For example, as indicated in the last row of Table 4.4, for the triple interaction effect (psr) the MS from the sample directly estimates the population VC for the psr effect. Therefore, by using this MS(psr) as an estimated variance component for psr ($\hat{\sigma}^2$(psr)) in the double interaction (ps, pr & sr) EMS equations, simple algebra permits one to isolate the estimated population VCs ($\hat{\sigma}^2$) for each of the double interactions (e.g. $\hat{\sigma}^2$(sr) = (2.47 − 0.94) / 10 = 0.153). Deriving the estimated population VCs ($\hat{\sigma}^2$) for the three main effects (σ^2(p), σ^2(s), σ^2(r)) is only slightly more complicated. For example, the VC for persons can be estimated by inserting the MSs from Table 4.4 into Equation 4.11. Similar equations exist for estimating each population VC with observed sample MS values. Brennan (Brennan, 2001) provides a complete description of the rules and methods used for estimating population VCs from MSs obtained from a sample. Fortunately, specialized statistical software (GENOVA, SAS and BMDP) is capable of computing estimated VCs for the user, and in practice, researchers are not required to manually derive VC estimates.

$$\hat{\sigma}^2_{(p)} = \frac{MS_{(p)} - MS_{(ps)} - MS_{(pr)} + MS_{(psr)}}{n_s \, n_r} \qquad (4.11)$$

APPENDIX 4.2: STATISTICAL FOUNDATIONS OF A DECISION STUDY

This appendix presents the logical and technical background for understanding the ratios used to compute G and Phi coefficients.

Again, employing the design used in the example problem, let us consider what the ratio for the G coefficient would be using various numbers of raters and stations. Equation 4.12 expresses the D study G coefficient as a ratio of VCs. Equation 4.13 expresses the D study Phi as a ratio of VCs. Estimated VCs can be used in Equation 4.12 and 4.13 to provide D study reliability estimates. The reader is encouraged to verify the results reported in Table 4.3 by using Equations 4.12 and 4.13 with the appropriate sample sizes and the VC estimates from Table 4.2. It should be noted that the denominator for the Phi (Equation 4.13) contains all sources of error, whereas the denominator for G (Equation 4.12) contains just the error sources impacting examinee rankings. The reader should additionally recognize that equations 4.12 and 4.13 are simply a more detailed version of equations 4.5 and 4.6 respectively.

$$G = E\rho^2 = \frac{\sigma^2(p)}{\sigma^2(p) + \sigma^2(ps) / n_s + \sigma^2(pr) / n_r + \sigma^2(psr) / n_s n_r} \quad (4.12)$$

$$Phi = \Phi = \frac{\sigma^2(p)}{\sigma^2(p) + \sigma^2(s) / n_s + \sigma^2(r) / n_r + \sigma^2(ps) / n_s + \sigma^2(pr) / n_r + \sigma^2(sr) / n_s n_r + \sigma^2(psr) / n_s n_r} \quad (4.13)$$

For each D study design there is an associated pair of G and Phi equations similar to Equations 4.12 and 4.13, but unique to the D study design. By inserting the appropriate values for n_r and n_s, the number of raters and stations, Equations 4.12 and 4.13 are appropriate for all [p x S x R] designs with any number of stations and raters. However, if the researcher would choose to examine other designs, such as a [p x (R : S)] design for example, a different D study equation would apply. A more detailed treatment of these equations can be found in G theory texts (Brennan, 2001; Shavelson & Webb, 1991). One of the primary strengths of G theory relates to the fact that it is easy to use G study results to calculate G and Phi for designs different from that employed in the G study.

Note

1. As the statistical estimation methods used in a G study are derived from analysis of variance, G theory also shares much in common with analysis of variance. However, there are also important differences between analysis of variance and G theory. The most salient difference is G theory's reliance on variance components and the fact that hypothesis and significance testing does not play a role in a G study analysis.

References

Brennan, R.L. (2001). *Generalizability theory.* New York: Springer-Verlag.

Crick, J.E., & Brennan, R.L. (1982) GENOVA®—A generalized analysis of variance software system (Version 3.1) [Computer software]. University of Iowa, Iowa City, IA. Available from http://www.education. uiowa.edu/casma/GenovaPrograms.htm.

Colliver, J.A., Verhulst, S.J., Williams, R.G., & Norcini, J.J. (1989). Reliability of performance on standardized patient cases: A comparison of consistency measures based on generalizability theory. *Teaching and Learning in Medicine,* 1(1), 31–7.

Kirk, R.E. (1982). *Experimental design: Procedures for the behavioral sciences* (2nd ed.) Pacific Grove, CA: Brooks/Cole Publishing.

Norman, G.R. (2003). Generalizability theory. In D.L. Streiner & G.R. Norman, *Health measurement scales: A practical guide to their development and use* (3rd ed., pp. 153–171). New York: Oxford University Press.

Shavelson, R.J., & Webb, N.M. (1991). *Generalizability theory: A primer.* Newbury Park, CA: Sage.

van der Vleuten, C.P.M., & Swanson, D.B. (1990). Assessment of clinical skills with standardized patients: State of the art. *Teaching and Learning in Medicine,* 2(2), 58–76.

5

STATISTICS OF TESTING

STEVEN M. DOWNING

Introduction

This chapter discusses some of the statistics commonly utilized in testing. Since this book focuses primarily on tests and other types of measures which result in quantitative data, some statistics are inevitable. Many of the tools used to evaluate tests and other measures used in health professions education require the application of some basic quantitative methods or statistics applied to testing.

As in other chapters, this treatment of statistics in testing is general and applied, avoiding statistical proofs and theoretical explanations and derivations. The purpose of this chapter is to give the reader an overview of some commonly used statistical techniques, their purpose and rationale, together with examples of their computation and use.

Using Test Scores

Assessments in health professions education generally yield quantitative data. Thus, it is important to consider some basic uses of such data, including various types of scores and score scale properties, and correlation and some of its special applications in assessment. A few basic statistical formulas that are useful in health professions education settings will also be presented.

Basic Score Types

Test or assessment data can be expressed as many different types of scores or on many different types of score scales. Each type of score or score scale has its advantages and disadvantages and each has certain properties that must be understood in order to properly and legitimately interpret the scores. This section notes some basic information about various types of scores and score scales commonly used in health professions education.

Table 5.1 summarizes various types of scores used in assessment and their characteristics.

Number Correct Scores or Raw Scores   For all assessments that are scored dichotomously as right or wrong, such as written achievement tests, the most basic score is the *number correct score*. The number correct or raw score is simply the count of the number of test items the examinee answered correctly. The number correct score or raw score is useful for nearly all types of statistical analyses, score reporting to examinees, and research analyses. The raw score is basic and fundamental and it is therefore useful for nearly all testing applications.

Table 5.1 Types of Scores

Score	Definition	Advantages	Limitations
Raw Scores	Count of number correct; raw ratings	Straightforward; simple to compute, understand, interpret	No relative meaning; need to know total number of items, prompts, points
Percent-correct Scores	Percentage of raw number correct	Simple to compute; widely used and understood	Can not be used with all statistical calculations; may be misleading
Standard Scores	Linear transformed score in SD units	Easily computed and explained relative score; linear transformation; useful in all statistics	May not be familiar to all users
Percentiles	Score rank in distribution	Commonly used and reported; easily computed; traditional score	Easily misunderstood, misused; not useful in statistical calculations; non-equal intervals; often misinterpreted
Equated Scores	Score statistically adjusted to maintain constancy of meaning, score scale	Interchangeability of scores on different test forms, from different administrations	Complex statistical calculations; complex assumptions

Percent-correct Scores   Raw scores are frequently converted to or transformed to *percent-correct scores* in health professions education settings. The percent-correct score is a simple linear transformation of the raw or number-correct score to a percentage, using the formula:

Percent-correct score = (Raw Score / number of items) * 100

The percent-correct score is a linear transformation, which means that the raw scores and percent-correct scores correspond one-to-one and the basic shape of the underlying distribution does not change. Generally, if percent or percent-correct scores are reported and used, one should also report the raw score upon which the percent-correct score is based. (Percents can be misused and can be misleading in some applications, especially when they are presented as the only data.) Also, percent-correct scores do not work properly with all statistical formulas commonly used to evaluate tests (such as the Kuder-Richardson formula 21 used to estimate scale reliability), so it is usually best to use raw scores or linear standard scores in most statistical calculations.

Derived Scores or Standard Scores   Several types of derived or linear standard scores are used in assessment applications. The linear standard score scale is expressed in the standard deviation (SD) score units of the original score distribution. The basic linear standard score, the *z-score*, has a mean of 0 and an SD of 1, and is computed by the following formula:

z-score = (X − mean) / SD
$\quad$ where:
$\quad$ X = raw score
$\quad$ Mean = mean of the raw score distribution
$\quad$ SD = standard deviation of the raw score distribution

Table 5.2 gives an example of ten raw scores and their transformation to z-scores with a further transformation to *T-scores*, which are defined as having a mean of 50, with an SD of 10. Some users prefer T-scores, because T-scores eliminate negative values and a mean score

Table 5.2 Raw Scores, z-Scores, and T-Scores

Raw Score	z-Score	T-Score
41.00	−.30921	46.91
45.00	−.07584	49.24
50.00	.21587	52.16
55.00	.50758	55.08
60.00	.79929	57.99
74.00	1.61608	66.16
18.00	−1.65108	33.49
20.00	−1.53440	34.66
55.00	.50758	55.08
45.00	−.07584	49.24
Mean = 46.3 (SD = 17.1)	Mean = 0; SD = 1	Mean = 50; SD = 10

equal to zero, which the z-score transformation yields. (Some students may be discouraged to receive a negative score, for example.)

The T-score formula is 10 (z-score) + 50. But, you can create a standard score with any mean and SD you wish. Simply multiply the z-score by a desired SD and add the desired mean score to this quantity (SD*(z-score) + desired mean).

The main advantage of these types of derived or standard scores is that they put score data in the metric of the standard deviation of the original raw scores, and maintain the exact shape of the original score distribution. For example, if the original raw scores are skewed to the right (which means that more students score to the high side of the mean than the low side of the mean) the standard score will have exactly the same shape as the original scores. This is a desirable characteristic for most scores that are computed in assessment settings. Other advantages of standard scores such as z- and T-scores is that they can be used in all other statistical calculations such as correlations, t-tests, and ANOVA, plus they can provide easily interpretable absolute and relative score information.

Normalized Standard Scores   It is possible to carry out another type of score transformation which normalizes or forces the transformed distribution of scores to be normally distributed or to follow the normal curve. These normalized standard scores are sometimes used by large testing agencies for research purposes, but are rarely used in health professions education classrooms or reported at the local university level, since there is little benefit to normalizing scores for these ordinary applications. Standard scores, such as z- and T-scores, are not *normalized* scores, since such derived scores maintain the exact shape of the underlying raw score distribution. Simple z- and T-scores should therefore not be referred to as *normalized scores*.

Percentiles   Percentiles or percentile ranks are a favorite type of standard score in health professions education. Percentiles have several slightly different definitions, but generally a percentile refers to a score at or below which that percentage of examinees falls on some distribution of scores.

Percentiles are an inherently relative score, with some benefits and many limitations. The advantage of percentiles is that they are commonly reported and easily computed. Most users think they understand the proper interpretation of percentiles or percentile ranks, yet they are frequently misunderstood or misinterpreted.

Percentiles usually have very unequal intervals, so that, for instance, the 5-point interval between the 50th and 55th percentiles is most likely not the same as the 5-point interval between the 90th and 95th percentile. For example, for a student to increase her test score from the 90th to the 95th percentile typically requires answering many more items correct than to move from the 50th to 55th percentile, because of unequal intervals on the percentile scale. Also, if the underlying raw score distribution upon which percentiles are based is normally distributed, then percentile ranks can be used to make familiar standard score-type of interpretations such as "84 percent of scores fall below + 1 SD above the mean score." But, if the underlying score distribution is non-normal or skewed, as most classroom-type test score distributions are, this interpretation may be incorrect.

Also, percentiles have limited usefulness in other statistical calculations. For example, one cannot legitimately compute correlations of percentiles or use percentiles in inferential statistics, such as *t-tests* or *ANOVA*. Percentiles may be used only to report the rank of the examinee with respect to whatever reference group is used for percentile calculation. And, percentiles may be misunderstood by some users as simple percent-correct scores, which is an incorrect interpretation.

Because of all these limitations, caution is urged in the use and reporting of percentiles or percentile ranks. Linear standard scores, such as z- or T-scores or their variants, are preferred, because there are many fewer limitations for these types of scores and there may be less potential for misinterpretation, misuse, or misunderstanding. Standard scores can be used in almost all statistical calculations, including correlations, inferential statistics, and so on. Plus, standard scores also indicate relative standing using the standard deviation units of the underlying distribution. Generally, derived scores such as z- or T-scores are considered to have equal-interval properties, making the absolute (as opposed to relative) interpretation of these scores more straightforward.

Corrections for Guessing: Formula Scores   One of the persistent controversies in educational measurement concerns the use of so-called "corrections for guessing" or "formula scores" (e.g., Downing, 2003; Downing, Chapter 7, this volume.). These formula scores attempt to compensate for random guessing on selected-response test items, such as multiple-choice items, by either rewarding non-guessing behavior on tests or by punishing guessing behavior. Generally, neither approach works very well and may in fact be somewhat harmful. Since the tendency to guess on selected-response items is a psychological characteristic which varies across a group of examinees, any attempt to control or compensate for presumed guessing is likely to create some error in the measurement. In fact, since the tendency to guess is a psychological construct—which certain bold examinees may exhibit even if they are directed not to guess and threatened with loss of fractional score points—the so-called "corrections for guessing" may add construct-irrelevant variance (CIV) to the scores. CIV, as noted in Chapter 2, is the reliable measurement of some construct other than that which is intended to be measured by the assessment.

Generally, formula scoring or corrections for guessing are not recommended. Simple raw scores or derived or standard scores, in addition to percent-correct scores, are typically sufficient. The best defense against random guessing in selected-response test items is to present well written items in sufficient numbers to reduce any ill effect of random guessing on the part of some examinees.

Equated Scores Most high-stakes large scale testing programs use and report an *equated standard score*. This score may look similar to standard scores such as z-scores or some variant of the z-score. But, these equated scores can be interpreted differently than linear standard scores and are considerably more complex than simple linear standard scores. Equated scores statistically adjust the average difficulty of test scores up or down slightly in order to hold constant the exact meaning of the measuring scale over time and over various administrations of the test. If this statistical adjustment is carried out properly, equated scores maintain the same meaning over time and test forms and can be legitimately compared and interpreted across different test administrations and different time periods of test administration. In statistical jargon, if the test scores are successfully equated, it is a matter of indifference which test form (at which test administration) the examinee takes because the resulting scores are on the same scale (Kolen & Brennan, 2004).

Test score equating is beyond the scope of this chapter. The major consideration to note here is that equated scores, such as those reported by large-scale testing agencies like the National Board of Medical Examiners (NBME), the Medical Council of Canada (MCC), and the Educational Testing Service (ETS) permit more complex interpretations of scores than the simple z- and T-scores discussed here. Conversely, simple z- or T-scores can be interpreted as invariant with respect to mean difficulty, as are equated scores, only when the groups tested have approximately equal levels of ability, which rarely occurs in practice.

Composite Scores   The term *composite score* refers to a summary score that reflects multiple component scores. Commonly, a composite score is a total score (or grade) which is formed by adding scores from multiple scores generated during a course. For instance, a total composite score may be formed by adding together (and possibly differentially weighting) various individual component test or assessment scores for a class or a clerkship. A simple example of a composite score is a total score which is formed by averaging differentially weighted individual test scores collected during a semester-long class in which several different tests are administered to students. Instructors decide how much to weight each individual test score (and inform students of these weights), then apply these policy weights to test scores prior to summing in order to form an overall composite score, upon which the final grade is determined.

In order to ensure that the weights for each individual component score is exact, it is best to transform each component score to a linear standard score, using the mean and standard deviation of that score distribution, prior to multiplying by the assigned policy weight. If scores are not standardized, the effective weighting may be quite different from the weight applied to the raw scores, since the test score distribution with the larger standard deviation will contribute more weight to the final composite score than component scores with a lower SD (Stagnaro-Green, Deng, Downing & Crosson, 2004).

For composite scores in more complex settings, such as clerkships or other performance settings in health professions education, scores often display widely different scales, with widely different variances, so it is especially important to standardize component scores prior to weighting and summing to a composite. Each individual component score should first be transformed to a standard score, then multiplied by the desired weight (as determined by some rational, judgmental, or empirical process) and then summed or averaged to a final composite (which might be transformed to some other metric for convenience).

The determination of the reliability of the composite score is a special topic in reliability. In order to estimate the reliability of the composite score accurately, it is necessary to take into account the reliability of each individual component score and the weight assigned to that component. Several methods—such as the stratified alpha coefficient—are available to properly estimate the reliability of the composite score (Feldt & Brennan, 1989; Thissen & Wainer, 2001). If the differential policy weights are not considered, the reliability of the composite score will be underestimated.

Correlation and Disattenuated Correlation

Correlation coefficients are central to many statistical analyses used in assessment research. For example, correlation is a primary statistical method used in validity and reliability analyses and also for test item analysis. Various specialized types of correlation coefficients are used in test analysis and research, but all have the Pearson Product Moment Correlation as their basis. All correlations track the co-relationship between two variables, showing both the strength and the direction of any relationship. Correlation coefficients range from −1.0 to +1.0, with ±1.0 indicating a perfect relationship between the variables. A perfect negative correlation is just as strong a predictor as a perfect positive correlation. With a negative correlation, of course, the variables move in exactly opposite directions, such that as one variable increases the other variable decreases. In some test analyses which use correlation coefficients, such as the item discrimination index used in item analysis, it would be rare if the correlation of the item score (0,1) and the total test score were to reach ±1.0.

Correlation coefficients are attenuated or decreased by measurement error. For example, the correlation between test scores on two different tests, administered to the same examinees, is often used as one source of validity evidence for the test scores. But, we know that the observed correlation is lower than the "true" correlation, because unreliable measures reduce or disguise the underlying relationship between the variables. If we could know the perfectly reliable scores (the true scores) from one or both tests, we could correlate these so-called "true scores" and understand the true relationship between the underlying traits that the two tests measure.

Classical measurement theory allows us to estimate this true score correlation or, as it is often called, the disattenuated correlation coefficient. The disattenuated correlation formula is presented in more detail in the appendix of this chapter. This simple formula shows that the observed correlation is divided by the square root of the product of the reliability of each test. If the reliability of only one of the two tests is known, typically 1.0 is used for the value of the unknown reliability, since this will be the most parsimonious or conservative assumption. Obviously, the lower the reliabilities of the measures, the more correction will be observed in the disattenuated correlation coefficient.

The disattenuated correlation is a useful theoretical tool which is often reported in research studies because it helps to elucidate the underlying or true relationship between test or assessment scores and a criterion scores. But, it is important to emphasize that in actual practice, the errors of measurement—for example, the unreliability of the predictor test scores and/or the unreliability of some criterion measure—should be included in the validity coefficients, since this represents the state of nature and the actual or observed correlation of the two variables in the real world setting. Disattenuated correlation coefficients should be clearly labeled as such and always reported together with the observed correlations upon which they are based.

Item Analysis

Item analysis is a quality control tool for tests, providing quantitative data at the item-level, as well as some important summary statistics about the total test. Item analysis should be used extensively for selected-response tests such as multiple-choice tests, but can (and should) also be utilized for observational rating scale data, ratings used in performance assessment simulations, and so on. Careful review of item analysis data can help to improve the reliability and consequently the validity of scores generated by instruments. Item analysis can assist in the improvement of the quality and clarity of test items and other types of rating scale prompts. Item analysis data, which represents the history of past performance of an item, should be stored in an item bank or other secure file for development of future tests. Item analysis data is also frequently used to complete a final key validation step prior to final scoring (Downing, 2006).

In its most basic form, item analysis represents counts (and percentages) of examinee responses to the options that make up a selected-response item. In order to evaluate the performance of the item or rating scale prompt (e.g., Livingston, 2006), these counts are usually further evaluated in terms of groups of high-scoring examinees and low-scoring examinees with various statistics computed to summarize the item difficulty and item discrimination (how well the test item differentiates between high- and low-scoring students).

Item Analysis Report for Each Test Item

Table 5.3 presents a detailed annotated example of typical item analysis data for a single test item. The top portion of the table gives the text of the multiple-choice item. The middle portion of the table presents the item analysis data, followed by a description of each entry of the item analysis data. Software used to calculate item analyses differ in style, format and some of the specific statistics computed, but all are similar to the one displayed in Table 5.3. Common data entries for most item analyses are: test item number or other identifier, index of item difficulty and item discrimination, option performance usually grouped by examinee ability and a discrimination index for each option of the test item.

Looking at the detail in Table 5.3, under the heading of "Option Statistics," note a breakdown of how examinees responded to each MCQ option. The MCQ options are listed as A to E and *Other* refers to those who omitted or failed to answer this item. The column labeled "Total" is the total proportion marking each option. The keyed correct option or answer is indicated and its total is used to calculate the "Prop. Correct" for this test item. The "low" and "high" groups refer to the lowest scoring 27% and the highest scoring 27% of examinees on the total test, with the numbers in the columns indicating the proportion of examinees in each group who responded to each option. (Using the lowest and highest 27% of examinees is the minimum group size needed in order to maximize the reliable difference between these two extreme score groups, because we can be fairly

Table 5.3 Item Analysis Example

Where it is an absolute question of the welfare of our country, we must admit of no considerations of justice or injustice, or mercy or cruelty, or praise or ignominy, but putting all else aside must adopt whatever course will save its existence and preserve its liberty.

This quote is most likely from which of the following?

     A. Niccolo Machiavelli
     B. Attila the Hun
     C. King Henry VIII
     D. Vlad the Impailer
     E. Napoleon Bonaparte

Item Statistics   *Option Statistics*

Prop.[1] Correct	Disc.[2] Index	Point[3] Biser.	Option[4]	Total[5]	Low[6]	High[7]	Point[8] Biser.
0.70	**0.30**	**0.27**	A*[9]	0.70	0.55	0.85	0.27
			B	0.05	0.08	0.01	−0.14
			C	0.02	0.03	0.02	−0.01
			D	0.13	0.18	0.07	−0.13
			E	0.10	0.16	0.04	−0.15
			Other	0.00	0.00	0.00	0.00

Guide to Item Analysis Statistics

1. Proportion Correct (p-value): The total proportion (percentage) of examinees who marked the item correct. In this example, the p-value or item difficulty is 0.70, indicating that 70% of all examinees who attempted this question marked it correct.
2. Discrimination Index (D): This discrimination index is the simple difference between the percentage of a high and low group of examinees who mark the item correct. In this example, $D = (0.85 − 0.55) = 0.30$.
3. Point Biserial Correlation/Discrimination Index (r_{pbis}): Correlation between the item score (0,1) and the total score on the test.
4. Option: The item options (1–5 or A–E). Other refers to missing data or blanks.
5. Total: Total proportion (percent) marking each option or alternative answer.
6. Low (Group): Proportion marking each option or alternative answer in the lowest scoring group of examinees on the total test. In this case, the group of examinees scoring in the lowest 27% of the total score distribution.
7. High (Group): Proportion marking each option or alternative answer in the highest scoring group of examinees on the total test. In this case, the group of examinees scoring in the highest 27% of the total score distribution.
8. Point Biserial Discrimination Index: This is the r_{pbis} for each option of the item, including the correct option. Note that, for the keyed correct option, the r_{pbis} is the same as noted in #3.
9. * Answer Key: The keyed correct answer.

certain that there is no overlap in group membership between the upper and lower 27% proficiency groupings.)

Item Difficulty

Item difficulty refers to the proportion of examinees who answer an item correctly. This index is usually expressed as a proportion or percent, such as *0.60* which means that 60% of the group of test takers answered the item correctly. (This index might more accurately be called an item easiness index, since it reflects proportion correct but it is usually referred to as an item difficulty index.)

The item difficulty index is the most basic essential information to evaluate about the performance of the test item.

Item Discrimination

Effective test items differentiate high-ability examinees from low-ability examinees. (Ability means achievement proficiency in this context.) This is a fundamental principle of all educational measurement and a basic validity principle. For example, an achievement test in head and neck anatomy purports to measure this achievement construct in a unified manner. Theory posits that those students who are most proficient in the content should score higher than students who are less proficient or who have learned less of the content tested. For this particular construct, the best criterion variable available is probably the total score on this particular test of head and neck anatomy. It follows that highly proficient students should score better on individual test items than less proficient or accomplished students. This logic describes the basic conceptual framework for item discrimination.

Item discrimination is the most important information to evaluate about the performance of the test item, because the level of discrimination reflects the degree to which an item contributes to the measurement objective of the test.

Discrimination Indices

Several different statistics are used as discrimination indices for tests. The most basic discrimination index is given by the simple difference in proportions of examinees in a high-scoring group who get the item correct and those in a low-scoring group who get the item correct. This index (D) is easily computed and can be interpreted like all other discrimination indices, such that high positive values are best and very low, 0, or negative values are always undesirable. See note 2 in Table 5.3 for the example of D.

As an example, if 77% of a high-scoring examinee group gets an item correct, but only 34% of a low-scoring group of examinees gets the item correct, the simple discrimination index, D, is equal to $77 - 34 = 43$. This $D = 43$ (usually expressed as $D = 0.43$) indicates strong positive discrimination for this test item and shows that this particular item sharply differentiates between high- and low-achievers on this test. The D index should be interpreted like all other item discrimination indices such that a minimum acceptable value is about +0.20 or so.

Point Biserial Correlation as Discrimination Index

Special types of correlation coefficients are also used as item discrimination indices for test item analyses. The point biserial (r_{pbis}) index of discrimination is the correlation between student performance on the item (that is, getting the item correct or incorrect, where $1 =$ correct and $0 =$ incorrect) and performance on the entire test. As in all correlation, the (theoretical) values of the point biserial index of discrimination can range from -1.0 to $+1.0$, indicating the strength of statistical relationships. (Because one variable in the correlation is dichotomous, the upper and lower bound of this type of correlation is usually not actually ± 1.0.) Practically, point biserial correlations of about 0.45 to 0.65 or so are considered very high. See note 3 in Table 5.3 for an example.

A simple quantitative illustration of item discrimination calculation for a single test item is given in Table 5.4. This example shows how

Table 5.4 Correlation of One Test Item Score with Score on the Total Test

Student	Item Score (Right-Wrong)	Score on Total Test
1	1	41
2	0	45
3	0	50
4	1	55
5	0	60
6	1	74
7	1	18
8	0	20
9	1	55
10	0	45

Note: Correlation between item score (1, 0)—right or wrong—is $r_{iT} = +0.14$. This low correlation of the item and total scores indicates a low (but positive) item discrimination for this single test item.

10 students score on one test item. The middle column describes how each of these 10 students scored on this particular test item, with a *1* indicating that the student got the item correct and a *0* indicating that the student got the item incorrect. The third column gives the total score on this test. So, in this example, student 1 answered this item correctly and scored 41 on the total test. The discrimination index (r_{iT}) for this item equals +0.14; this shows the correlation between the item scores (1, 0) and the total score on the test for this group of examinees and indicates that this item differentiates high and low scoring examinees positively.

Biserial Correlation as Discrimination Index

Another type of correlation coefficient is sometimes used as an item discrimination index: the biserial correlation. This is similar to the point biserial, but uses slightly different assumptions. It is a matter of some personal preference whether to use the point biserial or biserial. Often, item analysis software computes both of these indices. The main practical difference is that the biserial index is always slightly higher than the point biserial, so the interpretation of this index must be adjusted upward somewhat relative to the interpretation of the point biserial. Either or both correlations are perfectly reasonable to use and both indices provide exactly the same information; the only difference is in the magnitude of the scale.

What is Good Item Discrimination?

High positive discrimination is always better than low or negative discrimination. But, how high is high? Typically, large-scale standardized test developers expect effective items to have point biserial discrimination indices of at least +0.30 or higher, but for locally developed classroom-type tests, one may be reasonably happy with a discrimination index in the mid to high 0.20s. At minimum, all discrimination indices should be a positive number, especially if there are any stakes involved in the assessment. (Negatively discriminating test items add nothing to the measurement and may detract from some of the important psychometric characteristics of the overall test and reduce the validity of the test scores.)

General Recommendations for Item Difficulty and Item Discrimination

Table 5.5 presents an overview of some general recommendations for ideal item difficulty and discrimination for most classroom-type achievement tests. All of these recommended values should be interpreted in terms of the purpose of the examinations, the types of instructional settings, the stakes associated with the tests and so on.

Table 5.5 Item Classification Guide by Difficulty and Discrimination[1]

Item Class	Item Difficulty	Item Discrimination (Point Biserial)	Description
Level I	0.45 to 0.75	+0.20 or higher	Best item statistics; use most items in this range if possible
Level II	0.76 to 0.91	+0.15 or higher	Easy; use sparingly
Level III	0.25 to 0.44	+0.10 or higher	Difficult; use very sparingly and only if content is essential – rewrite if possible
Level IV	<0.24 or >0.91	Any Discrim.	Extremely difficult or easy; do not use unless content is essential

Source: 1. Adapted from Haladyna (2004).

These recommended values for item difficulty and discrimination represent ideals. For most classroom type testing settings, especially those with a more "mastery" instructional philosophy, these recommendations will be too stringent and may have to be realistically adjusted downward somewhat.

These recommendations are based on theory which suggests that the most informative test items are those of middle difficulty which discriminate highly. For most achievement tests, we would like most items to be in this middle range of average item difficulty, with high discrimination. These are the Level I items noted in Table 5.5. The next best item statistical characteristics are those noted as Level II items: somewhat easier items than Level I, but with fair discrimination. Level III and Level IV items are either very easy, or hard with low item discrimination. These are the least effective items psychometrically, but it is certainly possible that such items measure important content and should therefore be used (if absolutely necessary) to enhance the content-related validity of the test scores.

In interpreting the recommendations in Table 5.5, where possible consider both item difficulty and item discrimination. Both item parameters are important, but item discrimination may be more important than difficulty (if you have to choose between the two parameters). It must be noted that item difficulty and item discrimination are not totally independent. Middle difficulty items have a better chance of discriminating well because of higher expected variance. But, be aware that very easy items and very difficult items sometimes have high discrimination indices as an artifact of their extreme difficulty. Since few examinees fall into the category groups for very hard or very easy items, a change of a few examinees can change the discrimination index greatly, but this may be an artifact of the small numbers of examinees in ability groups.

Item Options

The ideal item is one in which each distractor (incorrect option) is selected by at least some students who do not know the content tested by the question. An incorrect option that fails to attract any examinees is a dysfunctional distracter and adds nothing to the item or the test (psychometrically). The correct or best answer option should have a positive discrimination index—the higher the better; of course, this is the discrimination index for the item. Incorrect options—the wrong answers, should have negative discrimination indices because the less able examinees should be choosing the incorrect answers at higher frequency than the more able examinees.

Number of Examinees Needed for Item Analysis

Treat any item difficulty or item discrimination index cautiously if the statistics are based on a test administration with fewer than 100 examinees or so. (We really need about $N = 200$ examinees to have stable item analysis statistics.) However, even for small samples (e.g., $N \cong 30$) the results may still provide some useful guidance for item improvement. Usually some information is better than no information when one is trying to improve a test, realizing that the statistics based on small ns are unstable and may change at the next administration of the item. (In statistical terms, the smaller the sample size on which an item analysis is based, the greater the sampling error and the larger the standard errors around the sample statistics.)

Note that all item analysis data based on classical measurement theory are sample dependent such that all item difficulty and discrimination statistics are confounded with the ability or proficiency of the particular sample of examinees. If the sample of examinees is large and if the range of student ability is fairly consistent for each administration of the test, item difficulty and discrimination values are likely to be stable over time.

Summary Statistics for a Test

Table 5.6 illustrates an example of summary statistics computed as part of a complete item analysis. These statistics are for a total test, with all terms defined in the column on the right of the table.

These statistics describe the overall performance of the test and provide validity evidence useful for test score interpretation by providing

Table 5.6 Example of Summary Item Statistics for Total Test

		Definition of Terms
N of items	35	Number of items
N of examinees	52	Number of examinees
Mean Raw Score	26.56	Mean number-correct raw score
Variance	8.36	Variance, number-correct raw score ($= SD^2$)
S.D.	2.89	Standard Deviation, number-correct raw score
Minimum	21.00	Minimum, number-correct raw score
Maximum	32.00	Maximum, number-correct raw score
Median	27.00	Median, number-correct raw score
Reliability	0.35	Internal consistency reliability: KR 20 or Alpha
SEM	2.34	Standard error of measurement
Mean Difficulty	0.76	Mean proportion/percent correct
Mean r_{pbis} Discrimination	0.08	Mean point biserial item discrimination
Mean Biserial	0.13	Mean biserial item discrimination

guidance for using scores in making judgments about examinees and also provide useful evaluative information about the performance of the test. This summary (Table 5.6) presents the total number of examinees and the total number of test items, the average raw score (number correct score) with its standard deviation and variance (SD^2). We also see the minimum, maximum, and median raw score. These data give an overview of the shape of the score distribution and describe generally where on the distribution most examinees scored. The mean item difficulty, together with the two mean item discrimination indices, give us additional information about how hard or easy the items were on average and how well they discriminate. The reliability coefficient is the Kuder-Richardson Formula #20 (or Cronbach's Alpha) which is an index of the internal consistency of the measuring scale, indicating the precision of measurement. The standard error of measurement (SEM) is computed from the reliability coefficient, showing the precision of measurement on the raw score scale.

Useful Formulas

The appendix presents some useful formulas together with worked examples using synthetic data. These formulas can be found in any basic educational measurement text, such as Mehrens and Lehmann (1991) and also Thissen and Wainer (2001). These four formulas are frequently used in assessment settings and can be hand calculated, using readily available data. If computer software is unavailable, these formulas can provide some useful information about assessments, and assist health professions educators in evaluating assessment data and planning future assessments.

A formula is provided to estimate the internal consistency reliability of a test when only the mean of test scores, the variance (SD^2), and the total number of test items is known. The Kuder-Richardson formula number 21 (KR 21) typically underestimates the more precise Kuder-Richardson formula number 20 (KR 20) slightly, but can be computed by hand, from the limited data available. The KR 20 is usually computed by computer software (within item analysis software), because it is computationally complex, using item-level data to estimate the variances used in the calculation.

The standard error of measurement (SEM) is an important statistic, computed from the reliability coefficient and the standard deviation of scores. Most item analysis software applications compute the SEM, but it is easily computed by hand if software is unavailable. The SEM can be used to build confidence intervals around observed test scores and is a useful application of the reliability coefficient indicating the precision of measurement and the amount of measurement error in scores, expressed in the metric of the standard deviation of the test scores.

The Spearman-Brown Prophecy Formula (S-B) is useful to estimate the expected increase or decrease in test reliability resulting from increasing or decreasing the number of test items in the scale. The S-B formula assumes that items which are added or subtracted from a test are more-or-less identical to the original items with respect to mean item difficulty, mean item discrimination, content, and so on.

The formula for the disattenuated correlation coefficient or the correction for attenuation of a correlation coefficient is also presented in the appendix and was discussed in the text above. With all the cautions for its use noted above, the disattenuated correlation coefficient estimates the correlation of true scores (in classical measurement theory) and answers the theoretical question: "What is the estimated correlation between the two variables—usually test scores or assessment ratings—if the scores or ratings were perfectly reliable?" The disattenuated correlation coefficient should be reported only together with the observed or actual correlation coefficient and should always be clearly labeled as the disattenuated correlation coefficient or the correction for attenuation.

Summary

This chapter has summarized some of the basic statistics used for assessment. Raw scores, the basic number-correct scores which generally serve as the fundamental scoring unit, were discussed. Standard scores, which express assessment scores in the metric of the standard deviation of the raw score scale, were generally recommended as more useful than percentiles. The fundamentals of classical item analysis and summary test score analysis were discussed and item analysis was recommended for all assessments in health professions education as a basic tool to improve assessments. Finally, several statistical formulas which are frequently and usefully used in evaluating assessments were presented, such that the reader can easily compute many of the basic evaluative test statistics.

APPENDIX: SOME USEFUL FORMULAS WITH EXAMPLE CALCULATIONS

Kuder Richardson Formula #21: Reliability Estimate

Use: An estimate of the internal consistency reliability if only the total number of test items, mean score, and standard deviation (SD) are known. Note raw scores, not percent-correct scores, should be used for these calculations.

Note that the KR 21 usually slightly underestimates the more precise KR 20 reliability, but the KR 20 requires computer software for calculation.

KR 21 = (K / K – 1) (1 – (M*(K – M) / (K* Var)))
Where:

K = Number of test items (raw number of items)
M = Raw score mean
Var = Raw score variance (SD²)

Worked Example: A basic science test has 50 test items, with a mean score of 36.5 and a standard deviation of 10. What is the KR 21 reliability estimate for this test?

KR 21 Reliability = (50 / 49) (1 – ((36.5 * (50 – 36.5) /
$\qquad$ (50 * 100)))
$\qquad$ = (1.0204) (1 – (36.5 * 13.5) / 5000)
$\qquad$ = (1.0204) (1 – (492.75 / 5000)
$\qquad$ = (1.0204) (1 – (0.09855)
$\qquad$ = (1.0204) (0.90145)
$\qquad$ = 0.92

Standard Error of Measurement (SEM)

Use: To form confidence bands (CIs) around the observed score indicating the range of scores within which the "true score" falls, with known probability.

$$SEM = SD * \sqrt{1 - \text{Reliability}}$$

Where:

SD = Standard Deviation of the test
Reliability = Reliability estimate for the test

Worked Example: A test of 100 items has a mean of 73 and an SD of 12, with a KR 20 reliability of 0.89. What is the standard error of measurement?

$$SEM = 12 * \sqrt{1 - 0.89}$$

$$= 12 * \sqrt{0.11}$$
$$= 12 * 0.33$$
$$= 3.96$$

If a student has a raw score of 25 on this test, what is the 95% confidence interval for his true score?

95% CI = $\overline{X}$ ± 1.96 (SEM)
$$= 25 \pm 1.96 \ (3.96)$$
$$= 25 \pm 7.76$$
$$17.24 \geq T \leq 32.76$$

Spearman-Brown Prophecy Formula

Use: To estimate the reliability of a test that is longer (or shorter) than a test with a known reliability

Reliability of longer test = (N * Rel of Org Test) / (1 + Rel of Org Test)
Where:

N = Number of times test is lengthened (or shortened)

Worked Example: A test of 30 items has a reliability of 0.35. What is the expected reliability if the test is lengthened to 90 items?

SB Reliability, 90 item test = (3 * 0.35) / (1 + 0.35)
$$= (1.05) / (1.35)$$
$$= 0.77$$

Disattenuated Correlation: Correction for Attenuation

Use: To estimate the "true score" correlation between two variables; to estimate the (theoretical) correlation between two variables if one or both variables were perfectly reliable. The disattenuated correlation coefficient (theoretically) removes the attenuating effect on the correlation coefficient due to random errors of measurement or unreliability.

Disattenuated Correlation $= R_{tt} = R_{xy} / \sqrt{(R_{xx} * R_{yy})}$

Where:

R_{tt} = Estimated Disattenuated Correlation Coefficient
R_{xy} = The observed correlation coefficient between variables x and y
R_{xx} = The reliability of variable (test) X
R_{yy} = The reliability of variable (test) Y

Worked Example: Tests A and B correlated 0.48. The reliability of Test A is 0.70 and the reliability of Test B is 0.51. What is the disattenuated correlation between Test A and Test B?

$$R_{tt} = 0.48 / \sqrt{(0.70 * 0.51)}$$

$$= 0.48 / \sqrt{0.357}$$

$$= 0.48 / 0.597$$

$$= 0.80$$

If both Tests A and B were perfectly reliable, the expected true score correlation is 0.80. The disattenuated correlation should be reported only in conjunction with the observed correlation and the estimate of reliability for both measures.

Note that if the reliability for only one of the two measures is known, set the unknown reliability to 1.0 for this calculation.

References

Downing, S.M. (2003). Guessing on selected-response examinations. *Medical Education*, 37, 670–671.

Downing, S.M. (2006). Twelve steps for effective test development. In S.M. Downing & T.M. Haladyna (Eds.), *Handbook of test development* (pp. 3–25). Mahwah, NJ: Lawrence Erlbaum Associates.

Feldt, L.S., & Brennan, R.L. (1989). Reliability. In R.L. Linn (Ed.), *Educational measurement* (3rd ed., pp. 105–146). New York: American Council on Education and Macmillan.

Haladyna, T.M. (2004). *Developing and validating multiple-choice test items* (3rd ed.). Mahwah, NJ: Lawrence Erlbaum Associates.

Kolen, M.J., & Brennan, R.L. (2004). *Test equating, scaling, and linking: Methods and practices* (2nd ed.). New York: Springer-Verlag.

Livingston, S.A. (2006). Item analysis. In S.M. Downing & T.M. Haladyna (Eds.), *Handbook of test development* (pp. 421–441). Mahwah, NJ: Lawrence Erlbaum Associates.

Mehrens, W.A., & Lehmann, I.J. (1991). *Measurement and evaluation in education and psychology* (4th ed.). New York: Harcourt Brace College Publishers.

Stagnaro-Green, A., Deng, W., Downing, S.M., & Crosson, J. (2004, November). Theoretical model evaluating the impact of weighted percent versus standard scores in determining third year clerkship grades. Paper presentation at the Annual Meeting of the Association of American Medical Colleges, RIME, Boston, MA.

Thissen, D., & Wainer, H. (Eds.). (2001). *Test scoring*. Mahwah, NJ: Lawrence Erlbaum.

6

STANDARD SETTING

RACHEL YUDKOWSKY,
STEVEN M. DOWNING, AND ARA TEKIAN

Introduction

A standard determines whether a given score or performance is good enough for a particular purpose (Norcini & Guille, 2002). The term "standard setting" refers to a process used to create boundaries between categories such as pass | fail, or honors | proficient | needs remediation. Standard setting is "central to the task of giving meaning to test results and thus lies at the heart of validity argument" (Dylan, 1996). Establishing credible, defensible, and acceptable passing or cut-off scores for examinations in health professions education can be challenging (Friedman, 2000; Norcini & Shea, 1997; Norcini & Guille, 2002). There is a large literature of standard setting, much of which is devoted to empirical passing score studies and comparisons of various standard-setting methods which are appropriate for selected-response tests or performance tests used in K-12 educational settings (Cizek, 2001, 2006; Cizek, Bunch, & Koons, 2004; Livingston, 1982; Norcini, 2003). This chapter will discuss key issues and decisions regarding standard setting, identify ways to assess the quality and consequences of resulting standards, and address special situations such as combining standards across subtests, setting standards for performance tests, and multiple-category cut scores. At the end of the chapter we provide detailed instructions for conducting six standard setting methods commonly used in health professions settings: Angoff, Ebel, Hofstee, Borderline Group, Contrasting Groups, and Body of Work.

A cut score is an operational statement of policy. All standard setting methods require judgment; the object of a standard setting exercise is to capture the opinions of expert judges in order to inform a policy decision of "how much is enough" for a given purpose. There is no single correct or best method to set standards for an examination; nor is there a single correct or "true" cut score that must be discovered. All standards are, to some extent, arbitrary. Thus standard setting can best be viewed as "due process"—a procedure to be followed to ensure that the cut score is not capricious; that it is reasonable, defensible, and fair.

Standards can be categorized as either relative (norm-based) or absolute (criterion-based). Relative standards identify a group of passing and failing examinees *relative* to the performance of some well defined group; the cut score or standard will depend on the performance of the specific group tested—for example, the bottom 5% of the class, or those who score more than two standard deviations below the mean of first time test takers. Relative standards are most appropriate when a rank ordering of students is needed in order to distribute limited resources: for example, to give "honors" grades to the top 10% of the students in a surgery clerkship, to select top scoring applicants for entry to dental school, or to identify those pharmacy students most in need of remedial tutoring before progressing to the next stage of training. The placement of the cut score will depend on the resources available.

Absolute or criterion-based standards are based on a predetermined level of competency that does not depend on the performance of the group—for example, a score of 70%. Absolute standards reflect a desired level of mastery; the criterion stays the same whether all students pass or none do. In health professions education the purpose of most examinations is to confirm mastery of a domain of knowledge or skill, so in the past decades most professional schools in the US have moved to the use of absolute standards.

This chapter will focus on ways to obtain defensible and reasonable *absolute* standards. The term "absolute" implies that passing score judgments are made such that judges are blind to actual performance data, looking only at the content of the test or the performance prompts. This is the purist view, but the reality is that totally pure absolute standards rarely turn out to be realistic, acceptable, or useful in the real world of health professions education. Expert judges tend to expect even borderline examinees to know more and be able to do more than is realistic. Studies have demonstrated that judges, absent all performance data, tend to set unrealistically high passing scores, which will fail an unreasonably high proportion of students (Cizek, 2001; Kane, Crooks & Cohen, 1999). Experts almost always expect too much of novice learners.

The point of view adopted in this book is that judges must be "calibrated" to have a realistic expectation of actual student performance. Such calibration requires presenting some performance data to judges so that standard setting panels have a reasonable expectation concerning actual student performance on the assessment. Some experts in education disagree with this point of view and may label such methods biased. We prefer the efficiency of judge calibration to the inefficiency of repeating the standard setting exercise a second or third time if the first rounds result in unacceptably high standards.

Eight Steps for Standard Setting

Hambleton and Pitoniak (2006) divide the process of setting absolute or criterion-based standards into six critical steps: selecting a method, preparing performance category descriptions, forming a standard-setting panel, training panelists, providing feedback to panelists and evaluating and documenting the validity of the process. In this chapter we will use a modification of their scheme, slightly elaborated to include eight steps (see Figure 6.1). We will discuss the key issues involved in each of these steps in turn.

Step 1: Select a Standard Setting Method

There is no "gold standard" for a passing score. There is no perfect passing score "out there" waiting to be discovered. Rather, the passing score is whatever a group of content expert judges determine it is, having followed a systematic, reproducible, absolute, and unbiased process. The key to defensible and acceptable standards is the

Step 1: Select a standard setting method
Step 2: Select judges
Step 3: Prepare descriptions of performance categories
Step 4: Train judges
Step 5: Collect ratings or judgments
Step 6: Provide feedback and facilitate discussion
Step 7: Evaluate the standard setting process
Step 8: Provide results, consequences and validity evidence to final decision makers

Figure 6.1 Eight Steps for Standard Setting.*

Source: * Modified from Hambleton and Pitoniak (2006)

implementation of a careful, systematic method to collect expert judgments, preferably a method that is based on research evidence. Different standard setting methods will produce different passing scores, and different groups of judges, following exactly the same procedures, may also produce different passing scores for the same assessment. Such facts are troubling only if one expects to discover the perfect or "gold standard" passing score. Process is the key concept, remembering that *all passing scores are ultimately policy decisions,* which are inherently subjective (Ebel, 1972).

Methods for setting standards can be described broadly as either test-based or examinee-based. In *test-based methods* such as the Angoff (Angoff, 1971) and Ebel (Ebel, 1972) methods described at the end of this chapter, judges review test items or prompts and estimate the expected level of performance of a borderline examinee (one just at the margin between two categories) on a given task. In *examinee-based methods* (represented here by the Borderline Group (Livingston & Zieky, 1982), Contrasting Groups (Burrows, Bingham, & Brailovsky, 1999; Clauser & Clyman, 1994; Livingston & Zieky, 1982) and Body of Work (Kingston, Kahl, Sweeney, & Bay, 2001) methods) judges categorize the performance of individual examinees, either through direct observation, review of proxies of their behavior such as performance checklists, or review of examinee products such as chart notes written after a standardized patient encounter. In these methods, the scores of examinees in different performance categories are utilized in order to generate the final cut score. Finally, *compromise methods* such as the Hofstee method combine features of absolute and relative standards, asking judges to estimate both acceptable passing scores and acceptable fail rates.

At the end of this chapter we describe these six methods—Angoff, Ebel, Hofstee, Borderline, Contrasting Groups and Body-of-Work—all of which are potentially useful for establishing realistic and acceptable standards for examinations in the health professions (see Table 6.6). Choice of method depends on the type of assessment data, feasibility, resources available, and the preferences of decision makers at a given site.

Step 2: Select Judges

For the absolute methods discussed here, the choice of content expert judges is crucial. The passing scores established are only as credible as the judges and the soundness of the systematic methods used (Norcini & Shea, 1997). Content expertise is the most important characteristic of judges selected for the standard setting exercise. Judges must also know the target population well, understand both their task as judges and the content materials used in the performance assessment, be fair, open-minded, and willing to follow directions, be as unbiased as possible, and be willing and able to devote their full attention to the task. In some settings, it may be important to balance the panel of judges with respect to demographic variables, such as ethnicity, gender, geography, and subspecialization. For most methods and settings, five to six independent judges might be considered minimum, with 10 to 12 judges the maximum. Practical considerations must often play a major role in judge selection, the numbers of judges used, the venues for standard setting exercises, and the exact manner in which the procedures are implemented.

Step 3: Prepare Descriptions of Performance Categories

Standard setting results in one or more cut scores that divide the distribution of scores into two or more performance categories or levels such as Pass | Fail, or Basic | Proficient | Advanced. Judges must have a clear idea of the behaviors expected in each of the categories. What behaviors characterize graduating medical students who are ready for supervised practice as residents? How does an "Advanced" level nursing student differ from a "Proficient" student in the context of a pediatric rotation? Performance categories are narrative descriptions of the minimally acceptable behaviors required in order to be included in a given category. The cut points represent the boundaries between these performance categories on the exam score distribution. The performance category descriptions may be generated by the same judges who will set the cut points, or by a different group of persons familiar with the curriculum and the examinees.

Step 4: Train Judges

It is essential that every standard setting judge fully understands the relationship between passing scores and passing rates. The passing *score* is the score needed to pass the performance test, often expressed as a percent-correct score. The passing *rate* is the percentage of students who pass the test at any given passing score (sometimes expressed as the failure rate). The higher the passing score, the lower the passing rate. If standard setting judges confuse these two statistics, their judgments will confuse the passing score and become a threat to the validity of the standard.

Most absolute standard setting methods pivot on the idea of the borderline student or examinee. This concept originated with Angoff's original work on absolute passing scores (Angoff, 1971). The cut score separating those who pass from those who fail corresponds to the point that exactly separates those who know (or can do) just enough to pass from those who do not know enough (or cannot do enough) to pass. The borderline examinee is thus one who has an exactly 50–50 probability of passing or failing the test. The borderline examinee is the marginal student—one who on some days might just pass your assessment, but on other days might fail.

The definition of borderline examinee is straightforward, but operationalizing this definition can be challenging. Asking judges to describe borderline students they have known imparts a clear under-standing of what it means to be "borderline" and facilitates group consensus prior to beginning the standard setting work.

Step 5: Collect Ratings or Judgments

See the detailed instructions for each of the six methods provided at the end of this chapter. Quality control and documentation of collection processes are essential to provide "response process" type evidence for the validity of the standards obtained. The procedures described in this paper are examples of only one particular way to implement each method. Every setting is unique and minor (or major) modifications to these standard-setting procedures may be required in some settings.

Step 6: Provide Feedback and Facilitate Discussion

Many of the test-based methods include an iterative procedure in which outlier ratings are discussed and justified, performance data may be provided, and consequences (failure rates based on the judg-ments at that stage) may be revealed. The item rating procedure is then repeated, and judges may choose to revise their ratings, but are not required to do so. The cycle may be repeated one or two times. Iterative procedures tend to create more of a consensus among judges, but do not necessarily substantively change the resulting cut score (Stern, et al., 2005). Some educators forgo discussions and iterations for local low- to medium-stakes examinations.

We noted above that judges, absent data about actual examinee performance, tend to set unrealistically high passing scores. While proponents of iterative procedures tend to advocate the provision of performance data at the second iteration, few judges change their ratings once the initial mental effort has been expended (Kane, et al., 1999). To have a moderating impact on ratings performance data should be provided at the outset, before the first round of judgments (Clauser, Margolis, & Case, 2006; Kane, et al., 1999; Shea, Reshetar, Norcini, & Dawson, 1994).

Some judge panels wish to know, from time to time throughout the process, what passing score and/or passing rate they have established thus far in the process. Again, this is a matter for professional judgment and we take the position that, in general, more data is better than less data for all judgments.

Step 7: Evaluate the Standard Setting Procedure

No matter which standard setting method you choose, some evaluation of the resulting standard is appropriate. Is your cut score acceptable to your stakeholders? If not, is it because the test was not appropriately constructed, because your curriculum did not prepare students for the exam, or because your standard setting judges did not have (or use) information about the actual performance of the students?

Judges can provide information about whether they were sufficiently trained for the procedure, their ability to make the requested judgments and their confidence in the resulting cut scores. Positive answers to these questions from judges chosen for their content expertise provide an additional measure of credibility to the standards. Judges could be surveyed at two points—after training and after the entire procedure is complete. A sample survey is shown in Table 6.1.

Formal approaches to assessing the psychometric characteristics of standards can assist in the evaluation of the standard setting results. Generalizability coefficients can provide a measure of the reliability of the judgments and D-studies can suggest the number of judges needed to achieve a reliable standard. The standard error of the mean (SE Mean) passing score is the standard deviation (SD) of the passing score judgments across all judges, divided by the square root of the number of judges (n):

Standard Error of the Mean Cut Score = (SD of cut score) / $\sqrt{n}$

Computing two SEs of the mean in either direction allows us to build a 95% confidence interval around the cut score. Solving for n allows an estimate of the number of judges needed to reach a desired standard error of the mean. Jaeger (1991) suggests that the standard

Table 6.1 Standard Setting Feedback Questionnaire for Judges

After Orientation and Training:

1. How clear is the purpose of the test and the nature of the examinees?	Very clear	Clear	Not clear
2. How clear are the characteristics of a borderline examinee?	Very clear	Clear	Not clear
3. How clear is the rating task to be performed?	Very clear	Clear	Not clear

After the Completion of the Standard Setting Exercise:

4. How difficult was it to provide ratings?	Very difficult	Difficult	Not difficult
5. Was sufficient time provided for the rating task?	Too much time	Right amount of time	Not enough time
6. Was sufficient time provided for discussion?	Too much time	Right amount of time	Not enough time
7. How useful was the performance data provided?	Very useful	Useful	Not useful
8. Do you think the final passing scores are appropriate for the examinees?	Too high	Just right	Too low
9. How confident are you in appropriateness of the cut scores?	Very confident	Confident	Not confident

Comments:

error of the mean of the cut score should be no more than one-fourth of the standard error of measurement of the test. Cohen, Kane, & Crooks, (1999), perhaps more realistically, suggests that there is little impact if the SE of the cut score is less than half of the SE of the test. In a similar vein, Meskauskas (1986) suggests that the standard deviation of the judgments be small (no more than one-fourth) compared to the size of the standard deviation of examinee test scores. These recommendations may be difficult to achieve at a local level with typically small numbers of judges (Yudkowsky, Downing, & Wirth 2008).

Kane (1994) suggests three main sources of evidence to support the validity of standards. *Procedural evidence* includes explicitness, practicability, implementation, feedback from the judges, and documentation.

Internal evidence includes the precision of the estimate of the cut scores (such as the SEMean above), intra-panelist and inter-panelist consistency, and decision consistency. *External evidence* includes comparison to other standard setting methods, comparisons to other relevant criteria such as similar tests, and the reasonableness of the cut scores in terms of pass/fail rates.

Step 8: Provide Results, Consequences and Validity Evidence to Decision Makers

In the final analysis, standards are set not by content experts (judges) but by policy decision makers. They must consider the recommended cut scores, the consequences of applying these scores in terms of pass/fail rates, and evidence as to the credibility of the cut scores before reaching a decision whether to accept the recommendations. The consequences of different types of classification errors must be considered, especially in high stakes situations such as licensing or certification exams. False negative decisions are those in which someone who is qualified is categorized as "fail"; false positive decisions are those in which someone who is not qualified is categorized as "pass." A false positive error, licensing some unqualified practitioners, may pose patient safety risks; a false negative decision will result in a qualified practitioner being denied a license and may result in some patients being denied access to care. One way to minimize such errors is to increase or decrease the cut score by one standard error of measurement of the test, depending on the type of error deemed most salient (Clauser, et al., 2006).

At times, especially if no performance data was provided to the judges, the recommended standards may be unacceptably high; in that case the options are (1) to reconvene the panel of judges and ask them to repeat the exercise with performance data, (2) to convene a different panel of judges, and/or use a different standard setting method; or (3) to otherwise adjust the standards to be more acceptable. Since different standard setting methods are likely to produce different cut scores, some educators recommend using more than one method and taking a mean across the different methods to increase the credibility of the final cut score (Wayne, Barsuk, Cohen, & McGaghie, 2007).

Special Topics in Standard Setting

Combining Standards Across Components of an Examination: Compensatory vs. Non-compensatory Standards

Some assessments include several distinct components or stations—for example a written test that includes separate sections on physiology, pharmacology and pathology, a performance test composed of a series of standardized patient encounters, or a clerkship grade that encompasses a written exam, end-of-rotation faculty evaluations, and an OSCE. Can good performance on one component compensate for poor performance on another? If so, the overall standard can consist of the simple average of standards across encounters or components (compensatory scoring). Component scores (and standards) can be differentially weighted if desired—in the case of the clerkship grade, for example, the written test can comprise 50% of the final grade, with the faculty evaluations and OSCE each contributing another 25%. Component scores should be transformed to linear standard scores before weighting (see Axelson & Kreiter, Chapter 3, this volume and Downing, Chapter 5, this volume). Alternatively, a whole-test method such as Hofstee can be used to set a single cut score for the entire battery (Schindler, Corcoran, & DaRosa, 2007).

In some cases, however, a non-compensatory approach may be more appropriate, to ensure that students reach a minimum level of competence in several crucial but different domains. In this case standards must be set separately for each domain, and examinees must pass each component separately. Each component must include a sufficiently large sample of student behavior in order to be reliable, since very small samples of items—containing large sampling error—may result in incorrect decisions. Setting multiple hurdles to be passed will inevitably increase the failure rate.

In clinical cases, faculty often feel very strongly that a few crucial items must be accomplished for the student to pass, regardless of overall score. These items should be discussed at both the scoring and standard setting stages of exam planning.

Setting Standards for Performance Tests

Performance tests allow for direct observation of a particular competency in a contrived or simulated environment (see Yudkowsky, Chapter 9, this volume). An Objective Structured Clinical Examination or OSCE is a common example of a performance test, in which examinees rotate through a series of stations, each presenting a particular challenge. If content experts such as faculty observe and rate the performance of the examinees, the borderline group or contrasting groups method can be used. These methods are convenient and simple to implement; faculty are very comfortable with making judgments about an individual performance, and all judgments are made in the course of the exam so no additional faculty time is needed. If experts are not scoring the exam (for example when standardized patients provide checklist scores), methods involving judgments about the test items or test content (Angoff, Ebel, Hofstee) can be used.

The use of item-based methods such as Angoff to set standards for standardized patient cases, while very common, has been challenged on the basis that items within a case are not mutually independent (Ross, Clauser, Margolis, Orr, & Klass, 1996). One solution is to have judges work on the case level instead of the item level, estimating the total number of items a borderline examinee would obtain on the case (Stern, et al., 2005).

See Chapter 9 for additional discussion of standard setting in the context of performance tests.

Setting Standards for Clinical Procedures

The checklists used to assess procedural skills such as phlebotomy or lumbar puncture are often unique in that (1) they cover the *entire* set of behaviors needed to accomplish the procedure (rather than a sampling of salient items), and (2) the checklists are public—students are expected to use the checklist to learn and practice the procedure. Certain items on the checklist may be essential for patient safety. While in general pass/fail decisions should never be based on a single item because of the possibility of rater errors, in the interest of patient safety judges may require that an error on even one of these core items will trigger a retest on that procedure.

Setting Standards for Oral Exams and Portfolios

Standards for oral exams, essay papers and portfolios can be set using methods that combine expert global judgments with analytic scoring methods (i.e. Borderline Group or Contrasting Groups), or using whole test (Hofstee) or Body-of-Work methods for collections of items. Clear and explicit performance category descriptors can provide benchmarks for initial scoring purposes as well as for later standard setting efforts.

Multiple Category Cut Scores

Setting cut scores for multiple categories (e.g. honors | pass | fail, or expert | proficient | beginner) can be done using the same methods as for dichotomous pass/fail standards. The performance category descriptions provided to the judges must clearly differentiate the behaviors expected at each level. Other features of the pass/fail standard setting process may have to be modified somewhat to permit multiple outcome categories.

The accuracy of distinguishing cut score categories (e.g., pass | fail; high honors | honors; expert | proficient | needs remediation) is related to the reliability of the assessment scores and other characteristics of the data, such as the shape of the distribution of the scores, the location of the cut score(s), and the true base rates in the population (Clauser, et al., 2006). In general, the higher the reliability of the assessment scores and the lower the standard errors of measurement, the better classification accuracy can be expected. For example, Wainer and Thissen (1996) show that at a reliability of 0.50, we can reasonably expect scores to vary by at least one standard deviation

(SD) unit for about one-third of those tested. Even for relatively high reliabilities of 0.80, about 11 percent of students will have score changes of 1 SD or more.

False positive and false negative classification errors will occur more frequently when multiple cut points are used. In general, as expected, false negatives increase as the passing score increases and false positives decrease as pass scores are raised. The costs of false positives and false negatives must be considered as standard setting policies and procedures are selected and applied.

Setting Standards Across Institutions

Faculty at different schools setting standards for the same exam using the same standard setting method are very likely to come up with different cut scores. For example, faculty at five medical schools in the UK used the Angoff method to set passing scores for the same six OSCE stations and came up with widely varying cut scores; a student with a given level of competency might pass at one school and fail at another (Boursicot, Roberts, & Pell, 2006). If uniform standards are desired across schools, standard setting teams should include members across the participating schools as well as external experts if appropriate. Groups should be encouraged to reach consensus on the characteristics of minimally competent (borderline) students before beginning the exercise. If several (mixed) groups are convened, a single cut score can be obtained by taking the mean across groups. Stern, Friedman Ben-David, Norcini, Wojtczak, & Schwarz (2006) used the Angoff method creatively in a pilot study to set international standards for medical schools in China. In this study the concept of the "borderline school" was used to define school level outcome standards.

Six Methods for Setting Performance Standards

The Angoff Method

The Angoff method (Angoff, 1971) was the first of the absolute methods and thus has the longest history of successful use, even in high-stakes testing situations. In this method, content experts make judgments about every item, so it is fairly easy to defend the resulting passing scores.

Angoff Standard-Setting Procedures There are five steps in implementing an Angoff standard setting exercise:

1. The standard-setting judges discuss the characteristics of a borderline examinee and note specific examples of borderline students.
2. Judges come to a consensus agreement on the qualities of the borderline examinee, with specific examples in mind.
3. Each judge estimates the performance of the borderline examinee for each performance prompt, item or rating (0 to 100%).
4. These judgments are recorded (usually by a non-judge recorder or secretary).
5. Judgments are then systematically combined (totaled and averaged) to determine a passing score on the performance test.

Some actual performance data may be given to the judges. Summary data such as the mean and standard deviation of exam scores or scores on a standardized patient case will help to calibrate judges as to the difficulty of the test for real students. Alternately, more specific data may also be presented, such as the proportion of the total group of students who get an item correct.

Item Review and Rating Judgments are carried out at the item level. The item review begins with one of the judges reading the first item. First the reader and then the other judges on the panel give their estimate of how well a borderline candidate will score on that item; judges rotate clockwise for each new item. Each judge's estimate (judgment) is recorded on a recording sheet or a computer spreadsheet. For each item, the judges answer one of the following two equivalent questions:

1. How many individuals in a group of 100 borderline examinees *will accomplish* this item correctly? (0 to 100%),

or

2. What is the probability that one borderline examinee *will accomplish* this item correctly? (0 to 1.0)

Note that the Angoff question asks judges to estimate how well students *will* perform, not how well they *should* perform. The difference between "will" and "should" needs to be emphasized. If the judgments for an item differ by 20% or more, those judges who provided the high and low scores may lead a discussion of their ratings for that item. Throughout the process, judges can modify their ratings or judgments. The review and rating of prompts continues until the entire checklist has been completed.

Table 6.2 shows the Angoff ratings for a ten-item performance examination rated by seven Angoff judges. The case passing score (percent) is the simple average of passing scores for all items.

A variant of the Angoff method (actually Angoff's original method) is to ask judges to make a simple "yes" or "no" judgment about each item/prompt. The question becomes: "Will the borderline examinee respond correctly to this item?" All "yes" answers are coded as "1," with "no" answers coded "0." The simple sum of the 1's

Table 6.2 Sample Angoff Ratings and Calculation of Passing Score

Item	Rater 1	Rater 2	Rater 3	Rater 4	Rater 5	Rater 6	Rater 7	Mean
1	0.80	0.87	0.85	0.90	0.80	0.95	0.85	0.86
2	0.70	0.75	0.80	0.85	0.75	0.85	0.75	0.78
3	0.50	0.63	0.55	0.60	0.65	0.60	0.60	0.59
4	0.70	0.68	0.70	0.70	0.65	0.70	0.70	0.69
5	0.75	0.70	0.80	0.85	0.70	0.85	0.80	0.78
6	0.60	0.65	0.80	0.75	0.65	0.85	0.80	0.73
7	0.50	0.58	0.55	0.60	0.70	0.90	0.60	0.63
8	0.70	0.78	0.75	0.75	0.65	0.80	0.70	0.73
9	0.45	0.50	0.50	0.45	0.43	0.55	0.45	0.48
10	0.60	0.69	0.65	0.65	0.65	0.70	0.70	0.66
							Sum[1]	**6.93**
							Pass Score[2]	**69.30%**

Notes

1. Raw Passing Score = Sum of item means = 6.93
2. Percent Passing Score = 100% * (sum of item means / number of items) = 100% * (6.93/ 10) = 69.30%

becomes the raw passing score when averaged over all judges (see Table 6.3). This simplified Angoff method (Direct or Yes/No method) may be useful for some types of examinations, such as laboratory tests, for which use of the traditional Angoff method would be difficult (Downing, Lieska, & Raible, 2003; Impara & Plake, 1997).

A variant of the Angoff method called the Extended Angoff procedure can be used with a rating scale rather than a dichotomous item (Hambleton & Plake, 1995). Each judge independently estimates the rating that a borderline student will get on each item. For example, if the student is being rated on a 5-point scale, a borderline student might be expected to achieve a rating of "3" on item 1 and of "4" on item 2. Calculate the mean rating for each item across all judges and average over items to obtain the raw passing rating score.

Table 6.3 Sample Simplified/Direct Angoff Ratings and Calculation of Passing Score

Item	Rater 1	Rater 2	Rater 3	Rater 4	Rater 5	Mean
1	1	1	0	1	1	0.8
2	1	1	1	1	1	1
3	1	0	1	0	1	0.6
4	0	0	0	0	0	0
5	0	0	0	1	1	0.4
6	1	1	1	1	1	1
7	0	0	1	0	1	0.4
8	1	1	1	1	1	1
9	1	1	1	1	0	0.8
10	0	0	1	0	0	0.2
					Sum[1]	**6.2**
					Pass Score[2]	**62%**

Notes

1. Raw Passing Score = Sum of item means = 6.2
2. Passing Score Percent = 100% * (sum of item means / number of items) = 100% * (6.2/ 10) = 62%

The Ebel Method

The Ebel method (Ebel, 1972) requires judges to consider both the difficulty of the item and its relevance. This method gives standard setting judges more information about the test and its individual items, but also requires more work and time of the judges than some other methods.

Ebel Standard-Setting Procedures   There are two major tasks required to implement an Ebel standard setting procedure:

1. prepare a matrix of item numbers categorized by relevance and difficulty;
2. estimate the proportion of borderline examinees who will succeed on the type of item in each cell in this matrix.

Item difficulty is determined by calculating the average difficulty (percent correct) for each item, based on actual data from an administration of the exam to a (representative) group of examinees. Difficulty ranges (easy, medium, hard) are arbitrarily determined, but should have some rational basis in the empirical data.

Relevance ratings (essential, important, acceptable) for each item must be obtained from judges (see # 6 below). It is customary for the same judges used to give the final Ebel ratings to carry out the relevance ratings, but this is not essential. Also, since some time is needed to carry out various computations and to create rating forms once the relevance ratings are obtained, it may be necessary to divide the Ebel standard setting exercise into two separate sessions. A different group of judges could carry out relevance ratings, if circumstances warrant.

Here is a summary of steps to accomplish an Ebel standard setting exercise:

1. Familiarize the judges with the content of the test, performance cases and/or the checklists or rating scales.
2. Discuss specific definitions of the relevance categories used: "essential, important, and acceptable." For example, "essential to good patient care—if this item is not accomplished, the patient's health is at risk."
3. Have each judge rate each item as *essential, important, or acceptable*.

4. Compute summary statistics (average across judges) for the relevance ratings of each item.

5. Compute mean item difficulty (proportion correct) for each item or prompt of each case or station, based on actual performance data.

6. For each case, prepare a matrix of items sorted by relevance and difficulty (see Table 6.4).

7. Lead the judges in a discussion of borderline student performance.

8. Reach some common understanding of the characteristics of the borderline examinee.

9. Ask each judge to provide an answer to the following question for each set of items designated by a cell in the matrix: "If a borderline student had to perform a large number of items or prompts like these, what percentage (0 to 100%) would the student perform correctly?"

10. Each judge records the estimated percentage of students who will correctly perform items like those noted in the cell.

11. Average judgments across all judges are computed and recorded, as shown in Table 6.4.

12. A weighted mean is computed for each row of the matrix, defined as the number of items in the cell multiplied by the mean rating for that cell, and then summed.

13. Adding the total for each row of the matrix gives the raw passing score as determined by the Ebel judges.

The Hofstee Method

The Hofstee method is sometimes referred to as the "relative-absolute compromise method," because it combines features of both relative and absolute standard setting (De Gruijter, 1985; Hofstee, 1983). Judges are asked to define minimum and maximum acceptable passing scores and failure rates. The standard is determined by the midpoint of the cumulative frequency curve of the exam scores as it passes through this bracketing rectangle (see Figure 6.2). Since it considers the assessment as a whole, it can be used conveniently for complex

Table 6.4 Sample Ebel Ratings and Calculation of Passing Score

Matrix of Checklist Item Relevance by Difficulty

Item Relevance	Easy (0.80–0.99)	Medium (0.45–0.79)	Hard (0–0.44)	Weighted Mean
Essential	Items # 4, 5 93% correct[1]	Item # 1 81% correct	Item # 3 63% correct	2 (0.93) + 0.81 + 0.63 = 3.30
Important	Item # 2 89% correct	Item # 10 76% correct	Item # 9 59% correct	0.89 + 0.76 + 0.59 = 2.24
Acceptable	N/A	Item # 7 62% correct	Items # 6, 8 42% correct	0.62 + (2(0.42)) = 1.46

Notes: Raw Passing Score = Sum of Weighted Means = 3.30 + 2.24 + 1.46 = 7.0 raw points

Percent Passing Score = 100% × (sum of item means / number of items) = 100% × (7.0 / 10) = 70%

1. In this example, for items rated as essential and easy, 93% correct represents the mean judgment of all the Ebel judges.

assessments composed of multiple disparate elements (for example a clerkship grade composed of a written exam, faculty ratings and an OSCE). Like the Ebel method, the Hofstee method requires analyzing and summarizing performance data prior to collecting judgments. Alternatively performance data can be obtained from a sub-group of representative examinees or from a prior administration of the examination. If the judges do not take actual performance data under close consideration, the cumulative frequency distribution curve may not be included within the score boundaries they define. The Graphical Hofstee (see procedure step 6/alternate) avoids this problem and ensures that the standard setting exercise will result in judgments that are applicable to the specific group examined.

Some researchers discourage use of the Hofstee method for high-stakes examinations, perhaps feeling that it is less credible because the judgments are global rather than based on individual items (Norcini, 2003).

Hofstee Standard-Setting Procedures   A group of content-expert judges, who are familiar with the students and the performance examinations under consideration, are assembled and trained in the Hofstee method.

Before the Exercise

1. Based on actual performance data, compute the mean and standard deviation of the test and any other statistics (such as mean scores at quartile cutoffs) that would be helpful in describing the overall performance of students on the test.
2. Consider presenting graphical data showing the overall distribution of scores.
3. Optionally, calculate and present other examination data such as any historical data about student performance on the same or similar tests over time.
4. Calculate and graph the cumulative frequency distribution (as a cumulative percent) of the total performance test score for each case. (Statistical software such as SPSS can be used to plot the cumulative frequency percent.) See Figure 6.2 for an example.

During the Exercise

1. Present and discuss the data discussed above with the standard setting judges.
2. Review the cases and the items, the scoring methods, and other relevant details of the exam.

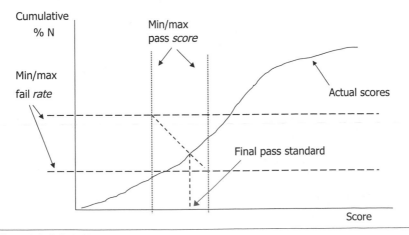

Figure 6.2 Hofstee Method.

3. Discuss the borderline examinee with the group of judges, coming to a consensus agreement on the characteristics of the examinee who just barely passes or just barely fails.

4. Present and discuss the four Hofstee questions, ensuring that each judge fully understands each question (see #6 below) and its implications.

5. Consider doing a practice run to be certain that judges fully understand the Hofstee procedures.

6. Have each judge answer each of the four questions, as noted here:

   a. The *LOWEST acceptable percentage* of students to **FAIL** the examination is: _____ percent (minimum fail rate).

   b. The *HIGHEST acceptable percentage* of students to **FAIL** the examination is: _____ percent (maximum fail rate).

   c. The *LOWEST acceptable percent-correct score* which allows a borderline student to pass the examination is: _____ percent (minimum passing score).

   d. The *HIGHEST acceptable percent-correct score* required for a borderline student to pass the examination is: _____ percent (maximum passing score).

6 (alternate). Alternatively, have judges draw lines designating the highest and lowest acceptable pass scores and fail rates *directly on the cumulative score graph*, with instructions to be sure to include the cumulative score line within the rectangle thus defined (Graphical Hofstee). Have judges specify and record the exact numerical value represented by their lines.

After the Exercise

1. Compute the mean percentage for each of the four questions, across all judges.

2. Plot the mean of the four data points (minimum and maximum acceptable fail percent and pass score) on the cumulative frequency distribution

3. The midpoint of the intersection of the minimum and maximum fail rates and pass scores represents the overall passing score for

the group of judges. See Table 6.5 and Figure 6.3 for a worked example.

If the cumulative frequency distribution curve does not fall within the score boundaries defined by the judges, and the judges cannot be recalled to run the exercise again, the standard can default to the minimum acceptable passing score or the maximum acceptable failure rate determined by the judges. Use of the Graphical Hofstee method (6 (alternate), above) will help prevent this problem since judges can immediately see the results of their judgments and whether the cumulative score line falls within the defined boundaries.

Table 6.5 Sample Hofstee Ratings and Calculation of Passing Score

	Rater 1	Rater 2	Rater 3	Rater 4	Mean
Minimum passing *score*	65	70	60	60	64
Maximum passing *score*	75	75	65	70	71
Minimum fail *rate*	5	0	10	7	6
Maximum fail *rate*	20	25	30	30	26

Note: Use Rater Means to obtain pass score by graphing onto cumulative percent graph, see Figure 6.3.

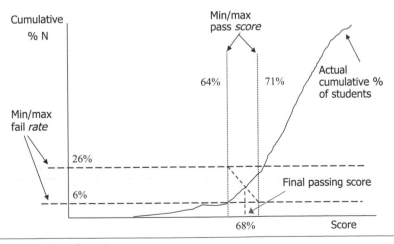

Figure 6.3 Hofstee Example.

Borderline Group Method

The Borderline Group method (Livingston & Zieky, 1982) is an examinee-centered rather than an item-centered method: judgments are made about individual test-takers, not test items or content. The method can be used when content experts who are qualified to serve as standard setters (e.g., faculty) have direct knowledge of the examinees or directly observe a performance test. (Appropriately trained standardized patients may be considered content experts in communication and interpersonal skills.) The judges' global ratings are used to determine the checklist score that will be used as the passing standard. One advantage of the method for performance tests is that it empowers clinician observers, who are familiar with the task of assessing student performance; all the necessary information can be obtained during the course of a performance test, eliminating the need to convene a separate standard setting meeting. A disadvantage of this method is that for small scale examinations there may be few students in the borderline group, possibly skewing the results. The related borderline regression method in which (checklist) scores are regressed on the global ratings uses all of the ratings instead of just those for the borderline group (Kramer, et al., 2003).

Borderline Group Standard Setting Procedures

1. Prepare judges by orienting them to the test, station or case and to the checklist or other rating instruments.
2. Judges may have prior classroom or clinical-setting knowledge of the examinees, or alternatively they may directly observe the test performance of each examinee. Each judge should observe multiple examinees on the same station rather than following an examinee across several stations. The test performance observed may, with appropriate training, consist of performance products such as individual checklist item scores or post encounter notes (in that case this method is similar to the body-of-work method).

3. The judge provides a global rating of [the overall performance of] each examinee on a three-point scale: Fail, Borderline, Pass.

4. The performance is also scored (by the judge or another rater) using a multiple-item checklist or rating scale.

5. The mean or median checklist score of those examinees rated "borderline" becomes the passing score for the test (See Figure 6.4). Alternatively, regress the checklist scores on the global ratings and use the resulting equation to obtain a cut score.

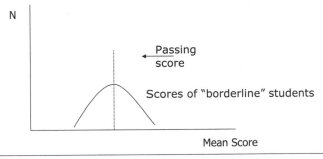

Figure 6.4 Borderline Group Method.

Contrasting Groups Method

The Contrasting Groups method (Burrows, et al., 1999; Clauser & Clyman, 1994; Livingston & Zieky, 1982) is another examinee-centered standard setting method, which requires using an external criterion or other method to divide examinees into two groups: experts vs. novices; passers vs. failers; or competent vs. non-competent. The standard is the score that best discriminates between the two groups. One of the advantages of this method is that the standard can easily be adjusted to minimize errors in either direction. Thus, if the error of greatest concern is mistakenly categorizing an examinee as a "pass" when they should have failed (for example, in certifying examinations), the standard can be moved to the right (see Figures 6.5 and 6.6).

Contrasting Groups Standard Setting Procedures

1. Examinee performance is scored by judges or other raters using a multiple-item checklist or rating scale.
2. Examinees are divided into expert and non-expert groups, based on an external criterion or by having expert observers provide a global Pass/Fail rating of the student's overall performance.
3. Graph the checklist score distributions of the two groups.
4. The passing score is set at the intersection of the two distributions if false-positive and false-negative errors are of equal weight, or moved to the right or the left to minimize the error of greater concern.

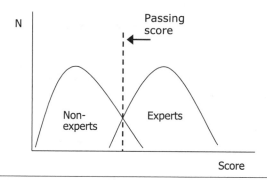

Figure 6.5 Contrasting Groups.

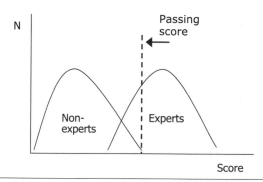

Figure 6.6 Minimizing Passing Errors.

Body of Work Method

Like the Hofstee, the Body of Work method (Kingston, et al., 2001) can be used to set standards for an assessment that is composed of multiple disparate components. The general approach is similar to that of Contrasting Groups, but the judgments are made about samples of examinee's durable work (such as essays, chart notes, or portfolios) rather than about the examinees and their directly observed performance. Work samples are typically scored by judges or other persons before the standard setting exercise takes place.

Body of Work Standard-Setting Procedures

1. Work samples are scored by judges or other raters using a multiple item checklist or rating scale.
2. Prepare judges by orienting them to the test, the examinees, and the definitions of any relevant categories.
3. Present judges with a large number of real, complete examinee work samples, spanning the range of obtained scores.
4. Judges assign each sample into one of the required categories (pass/fail, basic/proficient/advanced etc). This first *range-finding* round defines a "borderline region" where the scores of two categories overlap.
5. Additional work samples with scores from the borderline region only are categorized in a second *pinpointing* round.
6. The final cut score can be derived from the mean or median of scores in the borderline region, the intersection of adjacent distributions, or by use of a logistic regression procedure.

Conclusion

This chapter described the procedures for six different methods of setting standards. Which method should you choose for your examination? Frequently the choice will depend on the practical realities of the test. See Table 6.6 for a comparison of the six methods across several important dimensions.

Table 6.6 Comparison of Six Standard Setting Methods

	Judgment focused on:	Judgments require prior exam data?	Requires expert observers of performance?	Timing of Judgments
Angoff	Test items	No	No	Before exam
Ebel	Test items	Yes	No	After exam
Hofstee	Whole test	Yes	No	After exam
Borderline Group	Examinee performance	No	Yes	During exam
Contrasting Groups	Examinee performance	No	Yes	During exam
Body of Work	Examinee products	No	Yes	After exam

Different standard setting methods will produce different passing scores; there is no "gold standard." The key to defensible standards lies in the choice of credible judges and in the use of a systematic approach to collecting their judgments. Ultimately, all standards are policy decisions, reflecting the collective, subjective opinions of experts in the field.

References

Angoff, W.H. (1971). Scales, norms, and equivalent scores. In R.L. Thorndike (Ed.), *Educational measurement* (2nd ed., pp. 508–600). Washington: American Council on Education.

Boursicot, K.A.M., Roberts, T.E., & Pell, G. (2006). Standard setting for clinical competence at graduation from medical school: A comparison of passing scores across five medical schools. *Advances in Health Sciences Education*, 11, 173–183.

Burrows, P.J., Bingham, L., & Brailovsky, C.A. (1999). A modified contrasting groups method used for setting the passmark in a small scale standardized patient examination. *Advances in Health Sciences Education*, 4(2), 145–154.

Cizek, G.J. (2001). *Setting performance standards: Concepts, methods, and perspectives*. Mahwah, NJ: Lawrence Erlbaum.

Cizek, G.J. (2006). Standard setting. In S.M. Downing & T.M. Haladyna, (Eds.), *Handbook of test development* (pp. 225–258). Mahwah, NJ: Lawrence Erlbaum Associates.

Cizek, G.J., Bunch, M.B., & Koons, H. (2004). Setting performance standards: Contemporary methods. *Educational Measurement: Issues and Practice*, Winter, 31–50.

Clauser, B.E., & Clyman, S.G. (1994). A contrasting-groups approach to standard setting for performance assessments of clinical skills. *Academic Medicine*, 69(10), S42–S44.

Clauser, B.E., Margolis, M.J., & Case, S.M. (2006). Testing for licensure and certification in the professions. In R.L. Brennan (Ed.), *Educational measurement* (4th ed.). American Council on Education. Westport, CT: Praeger Publishers.

Cohen, A., Kane, M., & Crooks, T. (1999). A generalized examinee-centered method for setting standards on achievement tests. *Applied Measurement in Education*, 14, 343–366.

De Gruijter, D.N. (1985). Compromise models for establishing examination standards. *Journal of Educational Measurement*, 22, 263–9.

Downing, S.M., Lieska, N.G., & Raible, M.D. (2003). Establishing passing standards for classroom achievement tests in medical education: A comparative study of four methods. *Academic Medicine*, 78 (10, Suppl.), S85–S87.

Downing, S.M., Tekian, A., & Yudkowsky, R. (2006). Procedures for establishing defensible absolute passing scores on performance examinations in health professions education. *Teaching and Learning in Medicine*, 18(1), 50–57.

Dylan, W. (1996). Meaning and consequences in standard setting. *Assessment in Education: Principles, Policy and Practice*, 3(3), 287–308.

Ebel, R.L. (1972). *Essentials of educational measurement* (2nd ed.). Englewood Cliffs, NJ: Prentice-Hall.

Friedman, M. (2000). AMEE Guide No. 18: Standard setting in student assessment. *Medical Teacher*, 22(2), 120–130.

Hambleton, R.M., & Pitoniak, M.J. (2006). Setting performance standards. In R.L. Brennan (Ed.), *Educational measurement* (4th ed.). American Council on Education. Westport, CT: Praeger Publishers.

Hambleton, R.M., & Plake, B.S. (1995). Using an extended Angoff procedure to set standards on complex performance assessments. *Applied Measurement in Education*, 8, 41–56.

Hofstee, W.K.B. (1983). The case for compromise in educational selection and grading. In S.B. Anderson & J.S. Helmick (Eds.), *On educational testing* (pp. 107–127). Washington: Jossey-Bass.

Impara, J.C., & Plake, B.S. (1997). Standard setting: An alternative approach. *Journal of Educational Measurement*, 34(4), 353–66.

Jaeger, R.M. (1991). Selection of judges for standard setting. *Educational Measurement: Issues and Practice*, 10(2), 3–10.

Kane, M. (1994). Validating the performance standards associated with passing scores. *Review of Educational Research*, 64, 425–461.

Kane, M.T., Crooks, T.J., & Cohen, A.S. (1999). Designing and evaluating standard-setting procedures for licensure and certification tests. *Advances in Health Sciences Education*, 4, 195–207.

Kingston, N.M., Kahl, S.R., Sweeney, K., & Bay, L. (2001). Setting performance standards using the body of work method. In G. J. Cizek (Ed.), *Setting performance standards: Concepts, methods and perspectives* (pp. 219–248). Mahwah, NJ: Lawrence Erlbaum Associates.

Kramer, A., Muijtjens, A., Jansen, K., Düsman, H., Tan, L., & Van der Vleuten, C. (2003). Comparison of a rational and an empirical standard setting procedure for an OSCE. *Medical Teacher*, 37, 132–139.

Livingston, S.A., & Zieky, M.J. (1982). *Passing scores: A manual for setting standards of performance on educational and occupational tests*. Princeton, NJ: Educational Testing Service.

Meskauskas, J.A. (1986). Setting Standards. *Evaluation & the Health Professions*, 9, 188–203.

Norcini, J.J. (2003). Setting standards on educational tests. *Medical Education*, 37, 464–469.

Norcini, J., & Guille, R. (2002). Combining tests and setting standards. In G.R. Norman, C.P.M. van der Vleuten, & D.I. Newble (Eds.), *International handbook of research in medical education* (pp. 811–834). Dordrecht, The Netherlands: Kluwer Academic Publishers.

Norcini, J.J., & Shea, J.A. (1997). The credibility and comparability of standards. *Applied Measurement in Education*, 10(1), 39–59.

Ross, L.P., Clauser, B.E., Margolis, M.J., Orr, N.A., & Klass, D.J. (1996). An expert-judgment approach to setting standards for a standardized-patient examination. *Academic Medicine*, 71, S4–S6.

Schindler, N., Corcoran, J., & DaRosa, D. (2007). Description and impact of using a standard-setting method for determining pass/fail scores in a surgery clerkship. *American Journal of Surgery*, 193, 252–257.

Shea, J.A., Reshetar, R., Norcini, J.J., & Dawson, B. (1994). Sensitivity of the modified Angoff standard-setting method to variations in item content. *Teaching and Learning in Medicine*, 6(4), 288–292.

Stern, D.T., Ben-David, M.F., De Champlain, A., Hodges, B., Wojtczak, A., & Schwarz, M.R. (2005). Ensuring global standards for medical graduates: A pilot study of international standard-setting. *Medical Teacher*, 27(3), 207–213.

Stern, D.T., Ben-David, M.F., Norcini, J., Wojtczak, A., & Schwarz, M.R. (2006). Setting school-level outcome standards. *Medical Education*, 40, 166–172.

Wainer, H., & Thissen, D. (1996). How is reliability related to the quality of test scores? What is the effect of local dependence on reliability? *Educational Measurement: Issues and Practice*, 15(1), 22–29.

Wayne, D.B., Barsuk, J.H., Cohen, E., & McGaghie, W.C. (2007). Do baseline data influence standard setting for a clinical skills examination? *Academic Medicine*, 82 (10, Suppl.), S105–S108.

Yudkowsky, R., Downing, S.M., & Wirth, S. (2008). Simpler standards for local performance examinations: The Yes/No Angoff and Whole-test Ebel. *Teaching and Learning in Medicine*, 20(3), 212–217.

7

WRITTEN TESTS

Constructed-Response and Selected-Response
Formats

STEVEN M. DOWNING

Introduction

The purpose of this chapter is to provide an overview of the two
written testing formats most commonly utilized in health professions
education: the constructed-response (CR) and the selected-response
(SR) item formats. This chapter highlights some key concepts related
to the development and application of these testing modalities and
some of the important research evidence concerning their use. This
chapter is not intended to be a complete item writing guide or a
comprehensive and in-depth critical review of the current theoretical
and research literature on written testing or a scholarly defense of
written testing in either modality. Rather, the objective of this chapter
is to provide a practical summary of information about developing
and effectively using CR and SR methods to test cognitive achievement in health professions education, with some suggestions for
appropriate use.

Constructed-Response and Selected-Response Formats

The generic terms constructed-response (CR) and selected-response
(SR) are accurately descriptive of how these two testing formats work.
CR items require the examinee to produce a written response to a
stimulus, usually a question or a statement. In this chapter, CR items
are discussed as direct or implied open-ended questions or other types

of stimuli that require examinees to write (or type) responses or answers, which are then read and scored by content-expert human judges or raters. Essay tests are the most common application of the CR item form in health professions education. Such a narrow definition of CR tests—limited to essay questions alone—would be disputed by many educational measurement professionals who view CR testing as a type of performance testing (e.g., Haladyna, 2004). SR items require examinees to choose a correct or best answer from a fixed listing of possible answers to a question or other stimuli. Examinee answers to SR items may be computer-scored, using answer keys (listing of correct or best answers) developed by content experts. Multiple-choice items (MCQs) are a common example of the SR item form. Table 7.1 summarizes some characteristics of each format discussed in this chapter.

The prototypic CR item type is the essay question. For this chapter two general types of essays are discussed—those requiring long answers and those requiring short answers. A long-answer essay may

Table 7.1 Constructed-Response and Selected-Response Item Formats: Strengths and Limitations

	Constructed-Response	Selected-Response

Strengths	• Non-cued writing
	• Easy to create
	• Logic, reasoning, steps in problem solving
	• Ease of partial credit scoring
	• In-depth assessment
		• Broad representative content
		• Accurate, objective & reproducible scores
		• Defensibility
		• Accurate, timely feedback
		• Secure reuse of banked items
		• Efficient
		  o Time
		  o Cost
		  o Information

Limitations	• Subjective human scoring
	• Limited breath of content
	• Reproducibility issues
	• Inefficient
	  o Scoring time
	  o Testing time
	  o Information
	• Limited psychometrics and quality control
		• Difficult to write well
		• Bad public relations
		  o Guessing
		  o Memorable

require the examinee to write one, two or more pages in response to the question, while short-answer essay questions may require a one- to two-paragraph written response.

The multiple-choice item (MCQ) is the prototypic SR item type. All other examples of fixed-answer test item formats may be considered a variant of the multiple-choice item type. MCQ variants include: the true-false, alternate-choice, multiple-true-false, complex MCQ, matching, and extended matching item types. Table 7.2 lists some examples.

Assessment Using Written Tests

What are written tests good for? Written tests are useful in the measurement of cognitive knowledge or to test learning, achievement, and abilities. Referring to Miller's Pyramid, the "knows" and "knows how" level at the base of the pyramid are best measured by written tests. And, the ACGME toolbox suggests the use of written tests for measuring cognitive knowledge (Downing & Yudkowsky, Chapter 1, this volume). Most cognitive knowledge is mediated verbally, such that humans acquire cognitive knowledge through written or spoken words or by visual, auditory or other stimuli that may be translated or mediated verbally. Thus, written tests are ideally suited to test verbal knowledge. (The nature of "cognitive knowledge" and its acquisition is far beyond the scope of this book.) Many educational measurement texts discuss high-inference and low-inference written item formats, to distinguish the assessment of more abstract verbal knowledge from more concrete verbal knowledge (e.g., Haladyna, 2004; Linn & Miller, 2005).

Written assessments are best suited for the assessment of all the types of learning or cognitive knowledge acquired during courses of study in the health professions—through curricula delivered in classrooms, textbooks, lectures, library and internet research, student discussions in small learning groups, problem-solving group activities, on-line teaching/learning environments, and so on. Written tests are most often and most appropriately used to assess knowledge acquisition—as formative or summative assessments, to provide

Table 7.2 Examples of Constructed-Response and Selected-Response Items

1. **Constructed-Response: Short Answer (Three sentences maximum)**
   Name and describe the function of each of the bones of the human inner ear.

2. **Constructed-Response: Long Answer (Five pages maximum)**
   Discuss the human inner ear, describing in detail how the inner ear structures relate to hearing.

3. **Selected-response: Traditional Multiple-Choice (MCQ)**
   For a stable patient with a ventricular tachycardia of less than 150 beats per minute, which is the most appropriate first measure?

   A. Intravenous lidocaine hydrochloride
   B. Intravenous bretylium tosylate
   C. Synchronized cardioversion

4. **Selected-response: True-False (TF)**
   Random guessing is a major problem with the true-false testing format.

5. **Selected-response: Alternate-Choice (AC)**
   If the number of items on a test is increased from 40 items to 60 items, the reliability of the 60 item test will most likely be:

   A. Higher than the reliability of the 40 item test
   B. Lower than the reliability of the 40 item test

6. **Selected-response: Multiple True-False (MTF)**
   Which of the following increase the content-related validity evidence for an achievement test?   (Mark each option as True or False)

   A. Developing a detailed test blueprint
   B. Training test item writers in item writing principles
   C. Scoring the test using formulas that correct for guessing
   D. Using some test items that are very hard and some items that are very easy
   E. Selecting the most highly discriminating previously used test items

7. Selected-response: Traditional Matching

Match each term on the left (1–3) with a definitions (A–D) on the right.

Each definition can be used once, more than once, or not at all.

1. Hammer
2. Stirrup
3. Pinna

A. Smallest bone in human body
B. Passes sound vibrations from eardrum
C. Passes sound vibrations from malleus
D. Visible part of outer ear
E. Fluid-filled tubes attached to cochlea

8. Selected-Response: Extended Matching (EM)

Match each diagnosis (A–E) with the patient descriptions (1–3).

Each diagnosis can used once, more than once, or not at all.

A. Vasovagal reaction
B. Anaphylaxis
C. Lidocaine toxicity
D. Allergic contact dermatitis
E. Stroke

What is the most likely diagnosis for each patient who is undergoing or has recently undergone pure tumescent liposuction?

1. Immediately post op, a 49 year-old woman says that she "feels sick." Her blood pressure is normal and her pulse is difficult to palpate; her skin is pale, cool and diaphoretic.
2. Six hours post op, a 25 year-old man is agitated and has tingling around his mouth. His speech is rapid.
3. During surgery, a 34 year-old woman says she "feels sick." She has generalized pruritus, her blood pressure begins to decrease and her pulse rate is rapid. Her skin is red and warm.

(Continued Overleaf)

Table 7.2 Continued

9. Selected-Response: Complex Multiple-Choice (Type-K)

What is the best treatment for a common cold (URI)?

Mark A if 1, 2, and 3 only are correct

Mark B if 1 & 3 only are correct

Mark C if 2 & 4 only are correct

Mark D if 4 only is correct

Mark E if all are correct

1. Rest
2. Fluids
3. Antihistamines
4. Decongestants

10. Selected-Response: Testlets or Context-Dependent Item Sets

One month after returning from Mexico, a 22-year-old college student presents with jaundice and abdominal pain.

1. Which of the following will most likely develop in this patient?

   A. fulminant hepatic failure
   B. carrier state
   C. chronic hepatitis
   D. cirrhosis

2. What is the most likely route of transmission for this disease?

   A. inhalation of contaminated air droplets
   B. ingestion of contaminated food
   C. mucosal exposure to bodily fluids
   D. hematogenous spread

feedback on learning or to measure the sufficiency of learning in order to proceed in the curriculum. Written tests are not at all useful to test performance or "doing," unless that performance happens to be the production of writing (which can be tested only by written tests).

The primary guiding factor in determining the appropriateness of any testing format relates to its purpose, the desired interpretations of scores, the construct hypothesized to be measured, and the ultimate consequences of the test. The characteristics of the testing format should match the needs for validity evidence for some particular assessment setting and there should be a clear rationale for choice of the written format, given the validity needs of the assessment. For example, if the goal is to test student cognitive knowledge about the principles of effective patient communication or the understanding of various principles of effective communication with patients, a written test may match the purpose of the test and the required needs for specific types of validity evidence to support score inferences. But, in order to measure students' use of communication skills with patients requires some type of performance test—a simulation, a standardized oral exam, or a structured observation of student communication with patients in a real setting. A written test would be mismatched to the purpose of this test and the required validity evidence, given the intended purpose of the test.

Both the CR and the SR have some unique strengths and limitations, as noted in Table 7.1. Both testing formats have been researched and written about for nearly a century. Strong beliefs, long-held traditions, and vigorous opinions abound. In this chapter, we review some of the science and research evidence and summarize the best practice that follows from this research.

Constructed-Response Items

Constructed-response (CR) items, in some form, have been used to test students for centuries. In this chapter, CR items are discussed only as essay questions—either short- or long-answer essay questions.

CR formats have many strengths. For instance, the CR format is the only testing format useful for testing writing skills such as the adequacy of sentence and paragraph construction, skill at writing a persuasive argument, ability to organize logical thoughts, and so on. All CR items require non-cued written answers from examinees. The CR item format may permit the essay reader to score specific steps in working through a problem or the logic of each step used in reasoning or problem solving, which may facilitate partial credit scoring (as opposed to "all or nothing" scoring). CR formats may be most time efficient (for the instructor) in testing small groups of students, since less time will be spent writing essay questions or prompts than in creating effective SR items. Small groups of examinees also may make the essay scoring task time efficient. And, essay questions are usually easier to write than MCQs or other SR formats.

However, there are also many issues, challenges, and potential problems associated with essay tests. CR tests are difficult to score accurately and reliably. Scoring is time consuming and costly. Content-related validity evidence is often compromised or limited, especially for large content domains, because of sampling issues related to testing time constraints. And, there are many potential threats to validity for CR items, all related to the more subjective nature of essay scores and various biases associated with human essay readers. There are fewer psychometric quality-control measures, such as item analysis, available for CR items than for SR items.

The purpose of the CR test, the desired interpretation of scores, and hypotheses about the construct measured—validity—should drive the choice of which written format to use in testing cognitive knowledge. For instance, if the goals and objectives of instruction relate to student achievement in writing coherent explanations for some biochemical mechanism and in tracing each particular stage of its development, an essay test may be a good match. "Writing" is the key word, since only CR item forms can adequately test the production of original writing. (SR formats can test many of the components of writing, such as knowledge of vocabulary, sentence structure, syntax and so on.)

Anatomy of a Constructed-Response Prompt

CR items or questions are often referred to generically as prompts, since these stimuli can take many forms in performance testing: written questions, photographs, data tables, graphs, interactive computer stimuli of various types, and so on. These general stimuli serve to prompt a CR response, which can then be scored. In this chapter, we discuss CR items as essay questions only, since these are the most frequently used type of CR format in health professions education worldwide.

An essay question or prompt consists of a direct question on a specific focused topic and provides sufficient information to examinees to answer the question. All relevant instructions concerning answering the question, such as expected length of answer, time limits, specificity of answer, and so on must be clearly stated. See Table 7.2 for some examples.

Basic Principles of Writing Constructed-Response Items

"Writers of performance assessment items must adhere to the same rules of item writing used in the development of multiple-choice test items" (Welch, 2006, p. 312). Table 7.3 presents these item writing principles, as defined by the educational measurement textbooks and the empirical research on these principles (Haladyna, Downing, & Rodriguez, 2002).

CR item writing benefits from attention to these principles and revisions and editing based on independent review by other content experts (Downing, 2006). Clarity of meaning is an essential characteristic for all test items, since such text is highly scrutinized by examinees for subtle meaning. As in all testing, the content to be tested is the most fundamental consideration; the format selected for the test is always of secondary importance.

During the preparation of the essay-type question, a model or ideal answer to the question should also be prepared by the author of the question, just as a correct or best answer key should be designated by a SR item author. The specificity of the model answer must match the

Table 7.3 A Revised Taxonomy of Multiple-Choice Item Writing Guidelines[1]

Content

1. Every item should reflect specific content and a single specific mental behavior, as called for in the test specifications.
2. Base each item on important content; avoid trivial content.
3. Use novel material to test higher level learning. Don't use exact textbook language in test items, to avoid testing only recall of familiar words and phrases.
4. Keep the content of each item independent.
5. Avoid overspecific and over-general content.
6. Avoid opinion-based items.
7. Avoid trick items.
8. Keep vocabulary simple and appropriate for the examinees tested.

Formatting Concerns

9. Use the question, completion, and best answer versions of conventional MC, the alternate choice, true-false, multiple true-false, matching, and the context-dependent item and item set formats, but avoid the complex MC format.
10. Format the item vertically, not horizontally.

Style Concerns

11. Edit and proof items.
12. Use correct grammar, punctuation, capitalization, and spelling.
13. Minimize the amount of reading in each item.

Stem

14. Ensure that the directions in the stem are very clear.
15. Include the central idea in the stem, not in the options.
16. Avoid window dressing (excessive verbiage).
17. Word the stem positively, avoid negatives such as NOT or EXCEPT. If negative words are used, use the word cautiously and always ensure that the word appears capitalized and in bold type.

The Options

18. Develop as many effective choices as you can, but research suggests three is adequate.
19. Make sure that only one of these choices is the right answer.
20. Vary the location of the right answer according to the number of choices.
    Balance the answer key, insofar as possible, so that the correct answer appears an equal number of times in each answer position.
21. Place the choices in logical or numerical order.
22. Keep choices independent; choices should not be overlapping in meaning.
23. Keep choices homogeneous in content and grammatical structure.
24. Keep the length of choices about equal.
25. *None-of-the above* should be used carefully.
26. Avoid *All-of-the-above*.
27. Phrase choices positively; avoid negatives such as NOT.
28. Avoid giving clues to the right answer, such as:

    a. Specific determiners including *always, never, completely, and absolutely.*
    b. Clang associations, choices identical to or resembling words in the stem.
    c. Grammatical inconsistencies that cue the test-taker to the correct choice.
    d. Conspicuous correct choice.

    e. Pairs or triplets of options that clue the test-taker to the correct choice.
    f. Blatantly absurd, ridiculous options.
29. Make all distractors plausible.
30. Use typical errors of students to write your distractors.
31. Use humor if it is compatible with the teacher and the learning environment.

Source: 1. Quoted from and adapted from Haladyna, Downing, & Rodriquez, 2002, p. 312.

directions to examinees. This model or ideal answer will form the basis of a scoring rubric (the scoring key for CR items) used in the actual scoring of the response to the essay question (see Table 7.4 for example).

The CR item, including its specific directions for examinees, the ideal answer, and the actual scoring rubric should be prepared well in advance of the test administration, so that time for review, revision and editing is available.

Short-Answer versus Long-Answer Constructed-Response

Short-answer CR items require answers of a few words, a few sentences, or a few paragraphs, whereas long-answer CR items require written responses of several pages in length. The purpose of the assessment and the content-related validity requirements for broad sampling versus depth of sampling should drive decisions about CR length. In achievement assessment for most classroom settings, breath of sampling is important because the purpose of the test is to generalize to an examinee's knowledge of some large domain of knowledge from a limited sample. If CR tests are used, short-answer essays permit broader sampling of content than long-answer essays, because more questions can be asked and answered per hour of testing time.

If the purpose of the test is to sample a narrow domain of knowledge in great depth, long-answer essays may be the most appropriate format. Long-answer essays permit asking an examinee to produce answers of great detail, probing the limits and depths of knowledge about a single topic or content area. In some cases, long-answer essays may be appropriate, but generally these longer essays are poor samples of large domains and therefore lack generalizability and validity evidence.

Scoring Constructed-Response Items

Scoring is a major validity challenge for CR items. CR scoring is inherently subjective and therefore requires attention to a number of issues in order to reduce the negative effect of subjectivity on scoring validity. In this context, we discuss scoring methods and rater characteristics together with some basic recommendations to increase scoring accuracy.

Constructed-Response Scoring Methods

There are two different approaches to essay scoring: analytic or holistic ratings. In analytic methods, essays are rated in several different categories or for several different characteristics. For example, analytic scoring might require ratings of the accuracy of the answer to the question and the specificity of the answer, the organization of the written answer, the writing quality, and so on. Analytic methods require the rater to concentrate on several different aspects of the essay, all of which are presumably related to the quality of the essay answer and the construct intended to be measured by the essay question. Score points are assigned to each analytic segment or aspect of the essay, based on some rationale. Holistic or global ratings require the essay reader to make only one single rating of the overall quality of the written answer.

Which is the best method, analytic or holistic? The answer depends on the purpose of the CR test. Analytic scoring methods may permit feedback to examinees on more specific aspects of performance than do global methods. However, many of the separate characteristics rated in the analytic method may correlate highly with each other, thus reducing the presumed benefit of analytic scoring methods. Global or holistic ratings are generally more reliable than individual ratings, but the intended use of the CR rating data should be the major factor in deciding on analytic or holistic methods (see

McGaghie et al., Chapter 8, this volume). Analytic methods usually require more scoring time than global methods, so feasibility and practicality will also be a factor in the choice of method.

Analytic methods may permit the weighting or differential allocation of partial credit scores somewhat more easily or more logically than global methods. For an essay item in which several different essay traits are rated, it is possible to allocate the total score for the essay differentially across the rating categories. For example, the content and structure of the essay answer may be weighted more highly than the writing quality and the organization of the answer; score points for the answer would be allocated accordingly. Analytic methods may assist the essay reader in staying focused on the essential features of the answer.

Model Answers

Whichever scoring method is used, an ideal or model answer should be prepared for each essay question rated. This model answer should list all of the required components to the answer. Model answers are analogous to the scoring key for a SR test, so they should be reviewed by content experts for accuracy and completeness. Model answers strive to reduce the subjectivity due to human raters, by introducing some objectivity and standardization to the scoring process.

Essay Raters

Human readers or raters of essay answers are essential. The subjectivity of human raters creates a potential major scoring problem. Human raters bring biases and many other potential sources of rater error to the task, so counterbalancing efforts must be taken to try to reduce problems due to rater subjectivity.

It is recommended that two independent raters read every essay answer and that their separate ratings be averaged—especially for essays that have higher stakes or consequences for examinees. The expectation is that averaging the ratings from two independent readers will reduce bias. For example, if one rater tends to be a "hawk" or severe and the other rater tends to be a "dove" or lenient, their mean rating will offset both the severity and the leniency bias. On the other hand, if both raters are severe or both are lenient, the average rating will do nothing to offset these rating errors or biases and will, in fact, compound the problem.

It is also often suggested that essay raters read all the answers to one essay question for all examinees, rather than reading all answers to all questions for a single examinee. It is thought that essay raters do better if they can focus on one essay answer at a time, but there is little evidence to support this recommendation.

Scoring Rubrics

A scoring rubric is a detailed guide for the essay rater and attempts to reduce some of the inherent subjectivity of human raters by stating pre-specified behavioral anchors for ratings. Scoring rubrics can take many forms in providing anchors and specific detail for the scoring task; the specific forms will differ for analytic or global rating methods. See Table 7.4 for a simple example of an analytic scoring rubric, to be

Table 7.4 Example of Analytic Scoring Rubric for Short-Answer Essay on the Anatomy of the Inner-Ear

Scale	Scale Point Description	Factual Accuracy	Structural Relationships	Writing
5	Excellent	All facts presented completely accurately	All structural relationships accurately described	Writing well organized, clear, grammatical
4	Good	Most facts correct	Most structural relationships correct	Writing fairly well organized, good clarity, mostly grammatical
3	Satisfactory	Many facts correct, some incorrect	Many structural relationships correct	Moderate organization and clarity, some grammatical errors
2	Marginal	Few facts correct	Few structural relationships correct	Little organization or clarity of writing, many grammatical errors
1	Unsatisfactory	No facts correct	No structural relationships correct	No organization or clarity, many serious grammatical errors

used in the scoring of a short essay answer. Note that the use of essay scoring rubrics fits well with the recommendation to use model answers and two independent raters—all suggestions intended to reduce the idiosyncratic subjectivity due to human raters.

Threats to Validity of Constructed-Response Scoring

Both the content underrepresentation (CU) and the construct-irrelevant variance (CIV) validity threats are potential issues for CR tests (Downing & Haladyna, Chapter 2, this volume; Downing & Haladyna, 2004; Messick, 1989). For example, if only long-answer essays are used for classroom-type achievement assessment, content underrepresentation is a potential threat, especially for large achievement domains. Long-answer essays may undersample large domains, since only a few questions can be posed and answered per hour of testing time.

Construct-irrelevant variance (CIV) threats to validity abound in essay-type testing. Rater error or bias due to reader subjectivity is the greatest source of potential CIV for essay testing. Unless great care is taken to reduce or control this type of rater error, collectively known as rater severity error, components of the final score assigned to essay answers can be composed of reliable ratings of irrelevant characteristics. Raters are notoriously poor, even when well trained, at controlling their tendencies to assign biased scores to essays.

The well-known rater errors of halo, leniency, severity, central tendency, and idiosyncratic rating fully apply to essay readers (McGaghie et al., Chapter 8, this volume). Tracking of raters and providing frequent feedback to essay raters on their performance, especially relative to their peers, may help temper some of these CIV errors. And using the average rating of two independent raters, who have different biases, may diminish some of the ill effects of rater bias. Obviously, formal written model answers seek to lessen the subjectivity of ratings, as do the use of written scoring rubrics.

Another source of error concerns examinee bluffing, which is sometimes attempted by examinees who do not know the specific answer to the question posed. Some bluffing methods include: restating the question to use up required space; restating the question in such as way as to answer a different question; writing correct answers to different questions (which were not posed in the prompt); writing answers to appeal to the biases of the essay reader, and so on (e.g., Linn & Miller, 2005). If bluffing attempts are successful for the examinee, CIV is added because the scores are biased by assessment of traits not intended to be measured by the essay.

Other potential CIV issues relate to the quality of handwriting, which can be either a positive or negative bias, writing skill (when writing is not the main construct of interest); skill in the use of grammar, spelling, punctuation (when these issues are not the primary construct); and so on. All such extraneous characteristics of the written response can unduly influence the essay reader, in either a positive or a negative manner, adding CIV to the scores and thereby reducing evidence for validity.

Constructed-Response Format: Recommendations and Summary

The constructed-response (CR) format is good for testing un-cued written responses to specific questions. If the purpose of the assessment is to test student achievement of the relevant content in a written form—where components of writing are critical to the content—CR is the format of choice. The CR format is the only format to use to test the actual production of writing.

CR formats may be preferred if the number of examinees is small, since scoring essay responses may take less time than writing selected-response items. Also, it may be possible to assign partial credit to CR answers in a logical or defensible manner. Short-answer essays are preferred to long-answer essays for most classroom achievement assessment settings, because of the possibility for better content-related validity evidence.

Scoring of essay answers is a challenge, due to the inherent subjectivity of the human essay reader. Using at least two independent and well trained raters, who use model or ideal answers and clear scoring rubrics to anchor their scores, is recommended. The provision of specific and timely feedback to essay raters may help to reduce some rater bias. The choice of analytic or global and holistic methods of scoring depends on the purpose of the test, the content of the essays, the stakes associated with the scores and feasibility issues.

Selected-Response Items

> "*Any* aspect of cognitive educational achievement can be tested by means of either the multiple-choice or the true-false form." (Ebel, 1972, p. 103)

This quote from Robert L. Ebel, a scholar of the SR format, provides an appropriate introduction to this section.

Selected-response (SR) items, typified by multiple-choice questions (MCQ) as the prototypic form, are the most useful written testing format for testing cognitive knowledge in most health professions education settings. Some examples of commonly used SR item forms are presented in Table 7.2.

The SR item format was developed nearly a century ago to provide an efficient means of cognitive testing for large groups of examinees. Ebel (1972) presents a brief history of the early development of the MCQ format and its first major use by the U.S. military for recruit selection testing in the early twentieth century. In discussions of the relative merits of SR and CR testing, it may be instructive to remember that SR formats were introduced to overcome shortcomings of the CR format.

MCQs are useful for testing cognitive knowledge, especially at higher levels. MCQs are most efficient for use with large groups of examinees because the time spent in preparing test items prior to administering the test is generally less than the time required to read and score CR items after the test, because MCQs can be easily and rapidly computer scored. Effective MCQs can be re-used on future tests, if stored securely in a retrievable item bank. Also, MCQs are most efficient for testing large knowledge domains broadly, so that the test is a representative sample of the total content domain, thus increasing the content-related validity evidence, and permitting valid inferences or generalizations to the whole of the content domain. MCQs can be scored accurately, reliably, and rapidly. Meaningful

MCQ score reports—providing feedback to students on specific strengths and weaknesses—can be produced easily by computer and in a timely and cost effective way—thus potentially improving the learning environment for students. Sound psychometric theory, with a large research base and a lengthy history, underpins MCQ testing. Validity and reliability theory, item analysis and other test quality-control methods, plus an emerging theory of MCQ item writing, provide support for the use of well crafted MCQs in the testing of cognitive achievement (Downing, 2002a, 2006; Downing & Haladyna, 1997).

For a complete and in-depth scholarly treatment of the MCQ format and its variants, refer to *Developing and validating multiple-choice test items*, third edition (Haladyna, 2004). This book-length treatment is the best single source of current research on the MCQ form and its application in educational testing.

Anatomy of an MCQ

A multiple-choice item consists of a *stem* or lead-in, which presents a stimulus or all the necessary information required to answer a direct or implied *question*. The stem and question are followed by a listing of possible answers or *options*.

Basic Principles of Writing Effective MCQs

Over many years of development, research and widespread use, principles for creating effective and defensible MCQs have emerged. These evidence-based principles have been summarized by studies, which reviewed the advice to MCQ item writers by authors of the major educational measurement textbooks and the recommendations based on relevant empirical research concerning these item writing principles (Haladyna & Downing, 1989 a, b; Haladyna, Downing, & Rodriguez, 2002). Table 7.3 lists a summary of these 31 principles and is adapted from Haladyna, Downing, and Rodriguez (2002).

There are empirical studies supporting about one-half of these 31 principles of effective item writing and most major educational measurement textbook authors endorse most of these principles. Thus, these 31 principles offer the best evidence in practice for creating effective and defensible MCQs. But, these general principles alone are not sufficient to assist the MCQ item writer in creating effective test items. For an excellent and detailed item writing guide, aimed specifically toward the health professions educator, see Case and Swanson (1998) and the National Board of Medical Examiners (NBME) website (www.nbme.org). This item writing guide presents excellent suggestions and many relevant examples of effective and ineffective SR items.

MCQs which violate one or more of these standard item writing principles have been shown to disadvantage some students. In one study, flawed items were artificially more difficult for medical students and misclassified 14 percent of students as failing the test when they passed the same content when tested by non-flawed MCQs (Downing, 2005).

Overview of Principles for Effective MCQs

The most effective MCQs are well focused on a single essential or important question or issue. The single most important requirement is that the item's content is relevant, important, and appropriate. Most of the information needed to answer the question is contained in the stem of the item, which is worded positively, and concludes with a direct (or indirect) question. Options (the set of possible answers) are generally short, since most of the information is contained in the stem of the item. There is a good match between the cognitive level posed by the question and the instructional objective of the instruction. Generally, many items test higher-order cognitive objectives of instruction (such as understanding, application, evaluation) using novel content; few items test the lower levels of the cognitive domain such as recall and recognition. The set of options are homogeneous such that all possible answers are of the same general class and every option is a plausible correct answer. One and only one of the options is the correct (or best) answer to the question posed in the stem. Experts agree on the correct or best answer. The wording of the MCQ is extremely clear so that there are no ambiguities of language. No attempt is made to deliberately trick knowledgeable examinees into giving an incorrect answer. All clues to the correct answer are eliminated from the item, as are all unnecessary complexities and extraneous difficulty, and all other ambiguities of meaning (Baranowski, 2006). The MCQ is drafted by the item author—an expert in the content of the item—who asks another content expert to review the draft item and its form. Sufficient time is allowed for review comments to be considered and changes to be incorporated into the final item (Downing, 2006).

On the other hand, a poorly crafted or flawed MCQ may test trivial content, at a low level of the cognitive domain (recall or recognition only). The item may have an unfocused stem, so that the question is not clearly stated—so that the examinee must read all of the options in order to begin to understand the question. Such a flawed MCQ may be worded negatively and so ambiguously that examinees are confused about the question being asked. The stem may be a non-focused, open-ended statement that requires the examinee to read all the options first in order to understand what question is being asked. There may be no correct or best answer to the question or more than one correct answer, so that the correctness of the scoring key can not be defended. The flawed MCQ may incorporate inadvertent cues to the correct answer, so that uninformed examinees can get the item correct; or, the item may be so ambiguously written that examinees who actually know the content intended to be tested by the MCQ get the item wrong (Downing, 2002a).

Elimination of five common flaws in MCQs may greatly reduce the ill effects of poorly crafted MCQs. These flaws are: unfocused stems, negative stems, the "all of the above" and the "none of the above" options, and the so-called partial-K type item (Downing, 2005), which is discussed later in this chapter (see Complex Item Forms). This study and others (e.g., Downing, 2002b) suggest that classroom achievement tests in the health professions typically utilize many flawed items—up to about one-half of the items studied had one or more item flaws, defined as a violation of one or more of the 31 evidence-based principles of effective item writing. And, these item flaws negatively impacted student achievement measurement and biased pass-fail decisions made from scores of tests composed of flawed items.

Creative Item Writing

Writing effective MCQs is both art and science. The *science* is provided by the evidence-based principles noted in Table 7.3. The *art* is associated with variables such as effective item writer training, use of effective training materials, practice, feedback, motivation, item review and editing skills, writing ability and so on. Writers of effective MCQ items are trained not born. Content expertise is the single most essential characteristic of an effective item writer. But content expertise alone is not sufficient, since item writing is a specialized skill and, like all skills, must be mastered through guided practice and feedback on performance. There is no reason to suspect, for example, that an internationally recognized expert in some health sciences discipline will necessarily be an expert MCQ item writer, unless that individual also has some specialized training in the science and art of item writing.

The world is awash in poorly written MCQs (Downing, 2002c). Writing effective, creative, challenging MCQs—which test important knowledge at higher levels—is a difficult and time consuming task. Lack of time for already overburdened instructors may be one major reason that there are so many poorly crafted MCQs used in typical classroom tests in the health professions. But the weakness is not with the MCQ format itself; the issues result from the poor execution of the format and the consequent negative impact of such poor execution on students.

Some MCQs Issues

Many criticisms, issues, and questions arise about MCQs and the details of their structure and scoring. Some of these concerns are reviewed here, with recommendations for practice, based on the research literature.

Number of MCQ Options   Traditionally, MCQs have four or five options. The question of the optimal number of options to use for an MCQ item has been researched over many years. So, the recommendation to use a minimum of three options is based on solid research (see Table 7.3, principle #18). A meta-analysis of studies by Rodriquez (2005) on the optimal number of options shows that generally three options is best for most MCQs.

Most four- or five-option MCQs have only about three options that are actually selected by 5 percent or more of the examinees and have statistical characteristics that are desirable (Haladyna & Downing, 1993). Incorrect options that are selected by 5 percent or more of examinees and have negative discrimination indices are called functional distractors. (See Downing, Chapter 5, this volume, for a discussion of item analysis data and its use.)

Since few examinees typically choose dysfunctional options, the recommendation is to "develop as many effective choices as you can, but research suggests three is adequate" (Haladyna, et al., 2002, p. 312). Using more than three options may not do much harm to the test, but will add inefficiencies for item writers and examinees and permit the use of fewer total MCQs per hour. So, the best advice is to develop as many plausible incorrect options as feasible, noting that plausibility will ultimately be determined empirically by reviewing the item analysis data showing the number of examinees who actually chose the incorrect options. The use of three-option MCQs require a sufficient number of total MCQs be used on the test—the usual advice being a minimum of about 35–40 items total. Also, note that items on a test may have a varying number of options, such that some items may have three options while other items naturally have four, five or even more options.

Three-option MCQ critics suggest that using fewer than four to five options increases random guessing and reduces test score reliability. Of course, for a single MCQ, the probability of randomly guessing the correct answer is 0.33 for a three-option item and 0.20 for a five-option item. But, this random guessing issue is not usually a problem, for well written MCQs, targeted in difficulty appropriately, and used in sufficient numbers to overcome any meaningful gain from an occasional lucky guess. On the issue of reliability, it is true that three-option items will be slightly less reliable than four to five option items, but this slight decrease in scale reliability is rarely meaningful (Rodriguez, 2005).

Random Guessing   Random guessing on SR items is usually over-estimated and concerns about guessing may be overstated. If SR items are well written, targeted at appropriate difficulty levels, reviewed and edited to eliminate all cues to the correct answer, random guessing is usually not a major problem. Examinees may be able to get an occasional item correct using only a lucky random guess so it is important to use sufficient numbers of total SR items on the test. If items are too difficult, examinees may have no choice but to blindly guess, so using appropriate item difficulty levels is important.

Random or blind guessing differs from informed elimination of incorrect answers, in which examinees use partial knowledge to eliminate some options and narrow their selection to the correct answer. In real life, partial knowledge is frequently used to solve problems and answer questions. We rarely have complete knowledge for decision making, especially in the health professions. We do gain information about student ability or achievement even when students use partial knowledge to answer SR items.

Random guessing is not a good strategy to achieve a high or even a satisfactory score on an SR test. For example, consider a 30-item MCQ test in which each item has three options. The probability of getting one item correct is 0.33—a good chance of randomly guessing a correct answer on that single item. But, to get two items correct using chance alone, the probability falls to 0.11; and, to get three items correct using random guesses only, the chance falls to 0.04. Even for a fairly short test of 30 items, using three-option MCQs, the probability of getting a score of 70 percent correct is only 0.000036. When a more typical test length of 50 items, each with three options, is used, the probability of getting a good score of 75 percent correct falls to 0.00000000070. The odds of achieving a high score on a test using random guessing alone are not good and most students understand that random guessing is not a good strategy to optimize their test scores.

The best defense against random guessing on MCQs is to create well crafted items and to present those items in sufficient numbers to reduce any major impact resulting from some random guessing.

Correction-for-Guessing Scoring   Methods or formulas used to score MCQ tests have been researched and debated for many years. There are two basic methods used to score SR tests: count the number of correct items (number-correct score) or use a formula to try to "correct" the number-correct score for presumed guessing. Test users have disagreed about using such formula scores throughout the history of SR testing.

The simple count of the number of items marked correctly is usually the best score. Raw scores such as these can be converted to any number of other metrics, such as percent-correct scores, derived scores, standard scores, and any other linear transformation of the number-correct score (Downing, Chapter 5, this volume).

All correction-for-guessing formula scores attempt to eliminate or reduce the perceived ill effects of random guessing on SR items. These formulas usually work in one of two ways: they try to reward examinees for resisting the temptation to guess or they actively penalize the test taker for guessing (Downing, 2003). However intuitively appealing these guessing corrections may be, they do not work very well and they do not accomplish their stated goals. Both the corrected and uncorrected scores correlate perfectly (unless there are many omitted answers), indicating that both scoring methods rank order examinees identically, although the absolute values of scores may differ. Further, no matter whether examinees are directed to answer all questions or only those questions they know for certain (i.e., to guess or not to guess), savvy, testwise, or bold examinees know that they will usually maximize their score by attempting to answer every question on the test, no matter what the general directions on the test state or what formulas are used to derive a score. So, corrections for guessing tend to bias scores (e.g., Muijtjens, van Mameren, Hoogenboom,

Evers, & van der Vleuten, 1999) and reduce validity evidence by adding construct-irrelevant variance (CIV) to scores, because boldness is a personality trait, and not the achievement or ability construct intended to be measured by the test.

Testlets: Context-Dependent Item Sets

One special type or special use of MCQs is in the testlet or context-dependent item set (e.g., Haladyna, 1992). See Table 7.2 for an example of a testlet. Testlets consist of stimulus materials which are used for two or more independent items, presented in sets. For example, a testlet could consist of a paragraph or two giving a detailed clinical description of a patient, in sufficient detail to answer several different questions based on the same clinical information. One item in the testlet might ask for a most likely diagnosis, another question for laboratory investigations, another on therapies, another on complications, and final question on expected or most likely outcomes.

Testlets are excellent special applications of SR or MCQ items. Testlets are efficient, in that a single stimulus (stem, lead-in) serves multiple items. Several items can be written for the common stem and, for test security purposes, different items can be used on different administrations of the test. Testlets permit a more in-depth probing of a specific content area.

Some basic principles of testlet use must be noted. All items appearing on the same test with a common stem must be reasonably independent such that getting one of the items incorrect does not necessarily mean getting another item incorrect. Obviously, one item should not cue the answer to another item in the set. Each item in the testlet is scored as an independent MCQ, but the proper unit of analysis is the testlet score and not the item score, especially for reliability analysis (Thissen & Wainer, 2001; Wainer & Thissen, 1996). If all of these conditions are met, testlets can be an excellent way to test some types of cognitive knowledge, but some care must be taken not to oversample areas of the content domain because several items are presented on the same topic. Two to three independent items per testlet set appears to maximize reliability (Norman, Bordage, Page, & Keane, 2006).

Other Selected-Response Formats

Extended-Matching

The extended-matching SR format extends the traditional matching format, making this item form useful to test higher-order knowledge (Case & Swanson, 1993). See Table 7.2 for an example. All matching items may be thought of as MCQs turned upside down, so that a common set of options is associated with a fixed set of items or questions. Each separate item of the EM set is scored as a free-standing item.

Like the traditional matching format, the extended-matching format is organized around a common set of options, all fitting the same general theme, and all providing plausible answers to a set of items designed to match this set of possible answers. See the NBME item writing guide (Case & Swanson, 1998) for good examples and discussion of this item type. As in traditional matching items, there should always be more options than items, so that a one-to-one correspondence is avoided. General directions for this form typically state: "Select each option once, more than once, or not at all."

Whereas traditional matching items generally test lower levels of the cognitive domain, like recall and recognition of facts, extended-matching items are ideal for testing higher-order cognitive knowledge relating to clinical situations such as clinical investigations, history taking, diagnoses, management, complications of therapy, outcomes of therapy, and so on. As a bonus, item writers, once they master the basics, may find EM items somewhat easier to create, since several related items are written around a common theme and at the same time. Also, EM items lend themselves to "mixing and matching" over different administrations of a test, since sometimes more item-option pairs than can be used on a single test are created for use on future tests.

For EM items of the clinical situation type, there must be a single common theme (e.g., diagnosis of related illnesses), with all the options fitting this common theme and all the items or questions relating to this theme, as in the example given in Table 7.2. Most EM items briefly describe a clinical situation, presenting all the essentials facts of a patient problem or issue and a single focused question related to these clinical facts or findings. The items should be relatively short (no more than two to four sentences) and the options should be a short phrase or a single word.

The total number of options to use in EM sets is limited only by the constraints of answer sheet design (if machine-scored answer sheets are used). Many standard answer sheets are designed for a maximum of ten or fewer options, so the number of EM options has to be limited to a maximum number of options available on the answer sheet.

Some cautions are in order about EM items. Overuse of this item type on a single test could lead to an oversampling of some content areas to the detriment of other content areas. Since the EM format demands a common theme, it is likely that each EM item in the set will be classified as sampling content from the same general area. Many EM items on the same test could, therefore, oversample some content areas, while other important areas are overlooked (leading to the CU threat to validity).

True-False Formats

The true-false (TF) item format appears to be a simple SR format, requiring the examinee to answer either true or false to a simple proposition (e.g., Ebel & Frisbie, 1991). See Table 7.2 for an example of a true-false item. The TF item form requires an answer that can be absolutely defended as being more true than false or more false than true.

In health professions education, there are many examples of true-false items used to test very low level cognitive knowledge. In fact, many educators believe that the TF item form can be used to test only low-level cognitive knowledge (facts) and that most TF items test trivial content. While this may be an unfair criticism, there are many examples of TF items to support such a belief.

Measurement error due to random guessing on TF items is also a frequent criticism. If true-false items are well written and used in sufficient numbers on a test form (e.g. 50 or more items), measurement error due to blind guessing will be minimized. If these conditions are not met, random guessing may be a problem on TF tests. Like MCQs, TF items are best scored as "right or wrong," with no formula scoring used to attempt to correct for guessing for most achievement testing settings in the health professions.

In fact, TF items can be used to test very high levels of cognitive knowledge (Ebel & Frisbie, 1991). The TF item has some strengths. For example, content-related validity evidence may be increased for TF items because many more TF items can be presented per hour of testing time compared to some other SR formats. Well written TF items can have sound psychometric properties, but TF items will almost always be less difficult than MCQs and the score reliability for TF items may be lower than for MCQs.

Creation of challenging, defensible TF items which measure higher-order knowledge is a challenging task. Some specialized skills pertain to TF item writing and these skills are rare.

Alternate-Choice Items (AC)

The Alternate-Choice (AC) item format (e.g., Downing, 1992) is a variant of the TF format. The AC form (see Table 7.2 for example) requires less absoluteness of its truth or falsity and may, therefore, be more useful in classroom assessment in the health professions. However, the AC format is not used extensively, probably because it has many of the same limitations of the TF item form or at least is perceived to have these limitations.

Multiple True-False Items (MTF)

The Multiple True-False (MTF) item format looks like an MCQ but is scored like a series of TF items. See Table 7.2 for an example. The MTF item consists of a stem, followed by several options, each of which must be answered true or false. Each item is scored as an independent item, as either correct or incorrect (Frisbie, 1992).

The strength of the MTF item is that it can test a number of propositions around a common theme (the stem) in an efficient manner. Some of the criticisms or perceived problems with TF items may apply to MTF items as well.

If MTF items are used together with other SR formats, such as MCQs or TF or EM item sets, it is important to consider how to fairly weight the MTF item scores relative to scores on other SR formats. The relative difference in time it takes to complete MTF items and MCQs is the issue. For example, if a test is composed of 40 MCQs and four MTF items each with five options (a total of 20 scorable units), what is the appropriate weight to assign these format scores when combining them into a single total test score? This weighting problem can be solved easily, but should be attended to, since—in this example—the 40 MCQs are likely to take at least at least twice as long to answer as the 20 MTF scorable units.

Other Selected-Response Formats: Key Features

The SR formats discussed thus far in this chapter all aim to sample an achievement or ability construct comprehensively and representatively, such that valid inference can be made from item samples to population or domain knowledge. The Key Features (KF) format (Bordage & Page, 1987; Page, Bordage, & Allen, 1995) is a specialized written format which aims to test only the most critical or essential elements of decision-making about clinical cases. Thus, the purpose of key features-type assessment and the construct measured by KF cases differs considerably from typical achievement constructs. Farmer and Page (2005) present a practical overview of the principles associated with creating effective KF cases.

The KF format consists of a clinical vignette (one to three paragraphs) describing a patient and all the clinical information needed to begin solving the patient's problem or problems. One or more CR and/or SR items follows this stimulus information; the examinee's task in these questions is to identify the most important or key elements associated with solving the patient's problem. The unique point of KF cases is that these items focus exclusively on only the most essential elements of problem solving, ignoring all other less essential elements. For example, KF items may ask the examinee to identify only the most critical working diagnoses, which laboratory investigations are most needed, and which one or more therapies is most or least helpful.

In some ways, the KF format is similar to the testlet format—a testlet with a unique purpose and form, that focuses in on the most critical information or data needed (or not needed) to solve a clinical problem. But, there are major differences also. KF items usually allow for more than one correct answer, and they often mix CR with SR item forms. In this context, research suggests that two to three items per KF case maximizes reliability; use of fewer items per KF case reduces testing information and lowers reliability while using more than about three items per KF case provides only redundant information (Norman, et al., 2006). Like MCQ testlets, the case score (the sum of all individual item scores in each KF case) is the proper unit of analysis for KF cases.

Development of KF tests is challenging and labor-intensive with specialized training and experience needed for effective development. When the purpose of the assessment matches the considerable strengths of the KF format, the efforts needed to develop these specialized items is worthwhile.

Selected-Response Formats and Forms to Avoid

Some SR formats fail to perform well, despite the fact that they may have some intuitive appeal. Some SR forms have systematic and consistent problems, well documented in the research literature (e.g. Haladyna, et al., 2002), and should be avoided. See the NBME Item Writing Guide (Case & Swanson, 1998) for a good summary of item forms that are problematic and not recommended. Most of the problematic SR formats have the same psychometric issues: Items are either more difficult or less difficult and have lower item discrimination indices than comparable straightforward item forms. These problematic items also tend to be of lower reliability than comparable SR forms. But, these psychometric reasons may be secondary to the validity problems arising from use of item forms that may confuse or deliberately mislead examinees or provide cues to correct answers.

Complex Item Forms

One example is the complex MCQ format, sometimes called the K-type item format, following NBME convention (Case & Swanson, 1998). This is a familiar format in which the complex answer set consists of various combinations of single options. See Table 7.2 for an example. It was believed that this complex answer arrangement demanded use of complex or higher-order knowledge, but there is little or no evidence to support this belief.

In fact, this complex item form has some less than desirable psychometric properties and may also provide cues to the testwise examinee (e.g., Albanese, 1993; Haladyna, et al., 2002). For example, once examinees learn how to take these items, they learn to eliminate some combined options readily because they know that one of the elements of the combination is false.

Variations of the complex format include the partial-K item which mixes some straightforward options and some complex options (Downing, 2005). Most testing organizations have eliminated these so-called complex formats from their tests.

Negative Items

Negation or the use of negative words is to be avoided in both item stems and item options. There are some legitimate uses of negative terms, such as the case of medications or procedures that are contra-indicated; this use may be legitimate in that "contraindication" is a straightforward concept in health care domains.

Negative items tend to test trivial content at lower cognitive levels. One particularly bad form is to use a negative term in the stem of the item and also in one or more options—making the item nearly impossible to answer. While finding the negative instance is a time-honored testing task, these items tend to be artificially more difficult than positively worded items testing the identical content and tend to discriminate less well—which lowers scale reliability (Haladyna, et al., 2002).

Some item writers are tempted to take a textbook sentence or some phrase taken directly from a lecture or other instructional material, place a "not" or other negative term in the sentence, and then apply this negation to an item stem. For true-false items, this is a particular temptation, but one that should be avoided for all SR item forms.

Unfocused-Stem Items

MCQ stems of the type: "Which of the following statements are true?" are a time-honored tradition, especially in health professions education. Such open-ended, unfocused stems are not really questions at all. Rather, such MCQs tend to be multiple-true false items disguised as MCQs. In order to answer the item correctly, the examinee must first decide what question is actually being posed (if any), and then proceed to attempt to answer the question. Research shows that these types of open-ended, unfocused items do not work well (e.g., Downing, 2005), especially for less proficient examinees.

One helpful hint to item writers is that one should be able to answer the question even with all the options covered. Clearly, this is not possible for stems such as "Which of the following statements are true?"

Selected-Response Items: Summary Recommendations

Selected-response items are typified by multiple-choice items (MCQs) and true-false (TF) items. The best advice, based on a long research history, is to create straightforward positively worded SR items, with each item having a clearly stated testing point or objective; adhere to the standard principles of item writing. Complex or exotic formats should be avoided, since the complex form often interferes with measuring the content of interest. SR items should test at the cognitive level of instruction and be presented to examinees in sufficient numbers to adequately sample the achievement or ability domain. Three options are generally sufficient for MCQs, if the items are well targeted in difficulty and used in sufficient numbers on test forms. Random guessing is not usually a serious problem for well written SR tests. Right-wrong scoring is usually best. Attempts to correct raw scores for guessing with formula scores do not work well and may distort validity or bias scores by adding construct-irrelevant variance (CIV) to test scores, although in some cases formula scoring increases test scale reliability (e.g., Muijtjens, et al., 1999).

Summary and Conclusion

This chapter has overviewed some highlights of written testing in the health professions. Constructed-response and the selected-response item formats are used widely in health professions education for the assessment of cognitive achievement—primarily classroom-type achievement. Each format has strengths and limits, as summarized in this chapter.

Overall, the SR format—particularly its prototypic form, the MCQ—is most appropriate for nearly all achievement testing situations in health professions education. The SR form is extremely versatile in testing higher levels of cognitive knowledge, has a deep research base to support its validity, is efficient, and permits sound quality control measures. Effective MCQs can be securely stored for reuse. The principles used to create effective and defensible SR items are well established and there is a large research base to support validity for SR formats. SR can be administered in either paper-and-pencil formats or by computer.

CR items—particularly the short-answer essay—are appropriate for testing uncued written responses. Scoring for CR items is inherently subjective and procedures must be used to attempt to control essay rater biases. CR formats, such as short essay tests, may be appropriate for small classes of students, but scoring procedures must be carefully planned and executed in order to maximize score validity.

References

Albanese, M. (1993). Type K and other complex multiple-choice items: An analysis of research and item properties. *Educational Measurement: Issues and Practice*, 12(1), 28–33.

Baranowski, R.A. (2006). Item editing and item review. In S.M. Downing & T.M. Haladyna (Eds.), *Handbook of test development* (pp. 349–357). Mahwah, NJ: Lawrence Erlbaum Associates.

Bordage, G., & Page, G. (1987). An alternative approach to PMPs: The key features concept. In I. Hart & R. Harden (Eds.), *Further developments in assessing clinical competence* (pp. 57–75). Montreal, Canada: Heal.

Case, S.M., & Swanson, D.B. (1993). Extended matching items: A practical alternative to free response questions. *Teaching and Learning in Medicine*, 5(2), 107–115.

Case, S., & Swanson, D. (1998). *Constructing written test questions for the basic and clinical sciences*. Philadelphia, PA: National Board of Medical Examiners.

Downing, S.M. (1992). True-False, alternate-choice and multiple-choice items: A research perspective. *Educational Measurement: Issues and Practice*, 11, 27–30.

Downing, S.M. (2002a). Assessment of knowledge with written test forms. In G.R. Norman, C.P.M. van der Vleuten, & D.I. Newble (Eds.), *International handbook for research in medical education* (pp. 647–672). Dordrecht, The Netherlands: Kluwer Academic Publishers.

Downing, S.M. (2002b). Construct-irrelevant variance and flawed test questions: Do multiple-choice item-writing principles make any difference? *Academic Medicine*, 77(10), s103–104.

Downing, S.M. (2002c). Threats to the validity of locally developed multiple-choice tests in medical education: Construct-irrelevant variance and construct underrepresentation. *Advances in Health Sciences Education*, 7, 235–241.

Downing, S.M. (2003). Guessing on selected-response examinations. *Medical Education*, 37, 670–671.

Downing, S.M. (2005). The effects of violating standard item writing principles on tests and students: The consequences of using flawed test items on achievement examinations in medical education. *Advances in Health Sciences Education*, 10, 133–143.

Downing, S.M. (2006). Twelve steps for effective test development. In S.M. Downing & T.M. Haladyna (Eds.), *Handbook of test development* (pp. 3–25). Mahwah, NJ: Lawrence Erlbaum Associates.

Downing, S.M., & Haladyna, T.M. (1997). Test item development: Validity evidence from quality assurance procedures. *Applied Measurement in Education*, 10, 61–82

Downing, S.M., & Haladyna, T.M. (2004). Validity threats: Overcoming interference with proposed interpretations of assessment data. *Medical Education*, 38, 327–333.

Ebel, R.L. (1972). *Essentials of educational measurement*. Englewood Cliffs, NJ: Prentice Hall.

Ebel, R.L, & Frisbie, D.A. (1991). *Essentials of educational measurement*. Englewood Cliffs, NJ: Prentice Hall.

Farmer, E.A., & Page, G. (2005). A practical guide to assessing clinical decision-making skills using the key features approach. *Medical Education*, 39, 1188–1194.

Frisbie, D.A. (1992). The multiple true-false item format: A status review. *Educational Measurement: Issues and Practice*, 5(4), 21–26.

Haladyna, T.M. (1992). Context-dependent item sets. *Educational Measurement: Issues and Practice*, 11, 21–25.

Haladyna, T.M. (2004). *Developing and validating multiple-choice test items* (3rd ed.). Mahwah, NJ: Lawrence Erlbaum Associates.

Haladyna, T.M., & Downing, S.M. (1989a). A taxonomy of multiple-choice item-writing rules. *Applied Measurement in Education*, 1, 37–50.

Haladyna, T.M., & Downing, S.M. (1989b). The validity of a taxonomy of multiple-choice item-writing rules. *Applied Measurement in Education*, 1, 51–78.

Haladyna, T.M., & Downing, S.M. (1993). How many options is enough for a multiple-choice test item. *Educational and Psychological Measurement*, 53, 999–1010.

Haladyna, T.M., & Downing, S.M. (2004). Construct-irrelevant variance: A threat in high-stakes testing. *Educational Measurement: Issues and Practice*, 23(1), 17–27.

Haladyna, T.M., Downing, S.M., & Rodriguez, M.C. (2002). A review of multiple-choice item-writing guidelines for classroom assessment. *Applied Measurement in Education*, 15(3), 309–334.

Linn, R.L., & Miller, M.D. (2005). *Measurement and assessment in teaching* (9th ed.). Upper Saddle River, NJ: Pearson/Merrill Prentice Hall.

Messick, S. (1989). Validity. In R.L. Linn (Ed.), *Educational measurement* (3rd ed., pp. 13–104). New York: American Council on Education and Macmillan.

Muijtjens, A.M.M., van Mameren, H., Hoogenboom, R.J.I., Evers, J.L.H., & van der Vleuten, C.P.M. (1999). The effect of a "don't know" option on test scores: Number-right and formula scoring compared. *Medical Education*, 33, 267–275.

Norman, G., Bordage, G., Page, G., & Keane, D. (2006). How specific is case specificity? *Medical Education*, 40, 618–623.

Page, G., Bordage, G., & Allen, T. (1995). Developing key features problems and examinations to assess clinical decision making skills. *Academic Medicine*, 70, 194–201.

Rodriguez, M.C. (2005). Three options are optimal for multiple-choice items:

A meta-analysis of 80 years of research. *Educational Measurement: Issues and Practice*, 24(2), 3–13.

Thissen, D., & Wainer, H. (Eds.). (2001). *Test scoring*. Mahwah, NJ: Lawrence Erlbaum Associates.

Wainer, H., & Thissen, D. (1996). How is reliability related to the quality of test scores? What is the effect of local dependence on reliability? *Educational Measurement: Issues and Practice*, 15(1), 22–29.

Welch, C. (2006). Item/prompt development in performance testing. In S.M. Downing & T.M. Haladyna (Eds.), *Handbook of test development* (pp. 303–327). Mahwah, NJ: Lawrence Erlbaum Associates.

8

OBSERVATIONAL ASSESSMENT

WILLIAM C. MCGAGHIE, JOHN BUTTER, AND MARSHA KAYE

This chapter has nine sections. *Section one* begins with a brief introduction about the use of observational methods for personnel assessment in the health professions. We point out that assessments based on observational data are used widely in health professions education yet the quality and utility of these assessments is rarely gauged. We also assert that observational assessment is chiefly formative, a type of *dynamic testing* (Grigorenko & Sternberg, 1998) where learner assessment and instruction coalesce. *Section two* addresses the purpose and focus of observational assessments. It answers two questions. "How can we describe the clinical performance of learners?" [and] "Are the behaviors we observe in learners similar to the behaviors needed for patient care?" *Section three* focuses on the social character of observational assessment. Here we assert that health professions education and assessment is an interpersonal enterprise, especially when done in clinical settings. Interpersonal behavior can yield accurate data yet always has room for subjectivity, selective perception, and measurement error. Observational assessments need to reduce these sources of bias. *Section four* presents an observational assessment toolbox as a table. Here we show how assessment goals and tools should be matched and identify advantages and problems of these pairings. *Section five* covers the acquisition of observational assessment tools either "off the shelf," from donation or purchase, or by means of constructing new measures. "Off the shelf" acquisition of measurement tools requires a hefty dose of *caveat emptor* [let the buyer beware]. Constructing new observational measures is hard work, yet yields large and lasting benefits if done correctly. *Section six* offers tips about how to administer an observational assessment, especially about standardization and control. *Section seven* is about data quality, arguing that data are useless for any purpose if their reliability and validity are suspect. *Section eight* talks about how to use observational assessment data toward the formative goal of learner improvement and also addresses mastery learning. *Section nine* reiterates a set of practical recommendations published earlier about how to improve the quality and utility of observational assessments in health professions education. There is a coda.

This chapter is long and ambitious. We believe that detail is important because observational assessments are used widely at all levels of education in the health professions. Our hope is that this chapter will help educators use observational assessments wisely.

Introduction

A century ago physician William Osler expressed the metaphor of the hospital as a college (1906). Osler argued that the hospital is not only a site for patient care but also a setting to educate doctors and other health care professionals. The primary source of medical teaching in the early twentieth century was the senior attending physician who lectured and supervised young house staff doctors. Attending physicians also judged their acolytes, chiefly by observing young doctors take patient histories, perform physical examinations, communicate with patients, formulate treatment plans, and provide clinical care. Observing, assessing, and improving learner performance in patient care settings has been a hallmark of health professions education for many years. Today, observational assessment toward the goal of learner improvement is as much a thread in the health professions education fabric as it was before the dawn of aviation and the internal combustion engine. The hospital (or clinic) as a college and observational assessment as a teaching tool are cornerstones of today's health professions education.

Observational assessment, usually guided by a structured checklist or a rating scale, is the most widely used approach to personnel evaluation in the health professions (Holmboe, 2004). Observational assessment is ubiquitous. It involves all health professions and covers all skills, dispositions, and character traits. The prevalence of observational assessment in professional education demands that clinical teachers understand its utility and strength, flaws and pitfalls. This chapter addresses such goals. The aim is to amplify another discussion about direct observation of students' clinical skills published recently (Holmboe, 2005) and several other general reviews about clinical competence evaluation in such health professions as nursing (Mahara, 1998), respiratory therapy (Cullen, 2005) and medicine (Epstein & Hundert, 2002; Waas, van der Vleuten, Shatzer, & Jones, 2001). We also offer some practical advice about how to improve observational assessments and better interpret their data.

Two key points need to be made plain at the start of this chapter. First, we view observational assessment as a form of *dynamic testing* (Grigorenko & Sternberg, 1998). This means that instruction and assessment are inseparable. The dynamic testing model (a) emphasizes the processes involved in learning and change, (b) features frequent feedback to learners based on observational data, and (c) "the test situation and the type of examiner–examinee relationship are modified from the one-way traditional setting of the conventional psychometric approach . . . to a form of two-way interactive relationship" (p. 75). Dynamic testing cast as observational assessment in the health professions is formative, focused on learner growth and change. It does *not* try to reach summative end points.

Second, we acknowledge the obvious by stating that observational assessment depends on the availability of skillful and motivated faculty educators. However, we disagree with the widespread myth that faculty status, seniority, or clinical experience automatically confers rating expertise. Clinical research (Herbers, Noel, Cooper, et al., 1989; Noel, Herbers, Caplow, et al., 1992) and practical experience show that teaching faculty need much preparation and frequent calibration to perform trustworthy observational assessments that yield reliable data (Williams, Klamen, & McGaghie, 2003). The health professions need to be just as diligent about training faculty evaluators to produce trustworthy assessment data as programs now in place to train judges for the Olympics (International Gymnastics Federation, 1989), the Miss America pageant (Goldman, 1990), and competitive dog shows (American Dog Show Judges, 2006).

Purpose and Focus

Purpose

Observational assessment of clinical learning assumes that earlier judgments have been made about learners' readiness for health professions education including their fund of scientific and clinical knowledge, patient care sentiments, and professional responsibility. Observational assessments are usually done after learners have passed muster at school admission and in basic science and professionalism courses. We assume, for example, that the student nurse in clinical training has survived a criminal background check. We expect that medical students in clinical rotations are free of alcohol and drug problems. Screening evaluations may find rare outliers. Yet nearly all students of the health professions who matriculate to clinical settings are prepared intellectually for work with patients and are personally fit for the challenge.

The principal purpose of observational assessments of learner behavior in the health professions is to *describe* what they are doing (Carnahan & Hemmer, 2005). Learners are evaluated in clinical context, embedded in the patient care environment where educational objectives are blurred by clinical priorities. The first personnel evaluation goal is to paint a portrait of each learner's clinical experience, performance, and the conditions under which they occur. Once the description is complete learners can be judged against developmental milestones that indicate how well educational objectives are reached. These evaluations are qualitative but no less rigorous than long quantitative tests.

The RIME framework, pioneered in the internal medicine clerkship at the Uniformed Services University of the Health Sciences (Pangaro, 1999) and amplified in other medical specialties (e.g., Ogburn & Espey, 2003) allows faculty judges to assess student learning developmentally, from "Reporter" to "Interpreter" to "Manager/Educator" (RIME). Described by Carnahan and Hemmer (2005) the RIME model has these elements.

Reporter

Students must: (1) accurately gather information about their patients, through an independent history and physical examination, chart review, and from other sources such as family or referring physicians; (2) use appropriate terminology to clearly communicate their findings, both orally and in writing; (3) interact professionally with patients and staff; and (4) consistently and reliably carry out their responsibilities. This stage requires that students have an adequate knowledge base, the basic skills to perform fundamental tasks, and core attributes of honesty, reliability, and commitment. Students who are Reporters can answer the "What" questions about their patients.

Interpreter

Students must: (1) demonstrate ability to identify and prioritize problems independently, (2) offer three *reasonable* explanations for new problems, and (3) generate and defend a differential diagnosis. This step requires a greater knowledge base, increased confidence and skill in selecting and applying clinical facts to a specific patient, and the ability to begin to pose clinical questions. Interpreters organize, prioritize, synthesize, and interpret problems. Students who are Interpreters can answer the "Why" questions about their patients.

Manager

Students must be more "proactive," suggesting diagnostic and therapeutic plans that include reasonable diagnostic options and possible therapies. This step takes even greater knowledge, more confidence, and the skill to select interventions for an individual patient. Managers understand their patients' needs and desires and can enter into "relationship-centered care."

Educator

Becoming a Manager is intricately tied to being an Educator.

Students must identify questions related to their patients that cannot be answered from textbooks, cite evidence that new or alternative therapies or tests are worthwhile, and share their acquired knowledge with other members of the health care team. Desire and ability to educate oneself and others is intrinsic to being a "manager" and reflects a desire not only to teach colleagues but also, and most importantly, to help the patient. A Manager/Educator answers the "How" questions, for themselves, and their patients. It is not simply a matter of "bringing in articles to the team."[1]

Practical implementation of the RIME model in clinical education involves frequent, tightly managed observational assessments of individual students by faculty using checklists and rating scales; faculty training in student assessment principles; regularly scheduled formal evaluation sessions by faculty to review and judge student progress data; and rigorous overall management (especially record keeping) by the program director. Descriptive student assessment using the RIME model is labor intensive and time consuming. However, the developmental profile the RIME format provides about each student's clinical skill and maturity is a solid return on investment. Students also value RIME based observational assessments for their professional feedback and opportunities for faculty contact (Carnahan & Hemmer, 2005; Holmboe, Yepes, Williams, & Huot, 2004; Ogburn & Espey, 2003).

Focus

The focus of observational assessment in health professions education is on the developmental increase in students' clinical knowledge, skill, patient care disposition, and professionalism as a result of instruction and experience. The focus is narrowed by thinking about student clinical learning in either or both of two outcome frameworks. The first, cast as a pyramid, was created by George Miller (1990). The second, a simple hierarchy, is Donald Kirkpatrick's (1998) invention. The two outcome frameworks are shown side-by-side in Figure 8.1.

The lowest level (least impressive) form of learner outcome assessment is Kirkpatrick's Level 1. Data in this category address customer satisfaction, e.g., "I attended an educational workshop and had a good time." Intermediate levels of the Miller pyramid and the Kirkpatrick hierarchy involve learner acquisition of increasingly complex clinical outcomes (e.g., knowledge and skill acquisition; ability to apply acquired knowledge and skill in classroom, laboratory, and clinical settings). The highest level of clinical learning outcomes is reached when student learning is linked directly to patient improvement (i.e., reduced mortality, improved activities of daily living) or better organizational life (e.g., lower absenteeism, boost in staff morale).

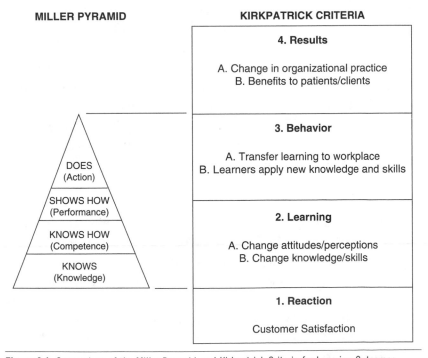

Figure 8.1 Comparison of the Miller Pyramid and Kirkpatrick Criteria for Learning Outcomes.

The levels of learning outcomes shown in the Miller (1990) pyramid and the Kirkpatrick (1998) hierarchy tell faculty evaluators that all descriptive student evaluations are not alike. Low-level expectations for beginning students are gradually raised as students grow in clinical experience, skill, and savvy. Assessments that rely on observations (or other data collection methods) should have a clear sense of the level at which the evaluations are focused using either the Miller (1990) or the Kirkpatrick (1998) scheme.

Social Character of Clinical Evaluation

Observational assessment of students in clinical settings involves watching them learning and delivering patient care, often in a semi-private hospital room or clinic location. Observational assessment by definition is an interpersonal activity and is subject to all of the potential pitfalls of human relations: subjectivity, false impressions, the three "isms" (ageism, racism, sexism), rumor, grudge, and misinterpretation. The goal, of course, is to reduce these potential sources of bias in observational assessments so that student evaluations are uniform, fair, and impartial. This is a big assessment challenge because observational data are always shaped subjectively—they are never fully objective. Informed practice of observational assessment stems from tolerance for error and ambiguity and acknowledgment that even seasoned clinical faculty are wrong sometimes. Decreasing incorrect evaluations is the practical aim because in an interpersonal context they can never be eliminated.

One of the major problems associated with observational assessments of health professions students is that they rarely happen. This is especially the case in medicine where many studies show that medical students and residents are almost never observed performing such basic tasks as taking patient histories and performing physical examinations (Holmboe, 2004). Similar educational research in other health professions including nursing (Darmody, 2005) and respiratory therapy (Cullen, 2005) has been reported less frequently yet shows patterns close to medicine. The practical message is that learner observational assessments must be scheduled regularly and recognized as an important part of faculty work. This work may be either delegated to selected faculty members or done as a shared educational responsibility.

Learners also shape the social character of clinical assessments. Students influence clinical evaluations by preceptors using subtle and overt forms of impression management. These are attempts to "look good," especially in public. To illustrate, qualitative research by Haas and Shaffir (1982, 1987) looked at the development and refinement of medical students' impression management skills over a range of educational experiences. They found that even new students develop a "*pretence* of competence even though one may be privately uncertain" (p. 142). Haas and Shaffir called this the students' "cloak of competence." They summarized their study by stating,

> A significant part of professionalization is an increased ability to perceive and adapt behavior to legitimators' (faculty, staff, and peer) expectations, no matter how variable or ambiguous. . . . In this context of ambiguity, students . . . accommodate themselves, individually and collectively, to convincing others of their developing competence by selective learning and by striving to control the impressions others receive of them. (p. 148)

We expect that students in other health professions are equally adept at managing faculty impressions in classroom and clinical settings. Faculty observational assessments should account for this potential source of bias.

Clinical faculty are not immune to social influences when they observe and record instances of student behavior and when they interpret data representing student learning and professionalism. Most often faculty observations and assessments of students are done one-on-one, usually including feedback and suggestions for improvement. However, several recent studies in clinical medical education present strong evidence that the quality and accuracy of formative decisions about learners is increased when done by faculty *groups* (Carnahan & Hemmer, 2005; Schwind, Williams, Boehler, & Dunnington, 2004). When based on recorded observational data, faculty group decisions about individual students and residents are less likely to be distorted by such sources of bias as students' personal characteristics

(Wigton, 1980), student "likeability" (Kalet, Earp, & Kowlowitz, 1992) or the "Mum Effect" (Tesser & Rosen, 1975), the widespread reluctance to transmit bad news (Carnahan & Hemmer, 2005).

Other research also endorses the importance of faculty observational assessments of students and residents working with real patients in genuine clinical settings (Holmboe, 2004; Holmboe & Hawkins, 1998; Norcini, Blank, Duffy, & Fortna, 2003). These and other investigators argue that evaluations using standardized patients (SPs) (Yudkowsky, Chapter 9, this volume) and other clinical simulations (McGaghie & Issenberg, Chapter 10, this volume) are necessary but not sufficient for completely valid assessment of clinical competence.

Psychologist Elizabeth Loftus, an expert on eyewitness testimony for legal proceedings and studies of judgment accuracy, teaches that even simple observations are done using a cascaded chain of events (Loftus & Schneider, 1987). This is clearly the case for observational assessment of clinical behavior. The chain of events has at least five links.

1. Learner emits the target *response* or *behavior*, e.g., chest percussion;
2. Response is *observed* by faculty;
3. Faculty observation is *interpreted* (e.g., correct–incorrect; superior, excellent, acceptable, marginal, poor);
4. Faculty interpretation is *recorded* as data; and
5. Recorded data are *judged* (e.g., competent–not competent)

The first link (behavioral response) is an objective event. The fifth link is a data-based assessment of the response. Links 2, 3, and 4 are points on the chain where error due to factors like bad eyesight (faculty observation), poor insight (incorrect interpretation) or flawed foresight (incorrect data file structure) can creep into the assessment scheme. The obvious answer is to calibrate the observational assessment mechanism to reduce the introduction of measurement error at links 2, 3, and 4. Since faculty members are the source of error at these locations it makes sense that faculty training and calibration is the best solution to the problem.

Faculty training to improve rating accuracy is rarely done in health professions education despite rigorous empirical demonstrations showing the need for such calibration (Herbers, et al., 1989; Noel, et al., 1992). A recent review on cognitive, social, and environmental sources of bias in clinical competence ratings (Williams, et. al., 2003) identifies four approaches to rater calibration and training that hold promise to improve the quality of observational data: (a) *rater error training*, (b) *performance dimension training*, (c) *frame of reference training*, and (d) *behavioral observation training* (Woehr & Huffcutt, 1994). However, despite published warnings and suggestions for improvement, faculty training and preparation for the work of observational assessment is one of the great unmet educational needs across the health professions.

Observational Assessment Toolbox

Student observational assessment in the classroom or clinic is a practical matter. The faculty evaluator needs to have a clear sense of the assessment goal (the *what* of assessment) and use an assessment tool (the *how* of assessment) for data collection. The proper fit of goals and tools is a key feature of quality observational assessment. A mismatch of goals and tools ("square peg, round hole") will produce measurement error (unreliability) and inaccurate faculty judgments about students.

Table 8.1 identifies ten assessment goals for student learning in the health professions ranging from conducting an interview to performing a physical exam, counseling skills, and professionalism. A set of optional assessment tools is presented beside each goal along with statements about their advantages and disadvantages. At least one citation to the professional literature is also given for each assessment goal for readers who seek more detailed information. The intent is not only to reinforce the idea of the goal–tool match but also to show the variety of ways the match can be made.

Faculty evaluators are urged to study the tabular entries carefully and to make informed choices about student assessment goals and tools.

Table 8.1 Observational Assessment Goals and Tools

Assessment Goal	Assessment Tools	Advantages	Limitations
Interview (History) (Norcini, Blank, Duffy, & Fortna, 2003; Orient, 2005)	Direct observation of clinical behavior	Observes learner over a range of activities; long behavioral record; opportunities for immediate feedback; live observer present	Role conflict; assumes equivalence of faculty; time consuming; impression management/manipulation by learners
	Mini-CEX*	Judgment about single, specific encounter; real patients; high reliability after four assessments	Task and patient specific; assesses only part of the clinical encounter
	SP†	Trained, experienced raters; other observers	Simulation; approximation to realism
	Videotape of clinical encounter	Realistic; capture clinical behavior	Time consuming; need consent; equipment needs; cost
Communication (Norcini, Blank, Duffy, & Fortna, 2003)	Direct observation of clinical behavior	Observes learner over a range of activities; long behavioral record; opportunities for immediate feedback; live observer present	Role conflict; assumes equivalence of faculty; time consuming; impression management/manipulation by learners
	Mini-CEX*	Judgment about single, specific encounter; real patients	Task and patient specific
	SP†	Trained, experienced raters; other observers	Simulation; approximation to realism
	Videotape of clinical encounter	Realistic; capture clinical behavior	Time consuming; need consent; equipment needs; cost
	Patient satisfaction survey	Increased reliability as database grows	Self-selection; positive response bias; no evaluation of patient care quality
	Self-assessment of clinical performance	Encourages learner reflection; convenience	Data usually unreliable; overestimates skill and knowledge levels
	Peer assessment of clinical performance	Practice and value peer review; encourages professionalism	Response bias without anonymity

Competency	Method	Strengths	Limitations
Physical Exam (Norcini, Blank, Duffy, & Fortna, 2003; Orient, 2005)	Direct observation of clinical behavior	Immediate feedback; correct problems quickly	Lack of a "gold standard;" more than one right way
	Mini-CEX*	Structured, focused; more reliable	Encounter specific; physical exam skills needing evaluation may not be present in available patients
	SP†	Standardized, uniform	SP may lack physical findings
	Medical record audit	Readily available; patient centered; written expression of learner's clinical reasoning	Documentation may not be reliable; reflects input from others beside learner
Patient Presentations (Green, Hershman, DeCherie, et al., 2005; Haber & Lingard, 2001)	Direct observation of patient presentations	Immediate feedback; correct problems quickly	Wide variation in evaluation without structured format
Clinical Reasoning (Orient, 2005; Wiese, Varosy, & Tierney, 2002)	Direct observation of episodes	Evaluates reasoning "in vivo"; immediate feedback; opportunities for correction	Wide variation in evaluation without structured format
	One minute preceptor	Structured, probes reasoning	Task and patient specific (narrow focus of evaluation)
Creating a Problem List (Weed, 1968)	Direct observation of events	Patient centered; realistic; promotes immediate feedback	Evaluation and feedback may be cursory due to time constraints
	Retrospective chart review	Patient centered; learner incorporates reading and deliberation to create a more polished product	Learner's skills are supplemented by others; time consuming
Procedures (Wayne, Butter, Siddall, et al., 2005a, 2006)	Direct observation of clinical behavior	Evaluates procedural skill "in vivo"	May involve unsafe practice with real patients
	Simulation-based clinical evaluation	Standardized; safe; forgiving; allows deliberate practice	Varies in realism; may be expensive

(Continued Overleaf)

Table 8.1 Continued

Assessment Goal	Assessment Tools	Advantages	Limitations
	Observational checklists	Structured; convenient	Requires rater training and calibration
	Objective Structured Assessment of Technical Skills (OSAT)	Structured, specific & focused; trained, experienced raters; other observers	Clinical simulation, approximates realism
Counseling Skills (Norcini, Blank, Duffy, & Fortna, 2003)	Direct observation	Realistic; immediate feedback; offers opportunities for patient education and correction	Time consuming for faculty; task specific
	Mini-CEX*	Focused task increases reliability	Time consuming; patient and task specific
	SP†	Trained, experienced raters; other observers	Simulation, approximation to realism
	Videotape of clinical encounter	Realistic; capture clinical behavior	Time consuming; need consent; equipment needs; cost
	Self-assessment of clinical performance	Encourages learner reflection; convenience	Data usually unreliable; overestimates skill and knowledge levels
Treatment Plan	Direct observation of clinical behavior	Patient centered; realistic; promotes immediate feedback	Time consuming for faculty
	Written exams of acquired knowledge	Best assessment of factual recall; large number of items increases reliability	Ability to apply information in clinical context is uncertain
Professionalism (Bracken, Timmreck, & Church, 2001; Norcini, 2006; Smither, London, & Reilly, 2005; Stern, 2006)	Direct observation of clinical behavior	Structured, focused observations yield reliable data; immediate feedback; opportunities for correction	Lack of a "gold standard"; behaviors most conspicuous by their absence; impression management/manipulation by learners

Method	Strengths	Limitations
"Physicianship" forms	Involves real patients; identifies behavioral extremes	Only egregious behaviors are reported; depends on faculty motivation to identify problem learners
Videotape of clinical encounter	Realistic; capture clinical behavior	Time consuming; need consent; equipment needs; cost
360° evaluation‡	Comprehensive evaluation surveys that allow data triangulation and multisource feedback	Time and labor intensive; requires much staff training and calibration; evaluations are unique to the organization and culture where they are done
Teamwork (Baker, Beaubien, & Holtzman, 2006; Hamman, 2004; Loughry, Ohland, & Moore, 2007; Thomas, Sexton, & Helmreich, 2004)		
Direct observation of clinical behavior	Evaluates team functioning "in vivo"; realistic, unconstrained assessment; assess shifts in team leadership	Team functioning may change as problem evolves; lack of a "gold standard"; wide variation in evaluation without structured format
Team surveys	Comprehensive; can cover many facets of teamwork; easy to complete	Usually retrospective; depends on unreliable, selective memory
Checklists	Simple, easy to use; focus and constrain evaluation responses	May oversimplify complex team performances

Notes

* "The mini-CEX was originally designed to evaluate residents [learners] in a setting reflective of day-to-day practice. Faculty observe a resident performing a *focused* history, physical, or counseling session during routine care experiences. . . . The mini-CEX facilitates multiple observations over time by different faculty members. . . . This longitudinal nature of the mini-CEX is its most important strength as an evaluation tool" (Holmboe, 2005).

† "Standardized patients (SPs) are laypersons who are trained and calibrated to present patient health problems uniformly for teaching or evaluation" (McGaghie, 2005).

‡ "360° evaluation is assessment of a learner [or practitioner] using rating data from a variety of sources, e.g., self, peers, supervisors, nursing staff, patients" (McGaghie, 2005).

Acquisition of Observational Assessment Tools

There are two sources of measurement tools that can be used for observational assessment of learners in the health professions. The first is to buy, borrow, or adapt measurement tools "off the shelf" from commercial vendors or colleagues. This is a common practice among educational program directors and faculty evaluators. Since there is no equivalent of *Consumer Reports* for users of professional education measures, "off the shelf" acquisition of these tools must be done with skill and care. We will offer some practical advice about these acquisitions. The second way to acquire observational assessment measures is to construct them yourself. This is hard work. However, evaluators who create assessment measures the right way will gain large and lasting benefits. We will also give practical advice about constructing assessment measures along with examples and references that provide detailed instructions. The bottom line is that trustworthy observational assessment data will only come from solid evaluation tools that are used properly.

General Advice

There are four general rules to follow whether observational assessment tools are selected "off the shelf" or developed locally.

1. Evaluation goals and tools must be matched. This is the clear message of Table 8.1, repeated here for reinforcement.
2. Faculty evaluators must be well-read about student assessment procedures in their profession. Learner assessment is a key professional duty that should be informed by knowledge of the literature.
3. Consult with an educational measurement expert if you have questions or problems. Clinicians in all fields consult with experts routinely about patient care problems. The same approach should be used for educational assessment issues.
4. Consult with a reference librarian for unmet information needs. Reference librarians are highly skilled at working with clinicians to address patient care *and* educational problems.

Selecting Assessment Tools

Educational evaluators who are in the market to buy or borrow observational assessment tools for local use should follow five simple steps before making an acquisition. Above all, they must be careful, smart shoppers.

1. Shop around. There are many commercial and not-for-profit sources of assessment instruments that may suit your needs so careful inspection is essential. A popular not-for-profit source is the *Health and Psychological Instruments* (HAPI) database which is accessible at health sciences libraries. It contains thousands of measurement tools, most reported in the peer-reviewed scientific literature. Instruments that are sold commercially through catalogs and websites rarely undergo rigorous peer review.

2. Critically appraise "off the shelf" assessment tools using textbook principles of clinical decision-making (Fletcher, Fletcher, & Wagner, 1996; Sox, Blatt, Higgins, & Marton, 1988). Potential users need to have a clear idea about the technical qualities of observational measurement tools and especially about the data they yield (i.e., reliability, validity).

3. Study the history of potential assessment tools to find out if they have been used successfully with learners and in settings similar to your own. Historical data should also be recent, not decades old.

4. Conduct pilot studies involving "off the shelf" assessment tools in your local setting. Measurement tools should survive a tryout phase before they are placed in general use.

5. Measure yourself. Place yourself in the role of a student or learner and undergo an observational assessment performed by a colleague. This experience will help you decide if the potential assessment tool truly fits your measurement purpose.

Constructing Assessment Tools

Instruction about how to construct measures that can be used for assessment of learning in the health professions is available from several sources. General advice is found in Wilson (2005). Practical suggestions about creating measures of acquired knowledge are found in Case and Swanson (2002) and Linn and Gronlund (2000). Approaches to creation of attitude measures are described by Robert DeVellis (2003). Development of health status scales is taught by Streiner and Norman (2003). Ronald Stiggins (1987) presents formulae for the design and development of performance assessments that are directly applicable to the health professions. Educational program directors and faculty evaluators are urged to study these sources.

Here are seven thoughts about constructing tools that can contribute to observational assessment of learners in the health care professions. The seven thoughts are grounded in experience and evaluation best practice.

1. Form a team that includes persons having clinical and educational measurement expertise. Clinical and educational skills are complementary. Both skill sets are needed to construct good assessment tools.

2. Planning and blueprinting are the essential first steps in constructing observational assessment tools. This involves clearly stating inclusion and exclusion criteria that structure a checklist, rating scale, or other assessment tool. What are the essential actions, for example, in an ACLS response to a patient with ventricular fibrillation? What actions can be omitted? Thinking through the details of the total assessment, from beginning to end, should be done before items or questions are written. See Chapter 10 (this volume) for an example of a test blueprint in clinical cardiology.

3. What is an item? Test, checklist, or attitude and survey questionnaire items are the building blocks of health professions observational assessments. Items should be discrete and uniform to increase the odds of error free (reliable) educational measurement. More items are usually better, within practical limits.

4. Measurement planning and blueprinting, and item writing and editing (refinement) should be done using a systematic plan.

Construction of assessment tools is a practical yet disciplined exercise, guided by an overall design.

5. Pilot studies should be done after early versions of observational assessments have been crafted. Small scale tryouts will reveal hidden flaws and content coverage failures. Improvements in the measures, informed by pilot test data, can be made before the assessment tools are placed in widespread use.

6. Health professions educators are urged to publish their work on instrument development. Creating assessment tools to serve local needs often has broad utility. A new and better measure of student nurses' proficiency at arterial puncture produced in Peoria will likely receive an eager reception in Portland, Paducah, and Poughkeepsie. Publishing reports about creating learner assessment tools also means the work will undergo rigorous peer review. It also means that the observational assessment tools are available for use by colleagues elsewhere.

7. Constructing assessment tools is hard work. However, there are many long-lasting benefits from these endeavors: Solid evaluations of learner competence, that can lead to educational feedback and improvement, publications, and an important contribution to one's field.

Examples of Constructed Measures

Three concrete examples of published instrument development reports in the health professions illustrate how this work can be done to systematically create assessment tools that measure knowledge, clinical skills, and attitudes.

Issenberg, McGaghie, Brown et al. (2000) used an eight step development procedure at the University of Miami to create a computer-based measure of clinical skills in bedside cardiology focused on knowledge acquisition and application. This work produced two interchangeable measures for use as a pretest and a posttest that are equivalent in content, difficulty, and data reliability. The measures have been used in several other research studies that produced published reports (Issenberg, McGaghie, Gordon et al., 2002; Issenberg,

Petrusa, McGaghie et al., 1999). The measures have also been adopted by medical teachers at other institutions as part of educational programs in bedside cardiology for students and residents.

A team of medical educators was responsible for teaching students and residents how to recognize and work up patients with musculo-skeletal (MSK) disorders. A key part of the educational program involved rigorous evaluations of the learners' clinical skills. Useful measures were not available from outside sources. Thus the team used a systematic, six step process to develop a set of four checklists (knee, shoulder, back, general) needed for observational assessment of the students' and residents' MSK examination skills (McGaghie, Renner, Kowlowitz, et al., 1994). The checklists were practical, useful, and produced reliable data.

The Nutrition Academic Award (NAA) Program was started by the NIH in the late 1990s to boost medical student, resident, and practitioner knowledge, attitudes, and clinical skills about nutrition in patient care. The NAA was a nationwide program with awards granted at scores of sites. Educational outcome measures addressing learner knowledge and clinical skills were available from several sources. However, there was no measure available to probe learners' attitudes about nutrition in patient care. A team of nutritionists, physicians, and behavioral scientists filled the gap by constructing a 45 item attitude measure with five subscales (nutrition in routine care, clinical behavior, physician–patient relationship, patient behavior/motivation, physician efficacy) derived from factor analysis (McGaghie, Van Horn, Fitzgibbon, et al., 2001). The subscales yield reliable data that are useful for learner feedback and research. Because it is published, the nutrition attitude measure is available for use by other educators and investigators at no cost.

Administration of an Assessment

An observational assessment needs to be administered according to a set of simple, practical rules to produce data that are useful for feed-back and learner improvement. Such rules are also imposed so that all learners are treated fairly, to underscore the seriousness of health care personnel evaluations, and to convey an expectation of professionalism to students, faculty, and college administrators.

Textbooks on educational measurement and evaluation (e.g., Linn & Gronlund, 2000) devote complete chapters to this topic. Health professions boards and certifying agencies administer examinations and other assessments under draconian conditions. However, health professions teachers and evaluators responsible for delivery of local observational assessments should administer the measures mindful of six simple principles.

1. Use *standardized procedures* throughout the assessment for all trainees. The uniformity gained by using such standardized procedures as the room or setting, time allocation, instruments, and minimum passing levels ensure that all learners are treated equally and fairly.

2. The assessment must be *managed tightly*. This is a part of standardized procedures but is listed separately to underscore the importance of people management: scheduling persons, facilities, and resources; advance preparation; attention to details.

3. Assessment administration needs to be mindful of *personnel control*, especially if multiple faculty members are used for identical observational measures. As measurement devices these faculty members should be calibrated via rater training. Faculty members need preparation (and updating) for this important work.

4. Data collection, entry into files, and storage must be done according to an *orderly plan*. Persons with clerical responsibility need to be competent at using widely available data base management programs (e.g., Microsoft Excel®).

5. Data analyses, summaries, and presentation as reports should be *simple and straightforward*. For individual learners the goal of giving feedback about progress toward professional milestones can be done in the form of a performance profile. The progress of learner groups can be gauged by aggregating individual profiles into a class or program report.

6. Administration of learner assessments should be done according to a *firm schedule* that is posted in advance. This will prevent

expressions of "surprise" that assessments will be done and clarify expectations among learners and their teachers.

Data Quality

The idea of data quality is a basic concept at all phases of health professions education. The quality of data derived from educational measurements is judged by two primary indexes: reliability and validity. *Reliability* refers to the accuracy and consistency of measurement data and is covered in detail earlier in this volume (Axelson & Kreiter, Chapter 3, this volume) and in many other writings (e.g., Downing, 2004). The idea of *validity* addresses the accuracy of permissible decisions or inferences that can be made from test data. Validity is not a property of tests or measurements themselves. Approaches to validity and its threats are also covered in an earlier chapter in this book (Downing & Haladyna, Chapter 2, this volume) and other scholarly writings (e.g., Downing, 2003). Specific validity threats for observational methods are noted in Table 8.2.

The basic point here is that data quality, judged in several ways, is *essential* for all assessment procedures in the health professions. High quality assessment data (high signal, low noise) are needed to ensure that educational feedback to learners is accurate and trustworthy. High quality data are also needed to fulfill research goals. Sound educational research in the health professions simply cannot be done without good outcome measures that yield reliable data that permit valid educational inferences.

Data used for observational assessments in the health professions are never perfect. The data are subject to many different sources of possible bias (Williams, Klamen, & McGaghie, 2003) and usually address a much more limited scope of professional behavior than evaluators intend (Boulet & Swanson, 2004). The aim is for evaluators to acknowledge the limits of observational data, take steps to reduce data flaws, and interpret the results of observational assessments with appropriate caution. While the measurement problems will never be eliminated, they can be addressed thoughtfully.

Table 8.2 Threats to Validity: In vivo Observational Methods

	Problem	Remedy
Construct Under-representation (CU)	Too few observations to sample domain adequately	Use multiple direct observations (e.g. mini-CEX, focused observations)
	Unrepresentative sampling of domain	• Blueprint the activities to be observed to ensure focused observations systematically sample the domain • Blueprint the rating scale to ensure competencies of interest are rated
	Too few independent ratings	• Use multiple raters • Use different raters for different observation events • Use raters from different disciplines with different perspectives (e.g. 360° or multi-source ratings)
Construct-irrelevant Variance (CIV)	Examiner bias	• Provide scoring rubric • Train examiners to use rubric
	Halo and Recency effects	Have examiners complete rating immediately after each direct observation (not at end of rotation)
	Systematic rater errors: Severity, Leniency, Central tendency	• Frame of reference training for examiners • Feedback to examiners showing their ratings compared to all other raters
Reliability Indicators		Generalizability Inter-rater reliability

How to Use Observational Data

The practical matter of educating and evaluating people to fulfill many different high-performance roles in the health professions begs the question of how to best use observational data in these contexts. We have stated several times that best educational practice would use observational assessment data chiefly for formative learner assessment aimed at description, feedback, and improvement. This aim is practical and achievable in most educational settings.

A more visionary goal is to carefully integrate observational data with focused, deliberate practice (Ericsson, 2004) of essential clinical skills; combined with very high standards of expected professional performance (Downing, Tekian, & Yudkowsky, 2006; Wayne, Fudala, Butter, et al., 2005b). This would lead to the ultimate goal of employing the *mastery model* of training and assessment in the health professions where all learners reach identical (and very high) educational outcomes with little or no outcome variation. The only educational feature that would vary among learners is the time needed to reach the high educational goal (McGaghie, Miller, Sajid, & Telder, 1978). This mastery model has been used successfully to educate internal medicine residents to achieve very high and uniform performance levels in advanced cardiac life support (ACLS) skills (Wayne, Butter, Siddall, et al., 2006) and to master thoracentesis (Wayne, Barsuk, O'Leary, et. al., 2008). A detailed description of the features and uses of the mastery model of education and assessment in the health professions has been published recently (McGaghie, Siddall, Mazmanian, & Myers, 2009).

The mastery model is the best available expression of *dynamic testing* (Grigorenko & Sternberg, 1998). This is an environment where learners and evaluators understand that educational activities and assessments coalesce—where assessment data are used as a tool, not as a weapon.

Practical Recommendations About Observational Assessment

We close this chapter by repeating a set of 16 practical recommendations for improving observational assessment practices in the health professions. The recommendations were first stated in a recent journal article (Williams, et al., 2003).

1. Assessments should cover a *broad range of clinical situations and procedures* to draw reasonable conclusions about learners' overall clinical competence.
2. Observational assessments should be done by *multiple raters* to balance the effects of rater differences.
3. Assessment instruments should be *short* and *focused*.

4. Formative assessments for teaching, learning, and feedback should be *separate* from assessments done for learner promotion or advancement.

5. Observational data must be *recorded promptly* to prevent distortion from memory loss or misplaced information.

6. Supplement formal observational assessments with *unobtrusive observations* to obtain a better estimate of trainees' normal clinical behavior.

7. Consider making promotion and grading decisions via a faculty *group review* rather than being the responsibility of a single evaluator.

8. Supplement traditional clinical performance assessments with *standardized clinical encounters* (e.g., standardized patients) and skills training and assessment protocols.

9. *Educate raters* to ensure familiarity with instruments and calibrated assessments.

10. Provide *sufficient time* for assessments so that ratings are thoughtful and candid, not rushed.

11. Be certain that evaluators observe and rate *specific learner performances*.

12. Use *no more than seven* quality rating categories (i.e., 1 = poor to 7 = excellent) on observational assessment instruments.

13. *Establish the meaning of ratings* through constant use and infrequent revision of rating instruments.

14. Give faculty raters *feedback* about their stringency and leniency to prevent formation of diverse groups of faculty "hawks" and "doves."

15. Learn about observational performance assessment from *other professions* (e.g., astronaut corps, business and industry, military) for ideas about how they address personnel evaluation.

16. Acknowledge the *limits of observational assessment* while working toward the goal of continuous quality improvement.

Coda

This chapter began by asserting that observational assessment is the most widely used approach to personnel evaluation in the health professions. We also cited several research studies that reached the uncomfortable conclusion that observational assessment is frequently done poorly, meaning that educational feedback is diluted and opportunities for improvement are lost. The ideas and suggestions given in this chapter are intended to improve the *status quo*. The goal is to help health science educators use observational assessments with wisdom and skill.

Note

1. Reprinted from Section 3, Descriptive Evaluation (authored by D. Carnahan & P.A. Hemmer); in Chapter 6, Evaluation and Grading of Students, L.N. Pangaro & W.C. McGaghie (Eds.). (2005) In R.E. Fincher et al. (Eds.), *The Guidebook for Clerkship Directors* (3rd ed., p. 156). Omaha, NE: Alliance for Clinical Education. Copyright © with permission from the Alliance for Clinical Education.

References

American Dog Show Judges, Inc. (2006). Advanced Institute. Retrieved January 2, 2008 from http://www.adsj.org/

Baker, D.P., Beaubien, J.M., & Holtzman, A.K. (2006). *DoD medical team training programs: An independent case study analysis.* AHRQ Publication No. 06–0001. Rockville, MD: Agency for Healthcare Research and Quality.

Boulet, J.R., & Swanson, D.B. (2004). Psychometric challenges of using simulations for high-stakes assessment. In W.F. Dunn (Ed.), *Simulators in critical care and beyond* (pp. 119–130). Des Plaines, IL: Society of Critical Care Medicine.

Bracken, D.W., Timmreck, C.W., & Church, A.H. (Eds.). (2001). *The handbook of multisource feedback.* San Francisco: Jossey-Bass.

Carnahan, D., & Hemmer, P.A. (2005). Section 3: Descriptive evaluation; in Chapter 6: Evaluation and grading of students. In R. Fincher et al. (Eds.), *Guidebook for clerkship directors* (3rd ed., pp. 150–162). Omaha, NE: Alliance for Clinical Education.

Case, S.M., & Swanson, D.B. (2002). *Constructing written test questions for basic and clinical sciences* (3rd ed.). Philadelphia: National Board of Medical Examiners.

Cullen, D.L. (2005). Clinical education and clinical evaluation of respiratory therapy students. *Respiratory Care Clinics of North America*, 11, 425–447.

Darmody, J.V. (2005). Observing the work of the clinical nurse specialist. *Clinical Nurse Specialist*, 19 (5), 260–268.

DeVellis, R.F. (2003). *Scale development: Theory and applications* (2nd ed.). Applied Research Methods Series No. 26. Thousand Oaks, CA: Sage Publications.

Downing, S.M. (2003). Validity: On the meaningful interpretation of assessment data. *Medical Education*, 37, 830–837.

Downing, S.M. (2004). Reliability: On the reproducibility of assessment data. *Medical Education*, 38, 1006–1012.

Downing, S.M., Tekian, A., & Yudkowsky, R. (2006). Procedures for establishing defensible absolute passing scores on performance examinations in the health professions. *Teaching and Learning in Medicine*, 18, 50–57.

Epstein, R.M., & Hundert, E.M. (2002). Defining and assessing professional competence. *Journal of the American Medical Association*, 287, 226–235.

Ericsson, K.A. (2004). Deliberate practice and the acquisition and maintenance of expert performance in medicine and related domains. *Academic Medicine*, 79 (10, Suppl.), S70–S81.

Fletcher, R.H., Fletcher, S.W., & Wagner, E.H. (1996). *Clinical epidemiology —The essentials* (3rd ed.). Philadelphia: Lippincott Williams & Wilkins.

Goldman, W. (1990). *Hype and glory*. New York: Villard Books.

Green, E.H., Hershman, W., DeCherrie, L., Greenwald, J., Torres-Finnerty, N., & Wahi-Gururaj, S. (2005). Developing and implementing universal guidelines for oral patient presentation skills. *Teaching and Learning in Medicine*, 17, 263–267.

Grigorenko, E.L., & Sternberg, R.J. (1998). Dynamic testing. *Psychological Bulletin*, 124, 75–111.

Haas, J., & Shaffir, W. (1982). Ritual evaluation of competence. *Work and Occupations*, 9, 131–154.

Haas, J., & Shaffir, W. (1987). *Becoming doctors: The adoption of a cloak of competence*. Greenwich, CT: JAI Press.

Haber, R.J., & Lingard, L.A. (2001). Learning oral presentation skills: A rhetorical analysis with pedagogical and professional implications. *Journal of General Internal Medicine*, 16, 308–314.

Hamman, W.R. (2004). The complexity of team training: What we have learned from aviation and its applications to medicine. *Quality and Safety in Health Care*, 13 (Suppl. 1), i72–i79.

Health and Psychological Instruments (HAPI). Database retrieved January 22, 2008 from: http://www.northwestern.edu/libraries/

Herbers, J.E., Noel, G.L., Cooper, G.S., Harvey, J., Pangaro, L.N., & Weaver, M.J. (1989). How accurate are faculty evaluations of clinical competence? *Journal of General Internal Medicine*, 4, 202–208.

Holmboe, E.S. (2004). Faculty and the observation of trainees' clinical skills. *Academic Medicine*, 79, 16–22.

Holmboe, E.S. (2005). Section 4: Direct observation of students' clinical skills; in Chapter 6: Evaluation and grading of students. In R.E. Fincher et al. (Eds.), *Guidebook for clerkship directors* (3rd ed., pp. 163–170). Omaha, NE: Alliance for Clinical Education.

Holmboe, E.S., & Hawkins, R.E. (1998). Methods for evaluating the clinical competence of residents in internal medicine: A review. *Annals of Internal Medicine*, 129, 42–48.

Holmboe, E.S., Yepes, M., Williams, F., & Huot, S.J. (2004). Feedback and the mini clinical evaluation exercise. *Journal of General Internal Medicine*, 19, 558–561.

International Gymnastics Federation (1989). *Code of points*. Indianapolis, IN: International Gymnastics Federation.

Issenberg, S.B., McGaghie, W.C., Brown, D.D., Mayer, J.D., Gessner, I.H., Hart, I.R., et al. (2000). Development of multimedia computer-based measures of clinical skills in bedside cardiology. In D.E. Melnick (Ed.), *The eighth international Ottawa conference on medical education and assessment proceedings. Evolving assessment: Protecting the human dimension* (pp. 821–829). Philadelphia: National Board of Medical Examiners.

Issenberg, S.B., McGaghie, W.C., Gordon, D.L., Symes, S., Petrusa, E.R., Hart, I.R., et al. (2002). Effectiveness of a cardiology review course for internal medicine residents using simulation technology and deliberate practice. *Teaching and Learning in Medicine*, 14, 223–228.

Issenberg, S.B., Petrusa, E.R., McGaghie, W.C., Felner, J.M., Waugh, R.A., Nash, I.S., et al. (1999). Effectiveness of a computer-based system to teach bedside cardiology. *Academic Medicine*, 74 (10, Suppl.), S93–S95.

Kalet, A., Earp, J.A., & Kowlowitz, V. (1992). How well do faculty evaluate the interviewing skills of medical students? *Journal of General Internal Medicine*, 7, 499–505.

Kirkpatrick, D.L. (1998). *Evaluating training programs* (2nd ed.). San Francisco: Berrett-Koehler.

Linn, R.L., & Gronlund, N.E. (2000). *Measurement and assessment in teaching* (8th ed.). Upper Saddle River, NJ: Prentice-Hall.

Loftus, E.F., & Schneider, N.G. (1987). Behold with strange surprise: Judicial reactions to expert testimony concerning eyewitness reliability. *University of Missouri-Kansas City Law Review*, 56, 1–45.

Loughry, M.L., Ohland, M.W., & Moore, D.D. (2007). Development of a theory-based assessment of team member effectiveness. *Educational and Psychological Measurement*, 67 (3), 505–524.

Mahara, M.S. (1998). A perspective on clinical evaluation in nursing education. *Journal of Advanced Nursing*, 28 (6), 339–346.

McGaghie, W.C. (2005). Section 1: General introduction; in Chapter 6: Evaluation and grading of students. In R.E. Fincher et al. (Eds.), *Guidebook for clerkship directors* (3rd ed., pp. 134–142). Omaha, NE: Alliance for Clinical Education.

McGaghie, W.C., Miller, G.A., Sajid, A., & Telder, T.V. (1978). *Competency-based curriculum development in medical education.* Public Health Paper No. 68. Geneva, Switzerland: World Health Organization.

McGaghie, W.C., Renner, B.R., Kowlowitz, V., Sauter, S.V.H., Hoole, A.J., Schuch, C.P., et al. (1994). Development and evaluation of musculoskeletal performance measures for an objective structured clinical examination. *Teaching and Learning in Medicine*, 6, 59–63.

McGaghie, W.C., Van Horn, L., Fitzgibbon, M., Telser, A., Thompson, J.A., Kushner, R.F., & Prystowsky, J.B. (2001). Development of a measure of attitude toward nutrition in patient care. *American Journal of Preventive Medicine*, 20, 15–20.

McGaghie, W.C., Siddall, V.J., Mazmanian, P.E., & Myers, J. (n.d.). Lessons for continuing medical education. From simulation research in undergraduate and graduate medical education. *Chest*, 135, in press.

Miller, G.E. (1990). The assessment of clinical skills/competence/performance. *Academic Medicine*, 65 (9, Suppl.), S63–S67.

Noel, G.L., Herbers, J.E., Caplow, M.P., Cooper, G.S., Pangaro, L.N., & Harvey, J. (1992). How well do internal medicine faculty members evaluate the clinical skills of residents? *Annals of Internal Medicine*, 117, 757–765.

Norcini, J. (2006). Faculty observations of student professional behavior. In D.T. Stern (Ed.), *Measuring medical professionalism* (pp. 147–157). New York: Oxford University Press.

Norcini, J., Blank, L.L., Duffy, F.D., & Fortna, G.S. (2003). The mini-CEX: A method for assessing clinical skills. *Annals of Internal Medicine*, 138, 476–481.

Ogburn, T., & Espey, E. (2003). The R-I-M-E method for evaluation of medical students on an obstetrics and gynecology clerkship. *American Journal of Obstetrics and Gynecology*, 189, 666–669.

Orient, J.M. (2005). *Sapira's art & science of bedside diagnosis* (3rd ed.). Philadelphia: Lippincott Williams & Wilkins.

Osler, W. (1906). The hospital as a college. In W. Osler (Ed.), *Aequanimitas* (2nd ed., pp. 329–342). Philadelphia: P. Blakiston's Son & Co.

Pangaro, L.N. (1999). Evaluating professional growth: A new vocabulary and other innovations for improving descriptive evaluation of students. *Academic Medicine*, 74, 1203–1207.

Schwind, C.J., Williams, R.G., Boehler, M.L., & Dunnington, G.L. (2004). Do individual attendings' post rotation performance ratings detect residents' clinical performance deficiencies? *Academic Medicine*, 79, 453–457.

Smither, J.W., London, M., & Reilly, R.R. (2005). Does performance improve following multisource feedback? A theoretical model, meta-analysis, and review of empirical findings. *Personnel Psychology*, 58, 33–66.

Sox, H.C., Blatt, M.A., Higgins, M.C., & Marton, K.I. (1988). *Medical decision making*. Boston: Butterworth-Heinemann.

Stern, D.T. (Ed.). (2006). *Measuring medical professionalism*. New York: Oxford University Press.

Stiggins, R.J. (1987). Design and development of performance assessments. *Educational Measurement: Issues and Practice*, 6 (3), 33–42.

Streiner, D.L., & Norman, G.R. (2003). *Health measurement scales: A practical guide to their development and use* (3rd ed.). New York: Oxford University Press.

Tesser, A., & Rosen, S. (1975). The reluctance to transmit bad news. In L. Berkowitz (Ed.), *Advances in experimental social psychology* (Vol. 8., pp. 193–232). New York: Academic Press.

Thomas, E.J., Sexton, J.B., & Helmreich, R.L. (2004). Translating teamwork behaviors from aviation to healthcare: Development of behavioral markers for neonatal resuscitation. *Quality and Safety in Health Care*, 13 (Suppl. 1), i57–i64.

Waas, V., van der Vleuten, C., Shatzer, J., & Jones, R. (2001). Assessment of clinical competence. *The Lancet*, 357, 945–949.

Wayne, D.B., Butter, J., Siddall, V.J., Fudala, M.J., Lindquist, L., Feinglass, J., et al. (2005a). Simulation-based training of internal medicine residents in advanced cardiac life support protocols: A randomized trial. *Teaching and Learning in Medicine*, 17, 210–216.

Wayne, D.B., Fudala, M.J., Butter, J., Siddall, V.J., Feinglass, J., Wade, L.D., et al. (2005b). Comparison of two standard setting methods for advanced cardiac life support training. *Academic Medicine*, 80 (10, Suppl.), S63–S66.

Wayne, D.B., Butter, J., Siddall, V.J., Fudala, M.J., Wade, L.D., Feinglass, J., et al. (2006). Mastery learning of advanced cardiac life support skills by internal medicine residents using simulation technology and deliberate practice. *Journal of General Internal Medicine*, 21, 251–256.

Wayne, D.B., Barsuk, J., O'Leary, K., Fudala, M.J., & McGaghie, W.C. (2008). Mastery learning of thoracentesis skills by internal medicine residents using simulation technology and deliberate practice. *Journal of Hospital Medicine*, 3, 48–54.

Weed, L.L. (1968). Medical records that guide and teach. *New England Journal of Medicine*, 278, 593–600; 652–657.

Wiese, J., Varosy, P., & Tierney, L. (2002). Improving oral presentation skills with a clinical reasoning curriculum: A prospective controlled study. *American Journal of Medicine*, 112, 212–218.

Wigton, R.S. (1980). The effects of student personal characteristics on the evaluation of clinical performance. *Journal of Medical Education*, 55, 423–427.

Williams, R.G., Klamen, D.A., & McGaghie, W.C. (2003). Cognitive, social, and environmental sources of bias in clinical competence ratings. *Teaching and Learning in Medicine*, 15, 270–292.

Wilson, M. (2005). *Constructing measures*. Mahwah, NJ: Lawrence Erlbaum Associates.

Woehr, D.J., & Huffcutt, A.I. (1994). Rater training for performance appraisal: A quantitative review. *Journal of Occupational and Organizational Psychology*, 67, 189–205.

9

PERFORMANCE TESTS

RACHEL YUDKOWSKY

A performance test is an examination designed to elicit performance on an actual or simulated real-life task. In contrast to observation of naturally occurring behavior "in vivo" (McGaghie, Butter, & Kaye, Chapter 8, this volume), the task is contrived for the purpose of the examination, and explicitly invites the examinee to demonstrate the behavior to be assessed. Thus a performance test is an "in vitro" assessment, at Miller's "shows how" level (Miller, 1990); see Figure 9.1. Since the examinees know they are being assessed, their performance likely represents their personal best or maximum performance, rather than a typical performance. Examples of performance tests include a road test to obtain a driver's license, an undersea diving test, and the Unites States Medical Licensing Exam (USMLE) Step 2 Clinical Skills Assessment. In this chapter we'll review some of the purposes, advantages and limitations of performance tests, and provide practical guidelines for the use of standardized patients (SPs), a simulation modality commonly used in health professions education. Focusing on the use of SPs for assessment rather than instruction, we'll discuss scoring options, multiple-station Objective Structured Clinical Exams (OSCEs), standard setting, and threats to validity in the context of SP exams; the same principles apply to performance tests using other modalities. There are several other types of simulations currently in use, such as bench models, virtual (computer-based) models, and mannequins. Many of the assessment issues addressed here also apply to these forms of simulation, which are discussed in greater detail in Chapter 10.

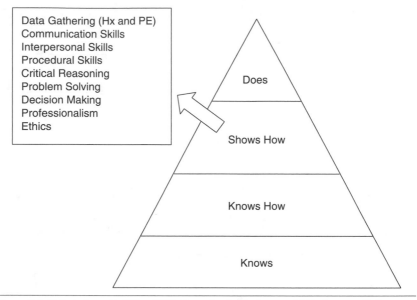

Data Gathering (Hx and PE)
Communication Skills
Interpersonal Skills
Procedural Skills
Critical Reasoning
Problem Solving
Decision Making
Professionalism
Ethics

Does

Shows How

Knows How

Knows

Figure 9.1 Miller's Pyramid (Miller, 1990): Competencies to Assess with Performance Tests.

Strengths of Performance Tests

Performance tests provide the opportunity to observe students in action as they respond to complex challenges, while controlling when, where, how and what will be tested. Performance tests are not limited to patients and problems that chance to present in clinical settings in a specific span of time. The simulation option provides a high degree of control over the examination setting, allowing standardization across examinees, advance training of examiners, and a systematic sampling of the domain to be assessed. When used formatively performance tests provide unique opportunities for feedback, coaching and debriefing, thus facilitating deliberate practice (Ericsson, 1993, 2004) and the development of skills and expertise. From a patient safety perspective, performance tests allow educators to ensure that learners have reached a minimal level of competency and skill before they are allowed to work with real patients. Disadvantages of performance tests are related to the complex logistics and difficulty of realistically modeling clinical tasks; simulations can be expensive, and the need for multiple stations or cases (see below) increases the resource cost in terms of both money and time.

Defining the Purpose of the Test

As with all assessments, faculty must be clear about the purpose of the test. What are the underlying constructs (competencies or skills) to be assessed?

Since performance tests are time consuming and expensive, they are best reserved for the assessment of skills that cannot be observed or assessed effectively elsewhere or by other means. Skills that involve interactions with patients are particularly amenable to performance tests. Communication and interpersonal skills with patients, family, staff and colleagues; data gathering by means of a history and physical exam (H&P); clinical reasoning and decision making; documentation in the patient chart; ethical and professional behavior and procedural skills all can be elicited and assessed effectively in simulated settings.

The choice of whether to assess individual skills or a complete clinical encounter depends in part on the level of the learner (Petrusa, 2002). Students early in training often learn discrete skills such as "examining the shoulder" or "taking a sexual history." These skills can be assessed by means of brief, five to seven minute stations in which they are instructed to demonstrate the particular skill: "please examine the shoulder of this patient." Intermediate learners must select salient history and physical exam items on their own when encountering a patient, and must construct a differential diagnosis and management plan. These learners are more appropriately tested in a longer, integrated patient encounter that elicits these competencies in the context of a given complaint. For more advanced learners, the ability to handle complex critical situations can be tested in an "error prone" environment that features staff blunders, non-functioning equipment, and distracting family members.

An observation of an actual (not simulated) clinical encounter can be part of a performance test if the encounter is taking place for the purpose of the exam: for example a mini-CEX (McGaghie, Butter, & Kaye, Chapter 8, this volume), the live interview in the

U.S. Psychiatry Board exam, or the first part of a traditional "viva," in which a preceptor rates the performance of a history and physical exam on an unknown patient. Note that a performance test does not require the subsequent oral examination or discussion of the patient— the encounter itself is the object of the rating. All of the principles discussed in this chapter, such as blueprinting, scoring the encounter, and standard setting, apply equally to performance tests based on real patients and to simulations.

Standardized Patients

Standardized patients (SPs) are persons who are trained to portray a given patient presentation in a consistent and believable manner, allowing the realistic simulation of patient encounters (Barrows, 1993; Barrows & Abrahamson, 1964). SPs can come from a range of backgrounds including professional actors, retired teachers, community volunteers, patients with stable physical findings, nurses, medical residents and students. "Hybrid" simulations use SPs in conjunction with bench models and mannequins (Kneebone, Kidd, Nestel, et al., 2005) to encourage a patient-centered approach to procedural skills. Unannounced SPs can be sent incognito into clinician offices and clinics to assess performance in actual practice (Rethans, Drop, Sturmans, & van der Vleuten 1991; Rethans, Gorter, Bokken, & Morrison, 2007). The SP methodology also has been extended to the portrayal of standardized students for faculty development (Gelula & Yudkowsky, 2003), and standardized family members, colleagues and staff.

"Simulated patient" is a generic term that includes portrayals that do not need to be highly consistent across encounters, for example patient simulation for the purpose of small group instruction. In contrast, the "standardized" aspect of the SP is crucial to the use of SPs for assessment. In a high-stakes assessment setting SPs must be able to keep the portrayal consistent across a large number of examinees, each bringing his or her own idiosyncratic questions and behaviors to the encounter. Consistent portrayal requires two elements: a highly specified script, and rigorous training of the SP.

The *SP script* contains the details of the portrayal. The script stipulates the age, gender, and other salient characteristics of the patient, and describes the patient's medical history and physical exam findings, their "backstory" (family, job, and life circumstances), their personality and affect. The script specifies information to be provided in response to open ended questions, information to be provided only if specifically elicited by the examinee, SP prompts for the examinee (e.g. questions such as: "Can I go home now?"), and the desired SP responses to different examinee behaviors. The extent and richness of the script depends in part on the length and nature of the expected interaction. A five-minute encounter in which a student examines the shoulder of the SP without gathering any historical information may require only a description of physical exam findings to be simulated (if any). A 30-minute encounter in which an examinee is asked to develop a differential diagnosis and treatment plan for a depressed elderly woman demands a highly detailed and elaborated script.

SP scripts should be written by teams of experienced clinicians, preferably based on their own experiences with an actual patient, with modifications to maintain patient confidentiality. Basing the script on a real patient provides the foundation for a rich backstory, supporting details such laboratory results, and the assurance that the script "hangs together" to present a plausible and realistic patient. Figure 9.2 lists suggested elements of an effective script and provides a template or scaffold for the needed information. SP scripts can also be found in published casebooks (The Macy Initiative, 2003; Schimpfhouser, Sultz, Zinnerstrom, & Anderson, 2000) and in online resource banks such as MedEd Portal (www.aamc.org/mededportal) and the Association of Standardized Patient Educators (www.aspeducators.org).

SP training: Once the script is available an SP can be trained to portray the patient accurately, consistently, and believably (van der Vleuten & Swanson 1990; Tamblyn, Klass, Schnabl & Kopelow, 1991; Colliver & Williams, 1993; Wallace, 2007). Training includes review, clarification and memorization of the case material, followed by rehearsal of the material in simulated encounters with the trainer and/or simulated examinees. The SP must be able to improvise

General Case Information
- ☐ Presenting complaint
- ☐ Diagnosis
- ☐ Case Author contact information
- ☐ Learning objectives, competencies addressed in case
- ☐ Target learner group (e.g. medical students, residents, nursing students, nurse practitioner students, other)
- ☐ Level of learner (year of training, advanced clinician, etc.)
- ☐ Duration of patient encounter

Case Summary and SP Training Notes
- ☐ SP demographics: name, gender, age range, ethnicity
- ☐ Setting (clinic, ER, etc.)
- ☐ History of present illness
- ☐ Past medical history
- ☐ Family medical history
- ☐ Social history and backstory
- ☐ Review of systems
- ☐ Physical examination findings (if indicated)
- ☐ Special instructions for the SP:
    - ☐ Patient presentation (affect, appearance, position of patient at opening, etc.)
    - ☐ Opening statement
    - ☐ Embedded communication challenges
    - ☐ Responses to open-ended questions
    - ☐ Responses to specific interviewing techniques or errors
- ☐ Special case considerations/props:
    - ☐ Specific body type/physical requirements
    - ☐ Props (e.g. pregnancy pillow)
    - ☐ Make-up (please include application guidelines if available)

Additional Materials
- ☐ Door chart information
- ☐ Laboratory results, radiology images (if indicated)
- ☐ Student instructions
- ☐ Student pre- or post-encounter challenge
- ☐ SP checklist or rating scale for scoring the encounter
- ☐ Observer checklist or rating scale
- ☐ SP feedback guidelines
- ☐ Other supporting documents (faculty instructions, etc.)

Figure 9.2 Essential Elements of a Standardized Patient Case.

Source: Adapted with permission from the Association of Standardized Patient Educators (ASPE) (Copyright 2008).

appropriately and in character when confronted with unexpected questions from the examinee. If more than one SP will be portraying the same case, training them together will promote consistency across different SPs. Video recordings of previous SPs portraying the case help provide consistency across different administrations of the test. If the SPs will be providing verbal or written feedback to the examinee, they should be trained to do so effectively (Howley, 2007). If the SPs will be rating the examinees, this requires training as well (see rater training, below). The entire training process can range from 30 minutes to eight hours and more, depending on the complexity of the script and the responsibilities of the SP. Once the SP is performing at the desired level, periodic assessment and feedback can help maintain the quality of the exam (Wind, Van Dalen, Muijtjens, & Rethans, 2004).

Scoring the Performance

Checklists and rating scales are used to convert the examinee's behavior during the SP encounter (or other observed performance) into a number that can be used for scoring. *Checklist* items are statements or questions that can be scored dichotomously as "done" or "not done"—for example, "The examinee auscultated the lungs." *Rating scales* employ a range of response options to indicate the quality of what was done—for example, "How respectful was the examinee?" might be rated on a four-point scale ranging from "extremely respectful" to "not at all respectful."

Case-specific checklists identify actions essential to a given clinical case, and are usually developed by panels of content experts or local faculty (Gorter, Rethans, Scherpbier, et al., 2000). Checklist items can also be derived by observing the actions of experienced clinicians as they encounter the SP (Nendaz, Gut, Perrier, et al., 2004). Ideally, items should be evidence-based and reflect best-practice guidelines. Since checklists are intended simply to record what took place in the encounter, completing the checklist does not necessarily require expert judgment. Nonetheless, to minimize disagreements between raters the checklist items must be very well specified, and raters must be trained to recognize the parameters of examinee behaviors that merit a score of "done" for a particular action. For example, the checklist item cited above "the examinee auscultated the lungs" might be more fully specified as "the examinee auscultated the lungs on skin, posteriorly, bilaterally, at three levels, while asking the patient to breath deeply through the mouth." If any one of these conditions is not met, the item is scored as "not done" or as "done incorrectly." The item could be split into individual items for each of the essential conditions (on skin, bilateral, three levels, etc.) if more detailed feedback is desired. Checklists may be completed by observers during the encounter or by the SP immediately after the encounter. Checklists of 12 to 15 items can be completed quite accurately by well-trained SPs (Vu, Mary, Colliver, et al., 1992). Some extensively trained SPs can complete much longer checklists, such as those required for a full head-to-toe screening physical exam (Yudkowsky, Downing, Klamen, et al., 2004).

While checklists can be used effectively with beginning learners to confirm that they followed all steps of a procedure or elicited a thorough medical history, comprehensive checklists are not always appropriate for more advanced examinees (Hodges, Regehr, McNaughton, et al., 1999). Expert clinicians often receive relatively low scores on history and physical exam (H&P) checklists that reward thoroughness; they tend to reach a diagnosis based on non-analytic processes such as pattern matching and thus perform a highly abbreviated H&P. When assessing more complex performance and/or advanced clinicians, rating scales completed by experts may be a more appropriate tool.

Rating scales provide the opportunity for observers to exercise expert judgment and rate the quality of an action. *Global* scale items rate the performance as an integrated whole; for example "Overall, this performance was: excellent | very good | good | marginal | unsatisfactory." *Analytic* scale items allow polytomous (multiple level) rating of specific behaviors: "Student followed up on patient non-verbal cues: frequently | sometimes | rarely | never." *Primary trait* rating scale items are used to assess a small number of salient features or characteristics of the overall performance; thus when assessing communication skills one might be asked to rate verbal communication, non-verbal communication, and English language skills. While checklists are usually case-specific, rating scales can be used to score behaviors or skills that are demonstrated across different cases, such as data gathering, communication skills, or professionalism. A variety of instruments for rating communication and interpersonal skills have been published (ACGME Outcome Project 2008: Tools from the field, Makoul, 2001a and b; Kurtz, Silverman, Benson, & Draper, 2003; Stillman, Brown, Redfield, & Sabers, 1977; Yudkowsky, Downing & Sandlow, 2006).

Because rating scales require the exercise of judgment, they are inherently more subjective than checklists. Providing anchors for the different rating options can improve agreement between raters (inter-rater reliability), especially if these anchors are behaviorally anchored (Bernardin & Smith, 1981). See Figure 9.3 for examples of different types of rating scale anchors.

Rubrics can be used to rate written products such as chart notes completed after an SP encounter. The rubric is, in effect, a behaviorally anchored rating scale providing detailed information about the performance expected at each score level (see Chapter 7 for more about rubrics in the context of written tests). A sample rubric for scoring a chart note is shown in Figure 9.4.

A. Likert-type Scales:

The student provided a clear explanation of my condition and the treatment plan.

1	2	3	4
Strongly disagree	Disagree	Agree	Strongly Agree

How clear were the student's explanations?

1	2	3	4	5
Not at all Clear	Somewhat Clear	Clear	Very Clear	Extremely Clear

B. Behaviorally Anchored Rating Scale (BARS)

Did the student provide a clear explanation of your condition?

1	2	3	4
Provided little or no explanation of my condition	Provided brief or unclear explanations of my condition	Provided a full and understandable explanation of my condition, pertinent findings, and important next steps	Provided a full explanation of my condition, his/her thinking about it and recommendation, and probed my understanding by asking me to summarize pertinent information

Figure 9.3 Rating Scale Anchors.

Please assess each component of the note	All key items present?		Any incorrect or dangerous items?	
History	Yes	No	Yes	No
Physical exam	Yes	No	Yes	No
Differential diagnosis	Yes	No	Yes	No
Plan for immediate workup	Yes	No	Yes	No

Please rate the overall quality of this patient note:

Rating	Example
1 = Not acceptable	Major deficiencies or disorganization in multiple sections
2 = Borderline acceptable	Major deficiencies or disorganization in one section but most essential points covered
3 = Acceptable	Minor deficiencies or disorganization in one or more sections.
4 = Excellent	Thorough, complete and well organized note. All four sections (History, PE, DDx and Workup) are complete.

Figure 9.4 Sample Rubric for Scoring a Student's Patient Chart Note.

Training Raters

Raters must be trained to use checklists and rating scales accurately and consistently. Training is best done with all raters in one group to facilitate consensus and cross-calibration. After reviewing the purpose of the exam and each of the items, frame of reference training (Bernardin & Buckley, 1981) can help ensure that all raters are calibrated and using the scale in the same way. The raters observe and individually score a live or recorded performance such as an SP encounter or chart note, then together discuss their ratings and reach a consensus on the observed behaviors corresponding to the checklist items and rating anchors. Ideally, raters should observe performances at high, middle, and low levels of proficiency and identify behaviors that are characteristic of each level.

Pilot-Testing the Case

Before deploying the case in an assessment, the station and rating instruments should be piloted with a few representative raters and examinees to ensure that the test will function as intended. Pilot tests frequently result in changes to the examinee instructions, specification of SP responses to previously unanticipated queries, and clarification of checklist items and rating anchors.

Multiple-station Performance Tests: The Objective Structured Clinical Exam (OSCE)

Performance on one clinical case or challenge is not a good predictor of performance on another case; this phenomenon is known as "case specificity" (Elstein, Shuman, & Sprafka, 1978). The ability to manage a patient with an acute appendicitis does not predict the ability to diagnose depression; demonstrating an appropriate history and physical exam (H&P) for a patient with chronic diabetes does not predict the ability to conduct an appropriate H&P for a patient with acute chest pain. Just as one would not assess a student's knowledge based on a single multiple-choice question, one cannot assess competency based on a single observation. One solution is the Objective Structured Clinical Examination or OSCE (Harden, Stevenson, Downie, & Wilson, 1975), an exam format that consists of a series or circuit of performance tests. Within an OSCE each test is called a "station"; students start at different points in the circuit and encounter one station after another until the OSCE is complete. A given OSCE can include stations of different types: SP-based patient encounters, procedures such as IV insertion, written challenges such as writing prescriptions or chart notes, interpretation of lab results, EKGs or radiology images, and oral presentations to an examiner (Figure 9.5). A larger number of stations allows for better sampling of the domain to be assessed, thus improving the reliability and validity of the exam—see the threats to validity discussion below.

The duration of an OSCE station can range from five minutes to 30 minutes or longer, depending on the purpose of the exam (Petrusa, 2002). Shorter stations allow the testing of discrete skills such as eliciting reflexes; longer stations allow the assessment of complex tasks in a realistic context—for example, counseling a patient reluctant to undergo colorectal screening. Ten to twenty minutes are usually

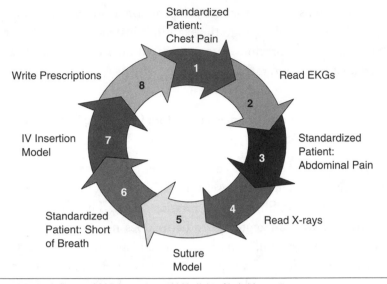

Figure 9.5 An 8-Station OSCE for an Internal Medicine Clerkship.

sufficient for a focused history and physical exam (Petrusa, 2002). For logistic convenience, all stations in a given OSCE should be of equal duration. "Couplet" stations consist of two linked challenges—for example, writing a chart note about the patient just seen in the previous station. The duration of the couplet station—the SP encounter plus note—will be equal to the combined time of two stations.

Scoring an OSCE: Combining Scores Across Stations

The unit of analysis in an OSCE is the station or case, not the checklist item, since items within a case are mutually dependent: whether a resident examines the heart depends on whether she elicited a history of chest pain. Checklist or scale items should be aggregated to create a station score. Subsets of the checklist can give information about performance on different aspects of the task, for example history taking vs physical exam, but these subscales rarely have enough items to stand on their own as reliable measures. However, skills subscales or primary-trait ratings of skills that are common to several cases can be averaged across cases to obtain an exam-level score for that skill. For example, communication and interpersonal skills (CIS) scores show moderate correlations across cases, so it is reasonable to average CIS rating scale scores across cases to obtain an exam-level score.

Compensatory vs non-compensatory or conjunctive scoring issues were discussed in Chapter 6 (Yudkowsky, Downing, & Tekian, this volume). Should good performance on one case or task compensate for poor performance on another? This is a policy-level decision. A skills-based compensatory approach would mean that good communication skills in one case could reasonably compensate for poor communication skills in another. On the other hand, decision-makers may feel that examinees should demonstrate competency in an absolute number of critical clinical situations such as chest pain, abdominal pain or shortness of breath—good performance on one would not compensate for poor performance on another. The ability to perform different clinical procedures is generally conjunctive—good performance inserting an IV does not compensate for poor performance obtaining an EKG.

Standard Setting

Many of the standard-setting methods described in Chapter 6, originally developed for written tests, have been adapted for use with performance tests (Downing, Tekian, & Yudkowsky, 2006). Item-based methods such as Angoff are commonly and easily employed to set cut scores for checklists, however the use of item-based methods for performance tests has been challenged since items on a checklist are not mutually independent (Ross, Clauser, Margolis, et al., 1996). Moreover, not all checklist items have equal clinical valence— the omission of one item may endanger a patient's life, while the omission of another may be of little import to the outcome of the clinical case. Standard setting methods based on the direct observation of examinees' performance, such as borderline-group (BG) and contrasting-group (CG), avoid these problems. Programs that use expert examiners (faculty) to observe and score SP encounters can easily use these examinee-based methods by having the examiners assign a global rating of fail, marginal pass, or pass in addition to completing the checklist for each examinee. The mean or median checklist score of examinees with a marginal pass rating is set as the cut score in the Borderline Group method, while the intersection of the passing and failing groups provides the basis for the cut score in the Contrasting-Group method (see Chapter 6 for details). Programs that use non-clinicians such as SPs to complete the checklists can have faculty experts rate the SP-scored checklists as proxies for examinee performance, use a compromise method such as Hofstee, or opt to fall back on item-based methods such as Angoff or Ebel while acknowledging their limitations. Case-level cut scores can be aggregated across cases to provide a compensatory-type standard for the whole test. Conjunctive standards will require that a specific number of cases be passed, or that two or more subscales be passed (for example, both data gathering and communication skills). Conjunctive standards will always result in a higher failure rate than compensatory standards, since each hurdle adds its own probability of failure.

Procedural skills testing brings a different set of challenges to standard setting. A mastery approach is especially appropriate in situations where the checklist is public and incorrect performance comprises a threat to patient safety or to the successful outcome of the procedure.

Logistics

Conducting an OSCE can be daunting. Some schools have full-time SP trainers, paid professional actors who serve as SPs, and a dedicated facility that includes several clinic-type rooms with audio-visual recording capability, affording remote observation and scoring of SP encounters. Online data-management systems facilitate checklist data capture and reporting, and allow both learners and faculty to view and comment upon digital recordings of encounters from remote locations. On the other hand, OSCEs also can be conducted on a more limited budget by using faculty as trainers and raters, recruiting students, residents, or community volunteers as SPs, and exploiting existing clinic space in the evening or weekend. Video-recording the encounters is helpful but by no means essential.

As an example of a high stakes OSCE, Figure 9.6 provides a summary description of the United States Medical Licensing Exam Step

The United States Medical Licensing Examination (USMLE) Step 2 CS*

Exam purpose	To ensure that new residents have the knowledge and skills needed to provide patient care under supervision.
Content domain	Patients and problems normally encountered during medical practice in the United States
Level of skill assessed (discrete skills vs full encounter)	Full encounter: Ability to obtain a pertinent history, perform a physical examination, and communicate findings to patients and colleagues.
Format	(1) Standardized patient encounters (15 minutes each) (2) Patient note written after each encounter (10 minutes), including pertinent history and physical exam findings, differential diagnoses, and plans for immediate diagnostic work up.
Number of stations (encounters)	Twelve
Skill section scores reported	(1) Integrated clinical encounter (ICE): Data gathering + patient note (2) Communication and Interpersonal Skills (CIS) (3) English language proficiency
Rating instruments	• Checklists for data gathering (Hx and PE) • Global rating scales for patient note and English proficiency • Primary trait rating scale for CIS
Raters	• SPs for Hx and PE checklists, CIS and English • Clinicians for patient note
Combining Scores across cases, cut scores	Compensatory within skill section (ICE, CIS, English) Conjunctive across skills—must pass each section separately

Figure 9.6 OSCE Case Example.
Note: * http://www.usmle.org/Examinations/step2/step2cs_content.html

2 Clinical Skills Assessment (USMLE Step 2 CS). Additional information about this OSCE is available at the USMLE website.

Threats to the Validity of Performance Tests

Threats to the validity of performance tests are summarized in Table 9.1. Our discussion will focus on the two main threats discussed in Chapter 2: under-sampling (construct under-representation) and noise (construct-irrelevant variance).

Construct under-representation, or under-sampling, can be a particular threat to the validity of performance tests since performance varies

Table 9.1 Threats to the Validity: Performance Tests

	Problem	Remedy
Construct Under-representation (CU) "Undersampling"	Not enough cases or stations to sample domain adequately	Use multiple stations (at least 8–10)
	Not enough items to reflect the performance in a given case	Use several checklist or rating scale items to capture the performance in each case
	Unrepresentative sampling of domain	Blueprint to be sure stations systematically sample the domain
Construct-irrelevant Variance (CIV) "Noise"	Unclear or poorly worded items	Pilot stations and rating instruments Train raters on items
	Station or item difficulty inappropriate (too easy/too hard)	Pilot stations and rating instruments with learners of the appropriate level
	Checklist items don't capture expert reasoning (mis-match of items to competencies)	Careful design of checklist and rating scale items to match level of examinee Use content-expert raters who can rate the quality of the response (vs done/not done)
	Rater bias	Provide behaviorally anchored scoring rubric Train raters to use rubric Use multiple raters across stations
	Systematic rater error: Halo, Severity, Leniency, Central tendency	Frame of reference training for raters
	Inconsistent ratings	Remove rater
	Language/cultural bias	Train raters Pilot and revise stations
	Indefensible passing score methods	Formal standard setting exercises
Reliability Indicators	Generalizability Inter-rater reliability Rater consistency Internal reliability of checklist or rating scale	

from station to station ("case specificity") but only a small number of stations or performances can be observed. A multiple-station performance test (OSCE) thus falls between the written test with hundreds of multiple-choice questions and the traditional viva or oral exam which may include only a single observation or questions about a single patient case.

The validity of an OSCE depends on its ability to sufficiently and systematically sample the domain to be assessed (Figure 9.7). Systematic sampling is supported by blueprinting and creating a table of test specifications (see Chapter 2). In the case of an SP-based OSCE, the blueprint should specify three C's: *content* subdomains, *competencies* to be assessed, and patient *characteristics;* the OSCE should include cases that comprise a systematic sampling of these elements. Figure 9.8 provides an example of blueprint elements for an SP-based assessment of psychiatry residents. A conceptual framework can assist in identifying salient elements to be sampled and assessed; examples of such frameworks are the ACGME competencies for residents in the US (ACGME outcome project: competencies), and the Kalamazoo consensus statement on medical communication (Makoul, 2001a and b); see Figure 9.9.

To be valid, OSCE stations must be long enough to allow the observation of the behavior of interest. If the behavior of interest is the ability to conduct a focused history and physical exam and generate a differential diagnosis and treatment plan based on that H&P, the OSCE will need to utilize longer (10–20 minute) stations and extend the testing time to allow for a sufficient number of encounters. Generally about 4–8 hours of testing time are needed to obtain minimally reliable scores (van der Vleuten & Swanson, 1990).

A potential disjunction between the exam and the clinical curriculum comprises an additional challenge to the content validity of the exam. An OSCE blueprint systematically maps the exam stations to the curriculum content and objectives. However, the clinical experiences of trainees are often opportunistic—the particular set of patient problems seen by a given student will depend on the patients who happen to be admitted to the hospital or seen in the clinic during the weeks of their clerkship. Comments from students that they have

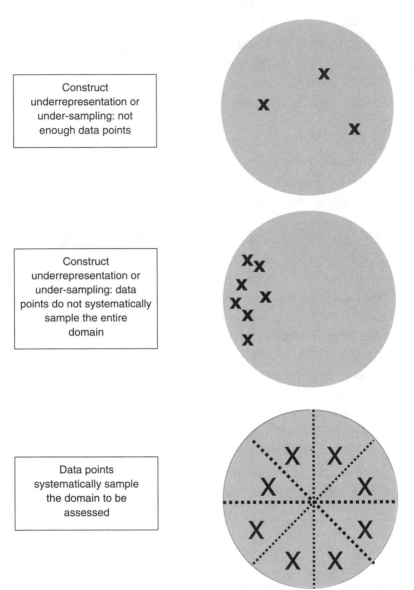

Figure 9.7 Construct Underrepresentation.

not encountered the clinical challenges included in the OSCE, or unusually low mean scores on a specific station, may provide valuable information regarding curricular gaps.

Another type of threat to validity is *construct-irrelevant variance*,

---

Content: *Identify the content subdomains to be assessed. For a psychiatry OSCE, these might include:*
- Psychotic disorders
- Affective disorders
- Anxiety disorders
- Substance abuse
- Child psychiatry

Competencies: *Identify tasks, competencies and skills to be assessed. For example:*
- History
- Physical exam
- Mental status exam
- Communication skills
- Differential diagnosis
- Writing a prescription
- Documentation in chart

Characteristics: *Identify patient demographics and other salient dimensions to be sampled. For example:*
- Age—child, adult, elderly
- Gender
- Ethnicity
- Chronic vs acute complaint
- Hospital vs outpatient clinic setting

Compile a set of cases or challenges that samples across the listed content, competencies and characteristics.

Sample stations for a psychiatry OSCE
- Interview a 25-year old woman who is in the emergency room complaining of panic attacks; write a chart note including pertinent findings and differential diagnosis.
- Perform and document a mental status exam for a 65-year old man hospitalized with chronic depression.
- Discuss medication changes and write a prescription for a 35-year old man with an exacerbation of hallucinations.
- Counsel a parent with an autistic child; document in the chart.

Figure 9.8 Creating Blueprint Specifications for an OSCE.

in which the spread of scores across students (score variance) reflects something other than differences in student ability. Any source of variance other than that due to actual differences of ability between students is considered error variance ("noise"). In SP-based performance tests the items, cases, SPs, raters, and occasion are all potential sources of measurement error. The Generalizability Coefficient G is a measure of the reliability of the exam as a whole (see Chapter 4); Generalizability analyses can help identify the

Accreditation Council for Graduate Medical Education: Six Competencies*
- Patient Care
- Knowledge
- Communication and Interpersonal Skills
- Professionalism
- System-Based Practice
- Practice-Based Learning and Improvement

The Kalamazoo consensus statement: Essential elements of communication in medical encounters**
- Build the doctor-patient relationship
- Open the discussion
- Gather information
- Understand the patient's perspective
- Share information
- Reach agreement on problems and plans
- Provide closure

Figure 9.9 Some Frameworks to Assist in Blueprinting OSCEs.

Source: *ACGME Outcome Project: Competencies. http://www.acgme.org **Makoul (2001a). Reprinted with permission from Lippincott Williams & Wilkins (Copyright 2001).

major sources of error for a given OSCE. Complementing the Generalizability analysis, Many Faceted Rasch Measurement (MFRM) analyses can identify any individual items, cases and raters that are problematic and the specific types of errors involved (Irama-neerat & Yudkowsky, 2007; Iramaneerat, Yudkowsky, Myford, & Downing, 2007). Case specificity, the variance due to cases and the interaction between cases and persons, is usually the greatest source of variance in performance tests, and is a much greater source of error than differences between raters. Thus it is much more effective to use one rater per station and increase the number of stations than to have two or more raters per station with a smaller number of stations (van der Vleuten, 1990). With proper training SPs contribute little error variance; repeated studies have shown that SPs can be trained to portray cases and complete checklists with a high degree of accuracy and consistency (van der Vleuten & Swanson 1990; Colliver & William, 1993). In general, if there is sufficient sampling of content via a sufficient sampling of cases or stations, and different raters and SPs are used across stations, then sampling across raters and SPs will also be sufficient to provide reproducible results.

Table 9.2 describes the sources of variance in a typical OSCE, along with typical errors and possible remedies.

Table 9.2 Sources of Error in an OSCE

Source of Variance	Reason	Result	Remedy
Person	Persons differ in their ability to do the behavior to be assessed	Differences in scores due to true differences in ability between persons	No remedy needed—this (and only this) is the desired score information
Item	Checklist or rating scale items or anchors not clear	Different raters will have different understandings of the item so will rate the same performance differently	Carefully word items Pilot the items Train raters
	Item-specific variance	Individual students find some items in a case more difficult than others (performance is variable across items within a case)	Use several items per case
Case	Case-specific variance	Individual students find some cases more challenging than others (performance is variable across cases within an exam)	Use many cases per exam
	Case situation or task is unclear or ambiguous	Students respond differently depending on their interpretation of the case	Pilot the case to be sure that it is clear and unambiguous
SP	SP portrays the case incorrectly	Students respond to a different case than authors intended	Train SP, Quality Assurance
	Different SPs vary in how they portray the case	Students respond differently to different SPs	Train SPs together
Raters	Systematic rater error: Halo, Severity, Leniency, Central tendency	Systematically biased ratings—e.g. an individual rater gives consistently high or low ratings	Provide behaviorally anchored scoring rubric. Frame of reference training for raters. Use different raters across stations. Statistical corrections for systematic errors. *(Continued Overleaf)*

Table 9.2 Continued

Source of Variance	Reason	Result	Remedy
	Rater bias	Ratings depend on irrelevant characteristics such as gender or race	Rater training Remove rater
	Inconsistent ratings	A given rater gives randomly inconsistent ratings—adds to the random noise in the system	Rater training Remove rater
Occasion	Occasion-specific factors environmental factors such as noise and temperature, individual factors such as illness or lack of sleep	Performance is affected by the occasion-specific factor	Control environmental factors Test on several different occasions

Consequential Validity: Educational Impact

One important aspect of an assessment is its impact on learning (van der Vleuten & Schuwirth, 2005). Adding an SP-based OSCE to the usual battery of MCQ written tests has been found to increase students' attention to clinical experiences and their requests for direct observation and feedback (Newble & Jaeger, 1983; Newble, 1988); testing procedural skills similarly leads students to seek opportunities for practicing these skills, a desirable result. However, the use of checklists in SP-based assessments can sometimes have unintended consequences. For example, if checklists require students to elicit a list of historical items and SPs are trained not to disclose the information unless specifically asked, students will learn to ask closed-ended questions in shotgun fashion instead of taking a patient-centered approach. Training SPs to give more elaborated and informative responses to open-ended questions can reduce this effect. Similarly, assessing the physical exam by means of a head-to-toe screening exam (Yudkowsky, Downing, Klamen, et al., 2004) ensures that students acquire a repertoire of PE maneuvers, but encourages students to learn these maneuvers by rote with no consideration of diagnostic hypotheses or potential physical findings. Using a hypothesis-driven

PE approach to assessment (Yudkowsky, 2007) can promote the development of clinical reasoning instead of rote learning. Educators should be alert to the potential for both positive and negative consequences of any assessment method, and ensure that the assessment experience encourages good habits of learning and practice.

Conclusion

Performance tests provide opportunities for examinees to demonstrate a particular competency or skill under controlled conditions. By utilizing standardized patients and other simulations, performance tests can control or manage many elements that are not predictable in live patient settings. Systematic sampling across cases, items and raters in performance tests is essential to minimizing sources of error and maximizing the Generalizability and validity of the score. The combination of systematic sampling, control and standardization afforded by performance tests allows for a valid, fair and defensible assessment of clinical skills.

Recommended Readings and Resources:

- For additional reading on standardized patients, see the excellent review papers by van der Vleuten & Swanson, 1990; Colliver & Williams, 1993; van der Vleuten, 1996; and Petrusa, 2002.
- For a look at the future of standardized patients see Adamo, 2003 and Petrusa, 2004.
- For a fascinating narrative of the history of standardized patients, see Wallace, 1997.
- To network with health professions educators working with standardized patients and simulations around the world, go to the websites of the Association of Standardized Patient Educators http://www.aspeducators.org/ and the Society for Simulation in Healthcare http://www.ssih.org/.

References

Accreditation Council for Graduate Medical Education: Outcome Project. Retrieved June 19, 2008 from: http://www.acgme.org

Adamo, G. (2003). Simulated and standardized patients in OSCEs: Achievements and challenges 1992–2003. *Medical Teacher*, 25(3), 262–270.

Barrows, H.S. (1993). An overview of the uses of standardized patients for teaching and evaluating clinical skills. *Academic Medicine*, 68, 443–451.

Barrows, H.S., & Abrahamson, S. (1964). The programmed patient: A technique for appraising student performance in clinical neurology. *Journal of Medical Education*, 39, 802–805.

Bernardin, H.J., & Buckley, M.R. (1981). Strategies in rater training. *The Academy of Management Review*, 6(2), 205–212.

Bernardin, H.J., & Smith, P.C. (1981). A clarification of some issues regarding the development and use of behaviorally anchored rating scales (BARS). *Journal of Applied Psychology*, 66, 458–463.

Colliver, J.A., & Williams, R.G. (1993). Technical issues: Test application. *Academic Medicine*, 68, 454–460.

Downing, S., Tekian, A., & Yudkowsky, R. (2006). Procedures for establishing defensible absolute passing scores on performance examinations in health professions education. *Teaching and Learning in Medicine*, 18(1), 50–57.

Elstein, A.S., Shuman, L.S., & Sprafka, S.A. (1978). *Medical problem solving: An analysis of clinical reasoning*. Cambridge, Massachusetts: Harvard University Press.

Ericsson, K.A. (2004). Deliberate practice and the acquisition and maintenance of expert performance in medicine and related domains. *Academic Medicine*, 79 (10, Suppl.), S70–S81.

Ericsson, K.A., Krampe, R.T., & Tesch-Römer, C. (1993). The role of deliberate practice in the acquisition of expert performance. *Psychological Review*, 100, 363–406.

Eva, K.W., Rosenfeld, J., Reiter, H.I., & Norman, G.R. (2004). An admissions OSCE: The multiple mini-interview. *Medical Education*, 38, 314–326.

Gelula, M., & Yudkowsky, R. (2003). Using standardized students in faculty development workshops to improve clinical teaching skills. *Medical Education*, 37, 621–629.

Gorter, S., Rethans, J.J., Scherpbier, A., van der Heijde, D., van der Vleuten, C., & van der Linden, S. (2000). Developing case-specific checklists for standardized-patient-based assessments internal medicine: A review of the literature. *Academic Medicine*, 75(11), 1130–1137.

Harden, R., Stevenson, M., Downie, W., & Wilson, M. (1975). Assessment of clinical competence using objective structured examinations. *British Medical Journal*, 1, 447–451.

Hodges, B., Regehr, G., McNaughton, N., Tiberius, R., & Hanson, M. (1999). OSCE checklists do not capture increasing levels of expertise. *Academic Medicine*, 74, 1129–1134.

Howley, L. (2007). Focusing feedback on interpersonal skills: A workshop for standardized patients. MedEdPORTAL: http://services.aamc.org/jsp/mededportal/retrieveSubmissionDetailById.do?subId=339.

Iramaneerat, C., & Yudkowsky, R. (2007). Rater errors in a clinical skills assessment of medical students. *Evaluation & the Health Professions 2007*, 30(3), 266–283.

Iramaneerat, C., Yudkowsky, R., Myford, C.M., & Downing, S. (2007). Quality control of an OSCE using generalizability theory and many-faceted rasch measurement. *Advances in Health Sciences Education*, published online, February 20, 2007.

Issenberg, S.B. (2006). The scope of simulation-based healthcare education. *Simulation in Healthcare*, 1, 203–208.

Kneebone, R.L., Kidd, J., Nestel, D., Barnet, A., Lo, B., King, R., et al. (2005). Blurring the boundaries: Scenario-based simulation in a clinical setting. *Medical Education*, 39, 580–587.

Kurtz, S.M., Silverman, J.D., Benson, J. & Draper, J. (2003). Marrying content and process in clinical method teaching: Enhancing the Calgary-Cambridge guides. *Academic Medicine*, 78(8), 802–809.

Makoul, G. (2001a). Essential elements of communication in medical encounters: The Kalamazoo consensus statement. *Academic Medicine*, 76(4), 390–393.

Makoul, G. (2001b). The SEGUE Framework for teaching and assessing communication skills. *Patient Education and Counseling*, 45, 23–34.

Miller, G. (1990). The assessment of clinical skills/competence/performance. *Academic Medicine*, 65 (Suppl.), S63–S67.

Nendaz, M.R., Gut, A.M., Perrier, A., Reuille, O., Louis-Simonet, M., Junod, A.F., et al. (2004). Degree of concurrency among experts in data collection and diagnostic hypothesis generation during clinical encounters. *Medical Education*, 38(1), 25–31.

Newble, D.I. (1988). Eight years' experience with a structured clinical examination. *Medical Education*, 22, 200–204.

Newble, D., & Jaeger, K. (1983). The effects of assessments and examinations on the learning of medical students. *Medical Education*, 17, 165–171.

Petrusa, E. (2002). Clinical performance assessments. In G.R. Norman, C.P.M. van der Vleuten, & D.I. Newble (Eds.), *International handbook of research in medical education* (pp. 647–672). Dordrecht, The Netherlands: Kluwer Academic Publishers.

Petrusa, E.R. (2004). Taking standardized-patient based examinations to the next level. *Teaching and Learning in Medicine*, 16, 98–110.

Rethans, J.J., Drop, R., Sturmans, F., & van der Vleuten, C. (1991). A method for introducing standardized (simulated) patients into general practice consultations. *British Journal of General Practice*, 41, 94–96.

Rethans, J.J., Gorter, S., Bokken, L., & Morrison, L. (2007). Unannounced standardized patients in real practice: A systematic literature review. *Medical Education*, 41(6), 537–549.

Ross, L.P., Clauser, B.E., Margolis, M.J., Orr, N.A., & Klass, D.J. (1996). An expert-judgment approach to setting standards for a standardized-patient examination. *Academic Medicine*, 71, S4–S6.

Schimpfhauser, F.T., Sultz, H., Zinnerstrom, K.H., & Anderson, D.R. (2000). *Communication cases involving standardized patients for medical student and resident training.* Buffalo, NY: The State University of New York at Buffalo School of Medicine and Biomedical Sciences.

Stillman, P., Brown, D., Redfield, D., & Sabers, D. (1977). Construct validation of the Arizona clinical interview rating scale. *Educational and Psychological Measurement*, 77, 1031–1038.

Stillman, P.L., Sabers, D.L., & Redfield, D.L. (1976). The use of paraprofessionals to teach interviewing skills. *Pediatrics*, 57, 769–774.

Stillman, P.L., Swanson, D.B., Smee, S., Stillman, A.E., Ebert, T.H., Emmel, V. S., et al. (1986). Assessing clinical skills of residents with standardized patients. *Annals of Internal Medicine*, 105, 762–771.

Tamblyn, R.M., Klass, D.J., Schnabl, G.K., & Kopelow, M.L. (1991). The accuracy of standardized patient presentation. *Medical Education*, 25, 100–109.

The Macy Initiative in Health Communication Casebook (2003). Referenced in and available from the authors: Yedidia, M.J., Gillespie, C.C., Kachur, E., Schwartz, M.D., Ockene, J., Chepaitis, A.E., et al. (2003). Effect of communications training on medical student performance. *The Journal of the American Medical Association*, 290, 1157–1165.

van der Vleuten, C.P.M. (1996). The assessment of professional competence: Developments, research, and practical implications. *Advances in Health Sciences Education*, 1, 41–67.

van der Vleuten, C.P., & Schuwirth, L.W. (2005). Assessing professional competence: From methods to programmes. *Medical Education*, 39, 309–317.

van der Vleuten, C.P., & Swanson, D.B. (1990). Assessment of clinical skills with standardized patients: State of the art. *Teaching and Learning in Medicine*, 2, 58–76.

Vu, N.V., Marcy, M.M., Colliver, J.A., Verhulst, S.J., Travis, T.A., & Barrows, H.S. (1992). Standardized (simulated) patients' accuracy in recording clinical performance check-list items. *Medical Education*, 26, 99–104.

Wallace, P. (1997). Following the threads of an innovation: The history of standardized patients in medical education. *CADUCEUS*, 13(2): 5–28.

Wallace, P. (2007). *Coaching standardized patients, for use in the assessment of clinical competence.* New York: Springer Publishing Company.

Welch, C. (2006). Item and prompt development in performance testing. In S.M. Downing & T.M. Haladyna (Eds.), *Handbook of test development* (pp. 303–328). Mahwah, New Jersey: Lawrence Erlbaum Associates.

William, R.G., Klaman, D.A., & McGaghie, W.C. (2003). Cognitive, social, and environmental sources of bias in clinical performance ratings. *Teaching and Learning in Medicine*, 15(4), 270–292.

Wind, L.A., Van Dalen, J., Muijtjens, A.M., & Rethans, J.J. (2004). Assessing simulated patients in an educational setting: The MaSP (Maastricht Assessment of Simulated Patients). *Medical Education*, 38(1), 39–44.

Yudkowsky, R., Downing, S., Klamen, D., Valaski, M., Eulenberg, B., & Popa, M. (2004). Assessing the head-to-toe physical examination skills of medical students. *Medical Teacher*, 26, 415–419.

Yudkowsky, R., Downing, S.M., & Sandlow, L.J. (2006). Developing an institution-based assessment of resident communication and interpersonal skills. *Academic Medicine*, 81, 1115–1122.

Yudkowsky, R., Bordage, G., Lowenstein, T., & Riddle, J. (2007, November). Can 4th year medical students anticipate, elicit, and interpret physical findings in a hypothesis-driven physical exam? [Abstract] *Annual Meeting of the Association of American Medical Colleges*, Washington D.C.

Ziv, A., Rubin, O., Moshinsky, A., & Mittelman, M. (2007). Screening of candidates to medical school based on non-cognitive parameters using a simulation-based assessment center. *Simulation in Healthcare*, 2(1), 69.

10

SIMULATIONS IN ASSESSMENT

WILLIAM C. MCGAGHIE AND
S. BARRY ISSENBERG

This chapter addresses the role of simulations in the assessment of health professionals. It amplifies, but does not duplicate, the lessons of Chapter 8 on Observational Methods and Chapter 9 covering Performance Examinations. Those chapters laid down an assessment foundation by describing methods including faculty ratings and simulated clinical encounters using standardized patients (SPs) as approaches to learner assessment. Here we focus on the utility of other health care simulation devices and procedures to contribute to personnel evaluation. In general, health care simulations aim to imitate real patients, anatomic regions, or clinical tasks, or to mirror the life situations in which care is delivered. These simulations range from static anatomic models and single task trainers (e.g., venipuncture arms and intubation mannequin heads) to dynamic computer-based systems that can respond to user actions (e.g., full body anesthesia simulators); from individual trainers for a single user to interactive role playing scenarios involving groups of people; and from low tech SP encounters to high tech virtual reality surgical simulators. All of these technologies *simulate* clinical contacts between health care providers, patients, and even patients' families with varying degrees of realism. This chapter is about how to choose and use these simulated encounters as tools to assess learner competence.

Simulations have a seductive allure in health professions education. They offer context in assessment settings by engaging learners in professional situations that resemble "in vivo" conditions. Simulations can be used in a variety of ways to evaluate individuals and health care teams including: (a) procedural skills; (b) critical thinking and responses to changing circumstances; (c) behavior under stress; and (d) teamwork. However, even high-fidelity simulations are never identical to real life. The idea is to use simulations as learner assessment tools that resemble patient care problems. Solutions to the simulated patient problems should match faculty evaluation goals for learners.

This chapter has seven sections. The first three sections are short and discuss key background matters: (a) What is a simulation? (b) The learner assessment skill set needed by simulation users [individuals or teams] from prior reading, or from practical experience; and (c) practitioner goals, being plain about assessment goals and how simulation tools can help you reach those goals. The next two sections give practical advice about designing a learner assessment plan grounded in clinical practice that features simulation technology. These sections include: (d) assessment design; and (e) measurement quality. The last two sections tackle tough issues that are now the focus of vigorous research and development. These are: (f) transfer of learning outcomes from the controlled simulation lab to the chaotic patient care clinic, and (g) present and future faculty development needs.

This chapter focuses on *assessment planning*, esp. the role of simulation as one of many tools for learner evaluation. The chapter is about *curriculum integration*, being sure that simulation used as an assessment tool matches educational goals. The importance of integrating simulation-based experiences into an overall curriculum plan is one of the key "lessons learned" from a 35-year systematic literature review on the features and uses of high-fidelity medical simulations that lead to effective learning (Issenberg, McGaghie, Petrusa, et al., 2005). The chapter differs from several other recent publications that address the use of simulations to evaluate health professionals (Dunn, 2004; Loyd, Lake, & Greenberg, 2004; McGaghie, Pugh & Wayne, 2007; Scalese & Issenberg, 2008). The differences are about emphasis and scope, not about the utility of simulation technology in personnel evaluation. For example, Dunn (2004) and Loyd, et al. (2004) give broad coverage to medical simulation for education and evaluation. McGaghie, et al. (2007) address simulation for assessing health professionals with an emphasis on educational research methods. Scalese and Issenberg (2008), by contrast, give detailed coverage to "bells and whistles" and technical features of an array of simulators now available in the health sciences.

What is a Simulation?

We begin this chapter with an operational definition of medical simulation given earlier (McGaghie, 1999).

> In broad, simple terms a simulation is a person, device, or set of conditions which attempts to present evaluation problems authentically. The student or trainee is required to respond to the problems as he or she would under natural circumstances. Frequently the trainee receives performance feedback as if he or she were in the real situation. Simulation procedures for evaluation and teaching have several common characteristics:
>
> - Trainees see cues and consequences very much like those in the real environment.
> - Trainees can be placed in complex situations.
> - Trainees act as they would in the real environment.
> - The fidelity (exactness of duplication) of a simulation is never completely isomorphic with the "real thing." The reasons are obvious: cost, [limits of] engineering technology, avoidance of danger, ethics, psychometric requirements, time constraints.
> - Simulations can take many forms. For example, they can be static, as in an anatomical model [for task training]. Simulations can be automated, using advanced computer technology. Some are individual, prompting solitary performance while others are interactive, involving groups of people. Simulations can be playful or deadly serious. In personnel evaluation settings they can be used for high-stakes, low-stakes, or no-stakes decisions (p. 9).

Health science simulations are located on a *continuum of fidelity* ranging from multiple-choice test questions (Boulet & Swanson, 2004) to more engaging task trainers (e.g., heads for intubation training) to full-body computer-driven mannequins that display vital signs and respond to drugs and other treatments (Issenberg & McGaghie, 1999). In most evaluation settings today's medical simulations rely on trained [faculty] observers to record learner response data, transform the data into assessment scores, and make judgments about trainees (e.g., pass/fail) from the scores. Some newer medical simulators automate data recording and scoring, which makes the process faster and less prone to observer error. However, in all situations the chain of events moves through a five step sequence: (a) stimulus presentation (e.g., simulator embedded patient problem or case); (b) examinee response; (c) data recording or capturing; (d) data transformation to a score; and (e) score judgment and interpretation. These are all parts of learner assessment. Our goal in this chapter is to show how medical simulation technology can make this cascaded enterprise efficient, effective, useful, fair, and feasible.

Two forms of medical simulation are not covered in this chapter. They are standardized patients (SPs) and computer games. Standardized patients are excluded because their use is covered extensively in Chapter 9 (Yudkowsky, this volume). Computer games are because at present time they have a limited role in the serious business of learner assessment in the health professions.

Learner Assessment Skill Set

We expect that health science educators who plan to use simulations for learner assessment have background knowledge in test development, administration, and use. For example, we anticipate that readers of this chapter have earlier covered the material in Chapter 1, Introduction to Assessment in the Health Professions. Readers should also have a good grasp of how written tests, observational methods, and performance examinations are developed and used from other chapters in this book. Familiarity with assessment principles given in these and other chapters will make it easier for educators to figure out the place of simulation in their assessment plans.

Practitioner Goals

Health science educators need to have one or more assessment goals clearly articulated before selecting and using simulation-based evaluation tools. *The goals–tools match is the most important message of this chapter.* A carpenter does not use a tape measure to pound nails. It's the wrong tool for the job. Similarly, educators should not acquire or build simulation devices for learner assessment without understanding their assessment goals, context, and consequences. Simulations are just one of many assessment options available to health science educators who are responsible for formative or summative trainee evaluation. Our aim is to help you match assessment goals and simulation tools to accomplish accurate and fair learner evaluations.

Table 10.1 presents 12 examples from the health professions of learner assessment goals matched with simulation assessment tools. All of the assessment goals in Table 10.1 are formative, i.e., in-progress tests and evaluations for the purpose of learner feedback and improvement. Of course, other assessment goals may be summative, i.e., final examinations or measures of professional competence like board examinations that have serious and lasting consequences or address selective professional school admission. The use of simulation technology for summative assessment in the health professions is currently rare but increasing gradually. Examples include the introduction of simulation into Israeli national board examinations in anesthesiology (Berkenstadt, Ziv, Gafni, & Sidi, 2006a, 2006b) and early feasibility research on the potential use of simulation combined with other modalities for high stakes medical testing in Canada (Hatala, Kassen, Nishikawa, et al., 2005; Hatala, Issenberg, Kassen, et al., 2007). Simulation technology has been used for selective medical school admission decisions in Israel where candidate interpersonal skills are evaluated using objective patient simulations rather than subjective letters of recommendation (Ziv, Rubin, Moshinsky, & Mittelman, 2007).

Table 10.1 is similar in purpose and format to Table 8.1 (McGaghie et al., Chapter 8, this volume) that addresses goals and tools for observational assessment. Education program directors and

Table 10.1 Simulation Based Assessment Goals and Tools

Assessment Goal	Example	Assessment Tool	Advantages	Limitations
Advanced Cardiac Life Support (ACLS)	Mastery assessment of medicine residents' responses to cardiac arrest scenarios (Wayne et al., 2006)	Simulated hospital "codes" in a laboratory setting using the METI life-size Human Patient Simulator (HPS®)	Very high-fidelity patient simulator and simulated "code" events. Assessment data are reliable and inferences about trainees are valid.	Simulator equipment and laboratory time are expensive and labor intensive.
Individual and Team Terrorism Training	"Assess individual and team skills acquired from an interactive training program to prepare emergency personnel to respond to terrorist acts" (Scott et al., 2006)	Scenario-based individual and team terrorist response exercises with faculty ratings of learning outcomes	Assessment data for individuals and teams are reliable and inferences about trainees are valid. EMT, paramedic, nurse, and physician trainees valued the training and assessment.	Individual and team training and assessment are time and labor intensive.
Anesthesia Acute Care	Assess acute care skills of anesthesiology residents and student nurse anesthetists (Murray et al., 2005)	Simulated acute care scenarios using the life-size patient mannequin developed by MEDSIM-EAGLE®	Acute care patient scenarios have very high realism. Assessment data are reliable and inferences about trainees are valid.	Simulator equipment and laboratory time are expensive.
Gynecological Laparoscopic Surgery	Evaluate basic laparoscopic surgical skills among three groups of gynecologic trainees based on surgical experience: novices, intermediate level, experts (Larsen et al., 2006)	Measurements of basic surgical skills were taken using the LapSimGyn virtual reality (VR) simulator	VR simulator provides a highly controlled, standardized measurement environment. Expected differences due to expertise groups were obtained.	Simulator-based assessment is costly yet very effective. Simulator training and assessment needs to be integrated into the surgical curriculum.
Pediatric Acute Care	Assess acute care management skills among pediatric residents using four simulated case scenarios: apnea, asthma, supraventricular tachycardia, sepsis (Adler et al., 2007)	METI high fidelity PediaSIM® mannequin human patient simulator with unweighted checklist data recorded by trained faculty raters	Controlled environment and rigorous rater training produced highly reliable data. Resident group differences due to clinical experience were found as expected.	Four simulated pediatric case scenarios are an insufficient sample for comprehensive resident assessment.

Nursing: General Introduction	"This qualitative study examined the [assessment] experiences of students in one nursing program's first term of using high-fidelity simulation as part of its regular curriculum" (Lasater, 2007)	Computerized human patient simulator of unspecified origin. Students' reactions to simulation-based training experiences were assessed using focus groups	"Simulator served as an integrator of learning . . . theoretical, psychomotor, laboratory and clinical practice skills." All enhanced acquisition of clinical judgment.	Engineering limitations of the simulator mannequin (e.g., lack of nonverbal communication; no reflexes, swelling, or color changes) limit generalizability.
Respiratory Therapy: Bronchoalveolar Lavage	To "evaluate simulation-based education for training and competency evaluation [among respiratory therapists—RTs] of the mini bronchoalveolar lavage (mini-BAL) procedure, with an emphasis on patient safety and procedure performance standards" (Tuttle et al., 2007)	Laerdal SimMan® computer-based full body patient simulator with checklist data recorded by trained faculty raters	Simulation setting allowed controlled, standardized trainee assessments that produced highly reliable data. Simulation-based training greatly increased RT's mini-BAL competence scores and score retention.	Further research will better link RT's clinical skills performance in the simulation setting to performance in real patient care.
Nursing: Global Clinical Competence	Evaluate nursing students' clinical skills and competence using a 15 station OSCE grounded [in part] on simulation-based assessment exercises; study the effects of a simulation-based nursing curriculum (Alinier et al., 2006)	Fifteen OSCE stations measuring theory on safety in nursing practice, clinical knowledge, technical ability, and communication skills using observational ratings by trained faculty	OSCE assessments of nursing students are reproducible and yield reliable evaluation data. Intermediate fidelity simulation-based assessment and training is realistic and well received by students. Scores improved with practice.	"Students and [faculty] facilitators need to be adequately prepared for the use of patient simulators as a teaching [and assessment] tool." OSCE assessments require much faculty preparation.
Paramedic Endotracheal Intubation	To "determine whether the endotracheal intubation (ETI) success rate is different among paramedic students trained on a human patient simulator versus on human subjects in the operating room (OR)." (Hall et al., 2005)	Following simulation-based OR ETI training, paramedic students "underwent a formalized test of 15 intubations in the OR" with measurements of success rate and complications	Simulation-based ETI training produced results statistically identical to training results using real patients in the OR. This reduces patient risk and allows training under controlled conditions.	Blinding of faculty assessors to the training condition of the paramedic students would further increase the objectivity of the outcome data.

(Continued Overleaf)

Table 10.1 Continued

Assessment Goal	Example	Assessment Tool	Advantages	Limitations
Carotid Angiography Competence	Document performance improvement in carotid angiography (CA) skills, measured by metric-based procedural errors, due to a virtual reality (VR) simulation course (Patel et al., 2006)	The Vascular Interventional System Trainer (VIST)-VR simulator recorded trainee CA skills at procedure time (PT), fluoroscopy time (FT), contrast volume, and composite catheter handling errors (CE)	Data recorded by the VIST-VR simulator had high internal consistency and test-retest reliability. CA scores increased with simulator practice and experience.	The study enrolled a relatively small sample of interventional cardiologists (n = 20). Research on a broader sample of [simulated] cases is also needed.
Acute Care Nurse Practitioner (ACNP) Clinical Skills	Assess acute care nurse practitioner (ACNP) clinical skills using high-fidelity human simulation (HFHS) technology (Hravnak et al., 2007)	Laerdal SimMan® computer-based full body simulator with faculty evaluations completed in real time and from video recordings	ACNP training and evaluation conducted in controlled environment where patient safety is not a concern. Many opportunities for learner debriefing with a variety of clinical problems.	Mannequin-based clinical simulation is never a perfect reproduction of real patient care. Costs of money and faculty time can be high.
Medical Student Basic Clinical Skills	Evaluate and educate volunteer medical students at two procedure scenarios (urinary catheter insertion, wound closure with sutures) using inanimate models attached to simulated patients. Qualitative documentation of study outcomes (Kneebone et al., 2005)	Inanimate models for urinary catheter insertion and wound closure assessed by observers. "Live" simulated patients amplified the clinical encounters	Learners' overall impressions of the evaluation and training scenarios were very positive. Study revealed ways to improve the simulation technology and its links with simulated patients.	Study was limited due to the relatively small number of clinical procedures. Expansion to other clinical education centers is also needed.

faculty should consider the goals-tools match thoughtfully as simulation-based learner assessment plans are formulated.

Assessment Design

Systematic and thoughtful test planning is needed to create and use assessment tools that yield reliable scores that permit valid decisions about trainee achievement. The assessment design is a step-by-step plan that increases the odds that assessment goals and simulation tools are matched. We endorse a six step plan for assessment design drawn from several sources to create an assessment program's architecture (Downing, 2006; Newble, et al., 1994; Scalese & Issenberg, 2008). The stepwise plan is a practical, useful guide for busy teachers and program directors who aim to match educational assessment goals and simulation tools. This will promote curriculum integration of simulation technology in the health professions.

Table 10.2 lists the six assessment planning steps. The following discussion amplifies each step.

Content and Organization

The content coverage of a test is a sample of the material in a course or unit, just as a professional school curriculum is a sample of professional work. Health science educators can neither teach all relevant content and skills nor test every educational objective. Thus test planning, like curriculum planning, aims to include a representative sample of the cases or problems that health professionals see clinically. Case selection for trainee assessment is often governed by frequency (e.g., respiratory infection), urgency (e.g., myocardial infarction) or importance (e.g., secure an airway) (Raymond & Neustel, 2006). Thoughtful case selection produces better assessments and lowers the chances that tests will contain obscure "zebras."

Clinical tasks embedded within cases also warrant attention. Routine tasks that span clinical cases (e.g., blood pressure measurement) are candidates for assessment due to their frequency and importance for patient care. Rare but critical clinical tasks (e.g., needle

Table 10.2 Simulation Based Assessment Planning Steps

1. **Content and Organization**
   - Content definition and level of resolution
   - Problems or cases
   - Tasks within problems
   - Blueprint or test specifications (Table 10.3 Test Blueprint for Clinical Cardiology)
2. **Assessment Methods**
   - Select test methods
   - Appropriate to clinical problems and tasks
   - Problems and tasks dictate test methods
   - Recognize simplicity, limits, and practical constraints
3. **Standardize Test Conditions**
   - Fixed conditions: "patient," examiner, setting
   - Variable condition: trainee
4. **Assessment Scoring**
   - Turn trainee responses into numbers
   - Data quality
5. **Standard Setting**
   - Derive a minimum passing score (MPS)
6. **Consequences**
   - Anticipate assessment aftermath or sequelae

aspiration for tension pneumothorax) are also assessment priorities. Rare and trivial clinical tasks (e.g., cerumen removal) are a much lower assessment priority.

The content and organization of a simulation-based assessment is best captured by a blueprint or set of test specifications. A test blueprint identifies the cases, tasks, or other content to be included (and, by inference, excluded) in an assessment and how they will challenge the trainee. Challenges might include diagnosis, perform a procedure, formulate a plan, or know when to get help. A test blueprint is an operational definition of the purpose and scope of an assessment (Downing & Haladyna, Chapter 2, this volume).

Table 10.3 presents an *example* blueprint of a simulation-based assessment in clinical cardiology using the "Harvey" cardiology patient simulator (CPS) (Gordon & Issenberg, 2006). The example is for a test of second year internal medicine residents who are completing a four week cardiology rotation. This illustrative blueprint shows that recognition of the 12 cardinal cardiac auscultatory findings can be

Table 10.3 Test Blueprint for Clinical Cardiology Using the "Harvey" CPS

Cardinal Auscultatory Findings	Evaluation Goals				
	Identify finding	Identify finding and correlate it with underlying pathophysiology	Identify finding and correlate it with underlying disease process and differential diagnosis	Identify finding and correlate it with the severity of the underlying disease process and clinical management	TOTAL
1. Second Sound Splitting	10%		5%		15%
2. Third Sound		5%	5%		10%
3. Fourth Sound				10%	10%
4. Systolic Clicks		5%	5%		10%
5. Innocent Murmur	5%			10%	15%
6. Mitral Regurgitation		5%		5%	10%
7. Aortic Stenosis					0%
8. Aortic Regurgitation	5%		10%		15%
9. Mitral Stenosis		10%			10%
10. Continuous Murmur					0%
11. Tricuspid Regurgitation	5%				5%
12. Pericardial Rub					0%
TOTAL	25%	25%	25%	25%	100%

assessed against four separate and increasingly complex evaluation goals. They range from identify finding to identify finding and correlate it with the severity of the underlying disease process and clinical management. Tabular cell entries show the distribution of test content for this example. The cell entries and marginal totals indicate that assessment of second sound splitting, innocent murmur, and aortic regurgitation are emphasized over other options. Cells and marginals also show that identifying findings is weighted equally with the other three more complex evaluation goals. Other health professions education programs (e.g., nursing, pharmacy, physical therapy) and levels of testing (i.e., beginner to advanced) may have very different evaluation weighting schemes.

The point of Table 10.3 is that health science educators who use simulation technology for learner assessment must make conscious decisions about what the tests will cover (and not cover) and with what emphasis. This involves professional judgment and choice shaped by reason, experience, and anticipation about future professional practice needs of today's learners. Test blueprint development and use, combined with clinical educators' judgment and choice, contributes content-related validity evidence to learner assessment practices. As Chapter 2 points out, this is a basic building block of an assessment program that makes valid decisions about learner competence.

Assessment Methods

Many assessment methods are available to health science educators who use simulation for learner evaluation. However, there is no formula or set of rules that tell teachers which assessment methods to use. Instead, these decisions should be shaped by two factors: (a) the clinical problem or tasks being assessed, and (b) simplicity and practical constraints.

To illustrate, Table 10.1 points out a variety of assessment methods embedded in the evaluation "goals and tools" framework. The bottom line is simple: assessment goals shape decisions about assessment tools. Complex clinical skills like responding to ACLS events require equally rich assessment tools such as computer-driven mannequins in a simulation laboratory environment (Wayne et al., 2005a, 2006). Simpler clinical skills such as suturing, intubation, and arterial puncture can be assessed using basic task trainers (Issenberg & McGaghie, 1999).

Standardize Test Conditions

The conditions for simulation-based learner assessment, like other approaches to personnel evaluation, need to be standardized to yield best results. Standardization means the situation, setting, procedures, and apparatus used for assessment are uniform for all learners. These are "fixed" conditions: (a) patient (mannequin, SP); (b) trained examiner; (c) assessment forms (checklist, rating scale); (d) room or laboratory space; (e) time allocation; (f) clinical equipment (bags, masks, drugs, sterile tray, etc.); (g) prompts or instructions (signs, cue cards, verbal or video orientation); and (h) dress code. Fixed conditions do not vary. All learners who undergo assessment operate in the same environment.

By contrast, the only "variable" element in this situation is the examinee. We assume that individual differences in knowledge, skill, attitude, reasoning, or other learning outcomes are being expressed and measured by the assessment. The reliability (signal) of assessment data depends on ruling-out extraneous error (noise) by standardizing test conditions. There are two distinct types of assessment noise: random error or unreliability (Axelson & Kreiter, Chapter 3, this volume) and systematic error or construct-irrelevant variance (CIV), which is discussed in Chapter 2 (Downing & Haladyna, this volume). The goal, of course, is to reduce both types of noise and boost the signal in assessment score data.

Assessment Scoring

How can health science educators turn trainee responses to a simulation-based exam into scores (numbers) that are useful for assessment? How can the educators be assured that the scores are quality assessment data?

Scores can be derived from examinee responses to simulation technology in at least five ways:

1. Keyboard or written responses to standardized questions embedded in the simulator or its associated software as a scenario unfolds (Issenberg, McGaghie, Brown, et al., 2000; Issenberg, McGaghie, Gordon, et al., 2002) or on subsequent post-encounter tests about simulated events (Williams, McLaughlin, Eulenberg, et al., 1999).
2. Item-by-item behavioral responses (*process* data) recorded on a checklist by trained and calibrated observers (Murray, Boulet, Kras, et al., 2005; Wayne, Barsuk, O'Leary, et al., 2008; Wayne,

Butter, Siddall, et al., 2005a, 2006) that capture procedural correctness. Checklist process data can also be recorded automatically by embedded software, capturing actions (e.g., carotid pulse check) that were taken without being mediated by an observer (Albarran, Moule, Gilchrist & Soar, 2006).

3. Judgments about behavioral *products* created in a simulation environment (e.g., dental amalgam) by trained and calibrated observers (Buchanan & Williams, 2004).

4. Global judgments about trainee performance recorded by faculty on rating scales (Hodges, Regehr, McNaughton, et al., 1999; Regehr, Freeman, Robb, et al., 1999).

5. Trainee responses captured by haptic sensors embedded in or near a simulator (Pugh, Heinrichs, Dev, et al., 2001; Pugh & Rosen, 2002; Pugh & Youngblood, 2002; Minogue & Jones, 2006).

Each of these scoring methods has strengths and limitations shaped by situation of use, level of required evaluation detail, and faculty training and calibration. Practical realities in health science education programs such as simplicity, ease of use, and time requirements limit decisions about scoring methods. The idea is to get high quality assessment data with low cost and effort. This is often a difficult tradeoff.

Standard Setting

Standard setting is important because it encourages the faculty to specify the minimum passing score (MPS) [standard] for each exam in the curriculum. Standards express faculty expectations for students. They tell learners for each assessment exercise "how much is good enough." Very high standards, seen in rigorous exam MPSs, send a message that excellence is expected from all learners, that the faculty will not accept mediocrity. High standards assert faculty academic values. Assessment standards are usually set using "seat of the pants" methods based on faculty judgments. However, improved and more thoughtful approaches are being used increasingly (see Chapter 6).

Professional approaches to setting academic performance standards in the health professions have been described recently (Downing, Tekian, & Yudkowsky, 2006; Norcini & Guille, 2002). They all rely on systematic collection of expert judgments about expected learner performance. Experts are usually panels of experienced practitioners in a health profession—frequently teaching faculty. Systematic collection of experts' judgments involves engaging faculty panelists in exercises that focus decisions about expected learner behavior. Two of many possible examples are: (a) item-by-item judgments about test questions or performance checklist items (Angoff); or, (b) judgments about an entire assessment (Hofstee). Both approaches have strengths and weaknesses. Some clinical educators have averaged the results of Angoff and Hofstee standard setting methods to offset differences in MPS stringency (Wayne, Fudala, Butter, et al., 2005b; Wayne, Barsuk, Cohen & McGaghie, 2007).

Consequences

All educational assessments have consequences ranging from professional school admission decisions to formative feedback to final high stakes judgments. Health science educators should carefully consider the consequences of their assessment plans for learners, faculty, and the sponsoring educational program.

Assessment sequelae for learners are usually obvious: (a) school admission or rejection; (b) pass and move ahead; (c) performance below standard, more work and reassess; (d) failure, short-run or final. Faculty assessment sequelae include feedback about teaching effectiveness, the burden of remediating failing students, and recognizing curriculum strengths and weaknesses. Assessment consequences for educational programs include those for learners, faculty, and also matters of cost, efficiency, and student selection. The point is that health science educators should anticipate the consequences of educational assessments to minimize their costs and maximize their benefits.

Measurement Quality

Assessment scores from simulation technology that are employed as either formative or summative outcome measures must be sound technically. The scores must be dependable, trustworthy, before they can be used for any educational purpose. *Reliability* is the technical term used to describe the dependability of assessment scores. Score reliability is like a signal-to-noise ratio where the "signal" is good information and "noise" is measurement error. Reliable scores have high signal and low noise. *Validity* is the term used to describe the accuracy of actions or decisions that are made from assessment scores. Valid educational actions and decisions depend on reliable assessment scores.

High quality, i.e., reliable trainee assessment scores are essential for at least three reasons: (a) accurate learner feedback; (b) valid decisions about learner advancement, promotion, or certification; and, (c) rigorous research on simulation-based health professions education. Educators know that learner feedback is useless, simply cannot be done, without reliable performance scores. Evaluators know too that accurate promotion or certification decisions about learners are impossible without reliable data. Educational scholars understand that data reliability must be reported in all research studies as a basic quality assurance index.

How can health professions educators working in a simulation-based context take steps to boost the reliability of assessment scores and the validity of actions and decisions? Time spent refining and pilot testing measurement tools, training and calibrating faculty raters, and simplifying data recording and management is always a good investment. This is especially the case when assessment scores are derived from ratings by faculty observers, a common situation in simulation-based learner evaluation. Inter-rater reliability (agreement) is essential here and should be established routinely as a continuous quality control mechanism.

Measurement quality expressed as score reliability and the validity of actions and decisions are everyday issues in simulation-based assessment. Downing (2003, 2004) provides a thorough discussion about reliability and validity in a pair of journal articles.

Chapters 2, 3, and 4 of this volume present detailed and practical discussions of measurement quality issues including validity, reliability, and generalizability of assessments in health professions education.

Transfer of Training—Lab to Life

How can clinical educators be sure that educational outcomes measured and assessed in a controlled, simulation laboratory setting transfer to trainee behavior in the chaotic clinical environment? Such transfer of training is difficult to evaluate for a variety of scientific and ethical reasons. However, the question is still legitimate in the current era of evidence based clinical practice and best evidence medical education (BEME) (Issenberg, et al., 2005). How can we generalize simulation-based assessments of learning—knowledge, skills, attitudes—from laboratory to life (Bligh & Bleakley, 2006)?

On scientific grounds this is a problem in *generalized causal inference* (Shadish, Cook, & Campbell, 2002). The scientific solution requires a thematic and cumulative series of controlled studies featuring tight experimental designs and highly reliable data. While several small experimental studies have been published (e.g., Rosenthal, Adachi, Ribaudo, et al., 2006; Seymour, Gallagher, Roman, et al., 2002) a large body of educational science work on simulation in healthcare is unlikely to be done in the near future. Instead, the clinical education community will rely on reason, experience, and quasi-experiments (e.g., Wayne, Didwania, Feinglass, et al., 2008b) to make a convincing case that simulation-based learning and assessment has a "payoff" in clinical practice.

Critics should be mindful that few important clinical or life innovations are verified scientifically via randomized controlled trials (RCT). For example, a recent article in the *British Medical Journal* informed readers that there has never been a RCT to evaluate the safety and utility of parachutes (Smith & Pell, 2003). Finding volunteers for the control group has been difficult. The alternative in clinical education is to rely on good sense and new techniques like statistical process control (Diaz & Neuhauser, 2007) to demonstrate that the learning and assessment effects of simulation-based technologies are too great to be dismissed. There are occasions when it would be foolish to ignore obvious and consistent outcomes.

Faculty Development Needs

Faculty training and development about effective use of simulation technology to promote learner achievement and assess learning outcomes must become a priority training goal. This is a key message of the recent Colloquium on Educational Technology sponsored by the Association of American Medical Colleges (AAMC, 2007). Simple or sophisticated simulation technology will be ineffective or misused unless health professions faculty are prepared as simulation educators.

The faculty development agenda is shaped, in part, by a discussion about the "scope of simulation-based healthcare education" authored by Issenberg (2006). The author argues that the best practice of simulation-based healthcare education is a *multiplicative product* of (a) simulation technology [e.g., task trainers, mannequins], (b) teachers prepared to use the technology to maximum advantage, and (c) curriculum integration. Issenberg (2006) asserts that the major flaws in today's simulation-based healthcare education and assessment stem from a lack of prepared teachers and curriculum isolation, not from technological problems or deficits.

There are at least five priority areas where faculty development activities are needed to insure that simulation-based education and assessment are efficient and effective.

1. *Simulation operation*, fluid use of high and low fidelity simulation technologies to promote learner education and assessment.
2. *Curriculum integration*, inserting simulation-based learning and assessment experiences as required curriculum features including many opportunities for deliberate practice by trainees (Ericsson, 2004).
3. *Recognition of the strengths and limits of simulation technology* for education and assessment in the health professions. Simulation is not a panacea. Its best use depends on the goals-tools match discussed earlier.

4. In assessment, recognition that best use of simulation will engage learners in *dynamic testing* (Grigorenko & Sternberg, 1998). Dynamic testing occurs when assessments not only yield evaluative data about trainees but also fulfill teaching goals.

5. Faculty must learn to combine simulation modalities in their education and assessment plans (Kneebone, et al., 2005). Lifelike and effective simulation experiences can involve a collection of electromechanical, human, and inanimate parts.

Conclusion

This chapter has covered the use of a variety of simulation technologies for learner assessment in the health professions. The emphasis has been on assessment planning, achieving a goals–tools match, with the intent of rational integration of simulation technology into health science curricula. We argue that simulation is not a panacea for assessment or instruction. Instead, simulation is one of many sets of tools available to health professions educators. Thoughtful use of these tools will increase the odds that educators will reach their assessment goals.

Simulation technology is rapidly increasing in sophistication, fidelity, and educational allure. Health professions educators must become thoughtful and critical consumers of simulation in its many forms to be clear about its practical utility and resist seduction by flashy gizmos and gimmicks.

References

AAMC Colloquium on Educational Technology (2007). *Effective use of educational technology in medical education* [summary report]. Washington, D.C.: Association of American Medical Colleges.

Adler, M.D., Trainor, J.L., Siddall, V.J., & McGaghie, W.C. (2007). Development and evaluation of high-fidelity simulation case scenarios for pediatric resident evaluation. *Ambulatory Pediatrics, 7*, 182–186.

Albarran, J.W., Moule, P., Gilchrist, M., & Soar, J. (2006). Comparison of sequential and simultaneous breathing and pulse check by health care professionals during simulated scenarios. *Resuscitation, 68*(2), 243–249.

Alinier, G., Hunt, B., Gordon, R., & Harwood, C. (2006). Effectiveness of intermediate-fidelity simulation training technology in undergraduate nursing education. *Journal of Advanced Nursing*, 54, 359–369.

Berkenstadt, H., Ziv, A., Gafni, N., & Sidi, A. (2006a). Incorporating simulation-based objective structured clinical examination into the Israeli national board examination in anesthesiology. *Anesthesia & Analgesia*, 102, 853–858.

Berkenstadt, H., Ziv, A., Gafni, N., & Sidi, A. (2006b). The validation process of incorporating simulation-based accreditation into the anesthesiology Israeli national board exams. *Israeli Medical Association Journal*, 8(10), 728–733.

Bligh, J., & Bleakley, A. (2006). Distributing menus to hungry learners: Can learning by simulation become simulation of learning? *Medical Teacher*, 28(7), 606–613.

Boulet, J.R., & Swanson, D.B. (2004). Psychometric challenges of using simulations for high-stakes assessment. In W.F. Dunn (Ed.), *Simulations in critical care education and beyond* (pp. 119–130). Des Plaines, IL: Society of Critical Care Medicine.

Buchanan, J.A., & Williams, J.N. (2004). Simulation in dentistry and oral surgery. In G.E. Loyd, C.L. Lake, & R.B. Greenberg (Eds.), *Practical health care simulations* (pp. 493–512). Philadelphia: Elsevier.

Diaz, M., & Neuhauser D. (2007). Pasteur and parachutes: When statistical process control is better than a randomized controlled trial. *Quality and Safety in Health Care*, 14, 140–143.

Downing, S.M. (2003). Validity: On the meaningful interpretation of assessment data. *Medical Education*, 37, 830–837.

Downing, S.M. (2004). Reliability: On the reproducibility of assessment data. *Medical Education*, 38, 1006–1012.

Downing, S.M. (2006). Twelve steps for effective test development. In S.M. Downing & T.M. Haladyna (Eds.), *Handbook of test development* (pp. 3–25). Mahwah, NJ: Lawrence Erlbaum Associates.

Downing, S.M., Tekian, A., & Yudkowsky, R. (2006). Procedures for establishing defensible absolute passing scores on performance examinations in health professions education. *Teaching and Learning in Medicine*, 18, 50–57.

Dunn, W.F. (Ed.). (2004). *Simulations in critical care education and beyond*. Des Plaines, IL: Society of Critical Care Medicine.

Ericsson, K.A. (2004). Deliberate practice and the acquisition and maintenance of expert performance in medicine and related domains. *Academic Medicine*, 79(10, Suppl.), S70–S81.

Gordon, M.S., & Issenberg, S.B. (2006). *Instructor guide for Harvey the cardiopulmonary patient simulator*. University of Miami School of Medicine, Gordon Center for Research in Medical Education.

Grigorenko, E.L., & Sternberg, R.J. (1998). Dynamic testing. *Psychological Bulletin*, 124, 75–111.

Hall, R.E., Plant, J.R., Bands, C.J., Wall, A.R., Kang, J., & Hall, C.A. (2005).

Human patient simulation is effective for teaching paramedic students endotracheal intubation. *Academic Emergency Medicine*, 12, 850–855.

Hatala, R., Issenberg, S.B., Kassen, B.O., Cole, G., Bacchus, C.M., & Scalese, R.J. (2007). Assessing the relationship between cardiac physical examination technique and accurate bedside diagnosis during an objective structured clinical examination (OSCE). *Academic Medicine*, 82(10, Suppl.), S26–S29.

Hatala, R., Kassen, B.O., Nishikawa, J., Cole, G., & Issenberg, S.B. (2005). Incorporating simulation technology in a Canadian internal medicine specialty examination: A descriptive report. *Academic Medicine*, 80, 554–556.

Hodges, B., Regehr, G., McNaughton, N., Tiberius, R., & Hanson, M. (1999). OSCE Checklists do not capture increasing levels of expertise. *Academic Medicine*, 74, 1129–1134.

Hravnak, M., Beach, M., & Tuite, P. (2007). Simulator technology as a tool for education in cardiac care. *Journal of Cardiovascular Nursing*, 22, 16–24.

Issenberg, S.B. (2006). The scope of simulation-based healthcare education. *Simulation in Healthcare*, 1, 203–208.

Issenberg, S.B., & McGaghie, W.C. (1999). Assessing knowledge and skills in the health professions: A continuum of simulation fidelity. In A. Tekian, C.H. McGuire, & W.C. McGaghie (Eds.), *Innovative simulations for assessing professional competence* (pp. 125–146). Chicago: Department of Medical Education, University of Illinois at Chicago.

Issenberg, S.B., McGaghie, W.C., Brown, D.D., Mayer, J.W., Gessner, I.H., Hart, I.R., et al. (2000). Development of multimedia computer-based measures of clinical skills in bedside cardiology. In D.E. Melnick (Ed.), *The Eighth International Ottawa Conference on Medical Education and Assessment Proceedings. Evolving assessment: Protecting the human dimension*. Philadelphia: National Board of Medical Examiners, pp. 821–829.

Issenberg, S.B., McGaghie, W.C., Gordon, D.L., Symes, S., Petrusa, E.R., Hart, I.R., et al. (2002). Effectiveness of a cardiology review course for internal medicine residents using simulation technology and deliberate practice. *Teaching and Learning in Medicine*, 14(4), 223–228.

Issenberg, S.B., McGaghie, W.C., Petrusa, E.R. Gordon, D.L., & Scalese, R.J. (2005). Features and uses of high-fidelity medical simulations that lead to effective learning: A BEME systematic review. *Medical Teacher*, 27, 10–28.

Kneebone, R.L., Kidd, J., Nestel, D., Barnet, A., Lo, B., King, R., et al. (2005). Blurring the boundaries: Scenario-based simulation in a clinical setting. *Medical Education*, 39, 580–587.

Larsen, C.R., Grantcharov, T., Aggarwal, R., Tully, A., Sørensen, J.L., Dalsgaard, T., et al. (2006). Objective assessment of gynecologic laparoscopic skills using the LapSimGyn virtual reality simulator. *Surgical Endoscopy*, 20, 1460–1466.

Lasater, K. (2007). High-fidelity simulation and the development of clinical judgment: Students' experiences. *Journal of Nursing Education*, 46, 269–276.

Loyd, G.E., Lake, C.L., & Greenberg, R.B. (Eds.). (2004). *Practical health care simulations*. Philadelphia: Elsevier.

McGaghie, W.C. (1999). Simulation in professional competence assessment: Basic considerations. In A. Tekian, C.H. McGuire, & W.C. McGaghie (Eds.), *Innovative simulations for assessing professional competence* (pp. 7–22). Chicago: Department of Medical Education, University of Illinois at Chicago.

McGaghie, W.C., Pugh, C.M., & Wayne, D.B. (2007). Fundamentals of educational research using simulation. In R. Kyle & W.B. Murray (Eds.), *Clinical simulation: Operations, engineering, and management* (pp. 517–526). Philadelphia: Elsevier.

Minogue, J., & Jones, M.G. (2006). Haptics in education: Exploring an untapped sensory modality. *Review of Educational Research*, 76(3), 317–348.

Murray, D.J., Boulet, J.R., Kras, J.F., McAllister, J.D., & Cox, T.E. (2005). A simulation-based acute care skills performance assessment for anesthesia training *Anesthesia and Analgesia*, 101, 1127–1134.

Newble, D., Dawson, B., Dauphinee, D., Page, G., Macdonald, M., Swanson, D., et al. (1994). Guidelines for assessing clinical competence. *Teaching and Learning in Medicine*, 6(3), 213–220.

Norcini, J., & Guille, R. (2002). Combining tests and setting standards. In G.R. Norman, C.P.M. van der Vleuten, & D.I. Newble (Eds.), *International handbook of research in medical education* (pp. 811–834). Dordrecht, NL: Kluwer Academic Publishers.

Patel, A.D., Gallagher, A.G., Nicholson, W.J., & Cates, C.V. (2006). Learning curves and reliability measures for virtual reality simulation in the performance assessment of carotid angiography. *Journal of the American College of Cardiology*, 47(9), 1796–1802.

Pugh, C.M., Heinrichs, W.L., Dev, P., Srivastava, S., & Krummel, T.M. (2001). Use of a mechanical simulator to assess pelvic examination skills. *Journal of the American Medical Association*, 286(9), 1021–1023.

Pugh, C.M., & Rosen, J. (2002). Qualitative and quantitative analysis of pressure sensor data acquired by the E-Pelvis simulator during simulated pelvic examinations. *Studies in Health Technologies and Informatics*, 85, 376–379.

Pugh, C.M., & Youngblood, P. (2002). Development and validation of assessment measures for a newly developed physical examination simulator. *Journal of the American Medical Informatics Association*, 9, 448–460.

Raymond, M.R., & Neustel, S. (2006). Determining the content of credentialing examinations. In S.M. Downing & T.M. Haladyna (Eds.), *Handbook of test development* (pp. 181–223). Mahwah, NJ: Lawrence Erlbaum Associates.

Regehr, G., Freeman, R., Robb, A., Missiha, N., & Heisey, R. (1999). OSCE performance evaluations made by standardized patients: Comparing checklist and global rating scales. *Academic Medicine*, 74(10, Suppl.), S135–S137.

Rosenthal, M.E., Adachi, M., Ribaudo, V., Mueck, J.T., Schneider, R.F., & Mayo, P.H. (2006). Achieving housestaff competence in emergency airway management using scenario based simulation training. *Chest*, 129, 1453–1458.

Scalese, R.J., & Issenberg, S.B. (2008). Simulation-based assessment. In E.S. Holmboe & R.E. Hawkins (Eds.), *Practical guide to the evaluation of clinical competence* (pp. 179–200). Philadelphia: Elsevier.

Scott, J.A., Miller, G.T., Issenberg, S.B., Brotons, A.A., Gordon, D.L., Gordon, M.S., et al. (2006). Skill improvement during emergency response to terrorism training. *Prehospital Emergency Care*, 10, 507–514.

Seymour, N.E., Gallagher, A.G., Roman, S.A., O'Brien, M.K., Bansal, V.K., Andersen, D.K., et al. (2002). Virtual reality training improves operating room performance: Results of a randomized double-blinded study. *Annals of Surgery*, 236, 458–464.

Shadish, W.R., Cook, T.D., & Campbell, D.T. (2002). *Experimental and quasi-experimental designs for generalized causal inference*. Boston: Houghton Mifflin.

Smith, G.C., & Pell, J.P. (2003). Parachute use to prevent death and major trauma related to gravitational challenge: Systematic review of randomized controlled trials. *British Medical Journal*, 327, 1459–1461.

Tuttle, R.P., Cohen, M.H., Augustine, A.J., Novotny, D.F., Delgado, E., Dongilli, et al. (2007). Utilizing simulation technology for competency skills assessment and a comparison of traditional methods of training to simulation-based training. *Respiratory Care*, 52, 263–270.

Wayne, D.B., Barsuk, J.H., Cohen, E., & McGaghie, W.C. (2007). Do baseline data influence standard setting for a clinical skills examination? *Academic Medicine*, 82(10, Suppl.), S105–S108.

Wayne, D.B., Barsuk, J., O'Leary K., Fudala, M.J., & McGaghie, W.C. (2008a). Mastery learning of thoracentesis skills by internal medicine residents using simulation technology and deliberate practice. *Journal of Hospital Medicine*, 3(1), 48–54.

Wayne, D.B., Butter, J., Siddall, V.J., Fudala, M.J., Feinglass, J., & McGaghie, W.C. (2006). Mastery learning of advanced cardiac life support skills by internal medicine residents using simulation technology and deliberate practice. *Journal of General Internal Medicine*, 21, 251–256.

Wayne, D.B., Butter, J., Siddall, V.J., Fudala, M.J., Lindquist, L., Feinglass, J., et al. (2005a). Simulation-based training of internal medicine residents in advanced cardiac life support protocols: A randomized trial. *Teaching and Learning in Medicine*, 17, 210–216.

Wayne, D.B., Didwania, A., Feinglass, J., Fudala, M.J., Barsuk, J.H., & McGaghie, W.C. (2008b). Simulation-based education improves quality of care during cardiac arrest team responses at an academic teaching hospital: A case-control study. *Chest*, 133, 56–61.

Wayne, D.B., Fudala, M.J., Butter, J., Siddall, V.J., Feinglass, J., Wade, L.D., et al. (2005b). Comparison of two standard setting methods for advanced cardiac life support training. *Academic Medicine*, 80(10, Suppl.), S63–S66.

Williams, R.G., McLaughlin, M.A., Eulenberg B., Hurm, M., & Nendaz, M.R. (1999). The Patient Findings Questionnaire: One solution to an important standardized patient examination problem. *Academic Medicine*, 74, 1118–1124.

Ziv, A., Rubin, O., Moshinsky, A., & Mittelman, M. (2007). Screening of candidates to medical school based on non-cognitive parameters using a simulation-based assessment center. *Simulation in Healthcare*, 2(1), 69.

11

ORAL EXAMINATIONS

ARA TEKIAN AND RACHEL YUDKOWSKY

The oral examination, sometimes known as a *viva voce*, is characterized by a face-to-face interaction between an examinee and one or more examiners. Test questions may be linked to a patient case, clinic chart, or other clinical material; exam sessions can range from focused five-minute probes to comprehensive "long cases" of up to an hour in length.

The stated purpose of an oral examination is to explore an examinee's thinking in order to assess skills such as critical reasoning, problem solving, judgment, and ethics, as well as the ability to express ideas, synthesize material and think on one's feet. The potential advantage of the oral exam over a constructed-response written exam lies in the examiner's ability to follow-up with additional probes that explore the examinee's response, and the ability to deepen or broaden the challenge in order to better define the limits of the examinee's abilities. The Accreditation Council for Graduate Medical Education (ACGME) lists oral exams as a candidate method for the assessment of competencies such as decision making, analytic thinking, use of evidence from scientific studies, and sensitivity to contextual issues such as age, gender, and culture (see also Chapter 1, this volume). Oral examinations should not be used primarily to assess knowledge, which is better assessed with a written exam, or to evaluate elements of the patient encounter, better assessed with simulations, performance exams or direct observational methods (see Figure 11.1).

Oral examinations are used both at undergraduate and postgraduate levels, as well as in many certification and licensure examinations. Orals were used as early as in 1917 with the foundation of the organized specialty boards in the US (Mancall, 1995). As of 2006, fifteen of 24 American Board of Medical Specialties (ABMS) member boards use some sort of oral examination as part of their evaluation or certification process, as do most specialties of the Royal College of Surgeons and Physicians of Canada, dentistry boards in the US and Canada, the Royal College of General Practice in Great Britain, and other certification bodies around the world.

The many threats to the validity of the oral exam as well as its cost in faculty time have been a source of controversy and concern over the usefulness of orals as an assessment strategy (Schuwirth & van der Vleuten, 1996; Wass, Wakeford, Neighbour, & van der Vleuten, 2003; Davis & Karunathilake, 2005; Yudkowsky, 2002). In this chapter we review these threats and suggest some ways to address them, primarily by means of *structured* oral exams. We'll also look at some examples of how oral exams are used around the world.

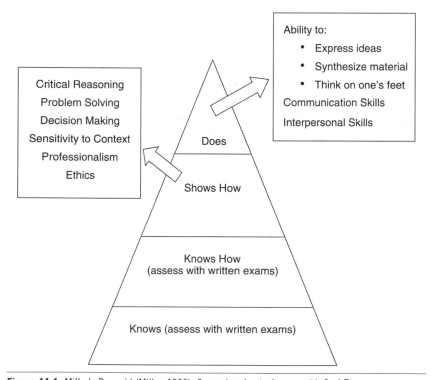

Figure 11.1 Miller's Pyramid (Miller, 1990): Competencies to Assess with Oral Exams.

Threats to the Validity of Oral Examinations

Concerns about the validity of traditional unstructured oral examinations have led to their gradual replacement by written tests, performance tests using simulations and standardized patients, and by structured oral exams, especially for high-stakes assessments. To understand this shift we will look at the vulnerability of oral exams to the two major threats to validity discussed in Chapter 2: construct underrepresentation (CU) and construct-irrelevant variance (CIV).

Construct underrepresentation (CU) or under-sampling is a major challenge for oral examinations. Like any other assessment, an oral exam must provide multiple data points that systematically sample the domain to be assessed. As with other tests of clinical skills, content specificity (Elstein, Shulman, & Sprafka, 1978) limits the ability to generalize from competency in one topic to competency in another. An oral exam that consists of questions about two or three topics or clinical scenarios is not likely to provide a broad and systematic sampling of the content domain (Turnball, Danoff, & Norman, 1996); an exam that assesses problem solving or clinical reasoning skills in only one or two scenarios is not sufficiently sampling that skill. Furthermore, if the oral exam is linked to encounters with real patients the content that can be assessed may be limited by patient availability, the patient's ability to cooperate, and his/her ability to consent to the exam (Yudkowsky, 2002). If learners are tested on different patients their tests may not be equivalent in either difficulty or content, compromising fairness and the ability to compare test scores across examinees.

Compounding the problem, early studies (Evans, Ingersoll, & Smith, 1996; McGuire, 1966) found that questions asked in oral examinations were not much different than questions in written examinations; Jayawickramarajah (1985) found that approximately two thirds of questions in an unstructured oral examination were simple recall. Regardless of the number of topics covered, these questions are not likely to elicit the higher-order thinking that is the appropriate focus of oral exams.

Construct irrelevant variance (CIV) refers to score variance due to factors that are irrelevant to the competency being assessed—for example, when characteristics such as politeness, demeanor, and dress impact the rating of clinical reasoning. CIV is a substantial threat to traditional oral examinations that use a small number of examiners per learner, since there are likely to be too few raters to compensate for stringency (hawk/dove) and bias effects (Linn & Zeppa, 1966; Schwiebert & Davis, 1993; Wass, et al., 2003, Weingarten, et al., 2000).

Construct-irrelevant variables that can impact the scores in oral examinations include mannerism and behavior, language and fluency, appearance and attractiveness (e.g., dress code—professional or non-professional), physical abnormalities/peculiarities or oddness, anxiety/stress level, and emotional status (Pokorny & Frazier, 1966). The level of confidence of candidates can have more influence on the score awarded by the examiners than what was actually said (Thomas, et al., 1992).

In an interesting experiment on the effect of communication style, Rowland-Morin and colleagues (1991) trained five actors and actresses to portray identical students with variations such as direct versus indirect eye-contact and moderate versus slower response rate. Examiners rated ten categories of performance (knowledge of facts, understands concepts, identified problems, integrates relevant data, makes proper decisions, is motivated, communicates effectively, is resourceful, has integrity, and is attractive in appearance). The study found that examiners were strongly influenced by the students' communication skills. Conversely, an examiners approving or disapproving facial expression can encourage or discourage an examinee's responses, introducing additional construct-irrelevant variance into the mix.

Structured Oral Examinations

The subjectivity, CU and CIV problems listed above led many educators to replace oral examinations with more objective and controllable methods such as written exams and performance tests using standardized patients and other simulations. Nonetheless, under controlled and standardized conditions as described below oral examinations can provide added value within a comprehensive assessment approach.

A *structured* oral examination offers significant benefits in combating CU and CIV. In a structured oral exam each examinee is exposed to the *same* or *equivalent tasks*, which are administered under the *same conditions*, in the *same amount of time*, and with *scoring as objective* as possible (Guerin, 1995). CU and CIV concerns can be addressed by assembling a series of oral exams, with careful blueprinting of the exam stations, standardization of questions and a rubric for scoring the answers; by utilizing multiple examiners with systematic training; by formal standard setting; and by systematic quality assurance efforts.

Structured oral examinations share many of the characteristics of performance tests such as standardized patient exams and Objective Structured Clinical Examinations (OSCEs) (Yudkowsky, Chapter 9, this volume). As with performance tests, increasing the number of tests or stations has a large impact on reliability/generalizability by increasing the sampling across content and raters, decreasing CU and allowing CIV to cancel out across tests/examiners. Daelmans, et al., (2001) investigated the effect of multiple oral examinations in an internal medicine clerkship, aiming for two 30-minute patient-based orals a day for five days. They found it would take ten 30-minute exams or about five hours of testing to reach a generalizability of 0.8, about comparable to the number of cases and time needed for a reliable OSCE (van der Vleuten & Swanson, 1990). Just as in OSCEs, increasing the number of exams with a single examiner at each "station" improves reliability more than doubling up examiners (Norman, 2000; Swanson, et al., 1995; Wass, et al., 2003).

Table 11.1 Characteristics of a Structured Oral Exam

- Multiple exam "stations"
- Content blueprinting
- Standardization of initial questions
- Rubrics to assist in scoring answers
- Multiple examiners
- Examiner training
- Formal standard setting
- Quality assurance efforts

Case Example 11.1: An Oral Exam "OSCE"

The McMaster University Admissions Multiple Mini-Interview (MMI) is a creative example of a structured oral (Eva, et al., 2004b). The traditional interview for admission to a health professions program can easily be conceptualized as an "oral examination"—a high stakes conversation between the interviewer and the applicant. The Multiple Mini-Interview is composed of an OSCE-like series of ten brief, structured interactions between students and faculty, community members and standardized "colleagues". Studies of the MMI confirm that applicant "performance" varied across interview contexts, and that the MMI predicted pre-clerkship and clerkship clinical performance better than did the traditional interview protocol (Eva et al., 2004a).

Blueprinting the Oral Exam

An exam blueprint ensures that the domain of interest is systematically and representatively sampled (Downing & Haladyna, Chapter 2, this volume; Haladyna, 2004; Downing & Haladyna, 2006). Use a specification table to identify the content area and skills to be assessed, and provide examples of questions to elicit the skills to be assessed (see Table 11.2 and the example in the MRCGP case study opposite).

Depending on the purpose of the exam, a variety of trigger materials may be used to provide a clinical context for the exam questions. An oral exam can be based on a live or simulated patient encounter, and serve as the probe for an OSCE station. At times the examiner himself may simulate a patient in order to assess a learner's data gathering or communication skills. In Chart-Stimulated Recall (CSR) (Maatsch, 1981) the examinee's own patients' charts serve as the trigger material for discussion with the examiner, allowing the examiner to probe deeply into the learner's clinical reasoning and decision making rationale in the context of care provided to his/her own patients.

Table 11.2 Blueprinting and Logistical Decisions

- Content domain and sub-domains to be sampled
- Skills/competencies to be assessed
  - Decision making
  - Patient management
  - Diagnostic interpretations
  - Sensitivity to contextual issues
  - Communication and interpersonal skills
  - Other
- Trigger materials (if any)
  - Real patients
  - Simulated patients
  - Written vignettes
  - Learner's own patient charts
  - Lab results
  - Examiner role play
- Desired breadth and depth of questions

Logistical Decisions:
- Number of oral exam stations
- Time/duration of each station
- Number of questions/cases per station
- Number of examiners per station

Case Example 11.2: Creative Blueprinting

The Examination for Membership in the Royal College of General Practitioners (MRCGP)

The MRCGP exam (United Kingdom) includes two consecutive 20-minute oral examinations, each conducted by a team of two examiners. Each candidate is assigned to two examiner teams linked as a quartet during a morning or afternoon session. To ensure a systematic sampling of candidate competencies, each quartet uses a blueprint grid to pre-plan ten topics that will be examined in all candidates that session. Topics are chosen that will enable candidates to demonstrate their decision-making skills in three competency domains (communication, professional values, and personal and professional development) and three contexts (patient care, working with colleagues, society and personal responsibility). For example, "Strategies for breaking bad news" is a topic that could assess the competency domain of "Communication" in the context of "Care of Patients"; the topic "Personal plans for re-accreditation" could assess the domain of "Personal and Professional Growth" in the context of "Society and Personal Responsibility" (Wass, et al., 2003). The three domains and contexts are the same for all examiner quartets. This somewhat unusual blueprint ensures that examiners focus their efforts on specific areas of interest to the RCGP that cannot easily be assessed in other ways.

The two examiners of each team alternate asking questions about one of the topics, spending no more than four minutes per topic, five topics per team. Each of the two examiners independently rates the candidate on all five topics using a nine-point categorical scale ranging from Outstanding through Bare Pass to Dangerous.

The RCGP is making a systematic effort to collect and disseminate validity evidence for their exam, resulting in a series of publications on the workings of a high stakes oral exam (RCGP website; Roberts, et al., 2000; Simpson & Ballard, 2005; Wakeford, et al., 1995; Wass, et al., 2003; Yaphe & Street, 2003).

Scoring and Standard Setting

Scoring issues for oral exams are similar to those for direct observation (McGaghie, et al., Chapter 8, this volume) and performance tests (Yudkowsky, Chapter 9, this volume), including instrument design for capturing and rating a performance and procedures for combining marks. Checklists and rating scales can encourage examiners to focus on the critical components of the exam, and behaviorally anchored scoring rubrics can help standardize ratings. As in performance tests, including global ratings helps to tap the unique judgment and experience of expert examiners.

Standard setting is a particular challenge for oral examinations. If left to the sole judgment of the individual examiner, pass/fail decisions could be legitimately attacked as both arbitrary and capricious. Pooling the judgments of several experts through a formal standard setting exercise will ensure that the cut scores are defensible and fair.

Any of the standard setting methods used for performance tests such as OSCEs can be adapted for structured oral exams with multiple "stations" and examiners. Examinee-based methods such as Borderline Group Method may be especially appropriate for oral exams in which different learners are questioned by different examiners. In this method the examiner scores or rates the examinee on several relevant items per the scoring rubric, and also provides a global rating ranging from definite pass to marginal pass to definite fail. The final pass/fail cut score is determined by the mean item score of all examinees with a "marginal pass" rating.

In an Angoff-type method, standards can be set either on the individual oral exam "station" level or on the test level. A panel of carefully selected judges reviews each item or exam station and each judge indicates the probability of the item or exam being successfully accomplished by a "borderline" examinee—an examinee just on the cusp of failure. The final cut score for the station or the test is the sum of the probabilities across items or stations.

See Chapter 6 (Yudkowsky, Downing, & Tekian, this volume) for a more complete discussion of standard setting issues, and Chapters 8 and 9 for discussion of scoring and standard setting in the context of observations and performance tests.

Preparation of the Examinee

Examinees taking an oral examination should know all the details involved in the process. Orient learners to the objectives, setting, duration, number of examiners, and the overall procedure in advance. Inform learners about the type of questions and criteria for passing, and provide opportunities to practice (particularly for high stakes examinations).

Selection and Training of the Examiners

Wakeford and colleagues (1995) suggest that selection criteria for examiners include appropriate knowledge and skills in the subject matter, "an approach to the practice of medicine and the delivery of health care that is within the limits of that acceptable to the examiners as a whole," effective interpersonal skills, demonstrated ability of a good team player, and being active in general practice. While selection of appropriate examiners is a critical step for any oral exam, one of the advantages of a structured oral exam is the opportunity to institute systematic training as well. For example, examiners can be trained to ask open-ended questions of higher taxonomic level, providing better assessments of the candidates' problem solving skills (Des Marchais & Jean, 1993). Frame-of-reference training, in which examiners practice rating exemplars of different levels of responses is an especially effective method for calibrating examiners to the rating scale (Bernardin & Buckley, 1981; and Yudkowsky (Chapter 9 this volume)). Newble, Hoare, & Sheldrake (1980) demonstrated that training tends to be ineffective for less consistent examiners, and suggested that inconsistent examiners and extremely severe or lenient raters be removed from the examiner pool. Systematic severity and leniency (but not inconsistency) can also be corrected by statistical adjustment of scores. Raymond, Webb, & Houston (1991) provide a relatively simple statistical procedure based on ordinary least squares (OLS) regression to identify and correct errors in leniency and stringency, resulting in a 6% change in the pass rate. In high-stakes exams, more complex statistical methods such as Many Faceted Rasch Measurement can help identify and correct for rater errors (Myford & Wolfe, 2003).

Quality Assurance

Quality assurance (QA) efforts can focus on preventing, checking for and remedying threats to the validity of the exam (Table 11.4), and on obtaining the five types of validity evidence described in Chapter 2. These might include activities such as reviewing the blueprint for content validity; ensuring that examiners' adhered to implementation

Table 11.3 Steps in Examiner Training for a Structured Oral Exam

1. Select examiners who are knowledgeable in the domain to be tested, familiar with the level of learners to be tested (e.g., 2nd year nursing students), and have good communication skills.
2. Orient examiners to the exam purpose, procedure, and consequences (stakes).
3. Explain the competencies to be assessed, types of questions to be asked and how to use any trigger material. Have examiners practice asking higher-order questions.
4. Review and rehearse rating and documentation procedures.
5. If possible, provide frame-of-reference training to calibrate examiners to scoring of different levels of responses.
6. Have new examiners observe an experienced examiner and/or practice via participation in a simulated oral examination.
7. Observe new examiners and provide feedback, after which an examiner is either invited or rejected. Examiners who are inconsistent or have clearly deviant patterns of grading (very lenient or very severe) should not be allowed to serve as examiners.
8. Continue ongoing calibration/fine-tuning of examiners, particularly in high stakes examinations.

Case Example 11.3: Assessing Examiners

The American Board of Emergency Medicine (ABEM) Oral Certification Exam

The ABEM five-hour oral certification examination (as of 2006) consists of seven structured oral simulations based on actual cases: five single-patient scenarios and two scenarios in which the candidate has to manage multiple patients concurrently. A single examiner scores each simulation, rating candidates on eight performance criteria based on critical actions relevant to that case. The examination blueprint (content specification) and pass/fail criteria can be found on the ABEM website: www.abem.org.

The ABEM expects their examiners to undergo six hours of training on case administration and scoring, achieving a high degree of inter-examiner agreement. Their examiners are monitored and evaluated on 17 criteria at each examination. Some of these are listed below.

- Established a comfortable tone of interaction with candidates

- Started cases on time
- Maintained control of case timing
- Finished cases on time
- Introduced cases according to guidelines
- Managed case material appropriately
- Administered cases according to agreed upon standards
- Played roles appropriately
- Cued appropriately
- Took comprehensive and readable notes

Examiners are assessed by senior examiners who rotate between rooms. Examiners who repeatedly deviate from training guidelines are not invited to return.

For more about the American Board of Emergency Medicine Exam see Reinhart, 1995 and Bianchi, et al., 2003.

guidelines for questions, scoring, and managing the exam; obtaining reliability indicators such as inter-rater reliability or generalizability estimates; investigating the relationship between scores on the oral exam and other assessments; and assessing the consequences of the cut-score standards set for the exam.

After the Exam

Planning for an oral examination includes consideration of post-examination issues common to all assessment methods. These include questions such as mechanisms for disseminating the results to examinees and other stakeholders; dealing with failing or marginal candidates, and whether there is an appeals process to review disputed scores.

Cost

There are many expenses involved in an oral exam: examination preparation and production cost (including item/case generation and scoring); costs associated with examiners' training, time and travel;

other reimbursements particularly if standardized or real patients are utilized; and venue/site expenses. The logistics of a structured oral exam are particularly complex, but are worth the extra cost and effort to be able to respond affirmatively to questions such as "Are we measuring what we intended to measure?" "Are the results reliable?" and "Is the exam worth the investment in time and money?"

Summary

Oral examinations remain the subject of debate and dispute, but when properly implemented orals can be credible contributors to the assessment toolbox. In the context of a low-stakes, formative assessment, an unstructured oral examination can provide an invaluable opportunity for faculty to engage in a conversation with learners, understand their thinking, and provide immediate feedback based on the encounter. In high-stakes settings, a structured, OSCE-like oral can provide a unique opportunity for in-depth probing of decision-making, ethical reasoning and other "hidden" skills.

When planning a structured oral examination, follow these evidence-based recommendations:

- Use multiple orals with multiple examiners
- Use a blueprint to guide question development
- Use a structured scoring system
- Select consistent, well-trained examiners
- Monitor the preparation, production, training, implementation, evaluation, and feedback phases of the examination process
- Use oral exams as one component of a comprehensive assessment system.

Table 11.4 Threats to Validity*: Oral Examinations

	Problem	Remedy
Construct Under-representation (CU)	Too few questions to sample domain adequately	Use multiple exams
	Unrepresentative sampling of domain	Blueprint to be sure exams systematically sample the domain
	Lower order questions (mis-match of questions to competencies)	Train examiners to use higher order questions
		Standardize the questions
		Use multiple examiners
	Too few independent examiners	Use one examiner per station
Construct-irrelevant Variance (CIV)	Flawed or inappropriate questions	Train examiners
	Flawed or inappropriate case scenarios or other prompts	Standardize questions
		Pilot test cases and prompts
		Provide scoring rubric
	Examiner bias	Train examiners to use rubric
	Systematic rater error:	
	Halo, Severity, Leniency, Central tendency	Frame of reference training for examiners
	Question difficulty inappropriate (too easy/too hard)	Train examiners
		Standardize questions
	Bluffing of examiners	Train examiners
	Language/cultural bias	Train examiners
	Indefensible passing score methods	Review and revise questions
		Use formal standard setting procedures
Reliability Indicators		Generalizability
		Inter-rater reliability
		Raterconsistency

Note: * For more about CU and CIV threats to validity, see Downing & Haladyna, Chapter 2, this volume.

References

Bernardin, H.J., & Buckley, M.R. (1981). Strategies in rater training. *The Academy of Management Review*, 6(2), 205–212.

Bianchi, L., Gallagher, E.J., Korte, R., & Ham, H.P. (2003). Interexaminer agreement on the American Board of Emergency Medicine Oral Certification Examination. *Annals of Emergency Medicine*, 41, 859–864.

Daelmans, H.E.M., Scherpbier, A.J.J.A., van der Vleuten, C.P.M., & Donker, A.B.J.M. (2001). Reliability of clinical oral examination re-examined. *Medical Teacher*, 23, 422–424.

Davis, M.H., & Karunathilake, I. (2005). The place of the oral examination in today's assessment systems. *Medical Teacher*, 27(4), 294–297.

Des Marchais, J.E., & Jean, P. (1993). Effects of examiner training on open-ended, higher taxonomic level questioning in oral certification examinations. *Teaching and Learning in Medicine*, 3, 24–28.

Downing, S., & Haladyna, T. (2006). *Handbook of test development*. Mahwah, NJ: Lawrence Erlbaum Associates.

Elstein, A., Shulman, L., & Sprafka, S. (1978). *Medical problem solving: An analysis of clinical reasoning*. Cambridge, MA: Harvard University Press.

Eva, K.W., Reiter, H.I., Rosenfeld, J., & Norman, G.R. (2004a). The ability of the multiple mini-interview to predict preclerkship performance in medical school. *Academic Medicine*, 79 (10 Suppl), S40–S42.

Eva, K.W., Rosenfeld, J., Reiter, H.I., & Norman, G.R. (2004b). An admissions OSCE: The multiple mini-interview. *Medical Education*, 38 (3), 314–326.

Evans, L.R., Ingersoll, R.W., & Smith, E.J. (1996). The reliability, validity, and taxonomic structure of the oral examination. *Journal of Medical Education*, 41, 651–657.

Guerin, R.O. (1995). Disadvantages to using the oral examination. In E.L. Mancall & P.H. Bashook (Eds.), *Assessing clinical reasoning: The oral examination and alternative methods* (pp. 41–48). Evanston, IL: American Board of Medical Specialties.

Haladyna, T. (2004). *Developing and validating multiple-choice test items*, (3rd ed.). Mahwah, NJ: Lawrence Erlbaum Associates.

Jayawickramarajah, P.T. (1985). Oral examinations in medical education. *Medical Education*, 19, 290–293.

Linn, B.S., & Zeppa, R. (1966). Team testing—One component in evaluating surgical clerks. *Journal of Medical Education*, 41, 28–40.

Maatsch, J.L. (1981). Assessment of clinical competence on the Emergency Medicine Specialty Certification Examination: The validity of examiner ratings of simulated clinical encounters. *Annals of Emergency Medicine*, 10, 504–507.

Mancall, E.L. (1995). The oral examination: A historic perspective. In E.L. Mancall & P.H. Bashook (Eds.), *Assessing clinical reasoning: The oral examination and alternative methods* (pp. 3–7). Evanston, IL: American Board of Medical Specialties.

McGuire, C.H. (1966). The oral examination as a measure of professional competence. *Journal of Medical Education*, 41, 267–274.

Miller, G. (1990). The assessment of clinical skills/competence/performance. *Academic Medicine*, 65 (Suppl.), S63–S67.

Myford, C.M., & Wolfe, E.W. (2003). Detecting and measuring rater effects using many-facet Rasch measurement: Part I. *Journal of Applied Measurement*, 4(4), 386–422.

Newble, D.I., Hoare, J., & Sheldrake, P.F. (1980). The selection and training of examiners for clinical examinations. *Medical Education*, 14, 345–349.

Norman, G. (2000). Examining the examination: Canadian versus US radiology certification exam. *Canadian Association of Radiologist Journal*, 51, 208–209.

Pokorny, A.D., & Frazier, S.H. (1966). An evaluation of oral examinations. *Journal of Medical Education*, 41, 28–40.

Raymond, M.R., Webb, L.C., & Houston, W.M. (1991). Correcting performance-rating errors in oral examinations. *Evaluation and the Health Professions*, 14, 100–122.

Reinhart, M.A. (1995). Advantages to using the oral examination. In E.L. Mancall & P.H. Bashook (Eds.), *Assessing clinical reasoning: The oral examination and alternative methods* (pp. 31–39). Evanston, IL: American Board of Medical Specialties.

Roberts, C., Sarangi, S., Southgate, L., Wakeford, R., & Wass, V. (2000). Oral examinations equal opportunities, ethnicity, and fairness in the MRCGP. *British Medical Journal*, 320, 370–375.

Rowland-Morin, P.A., Burchard, K.W., Garb, J.L., & Coe, N.P. (1991). Influence of effective communication by surgery students on their oral examination scores. *Academic Medicine*, 66, 169–171.

Schuwirth, L.W.T., & van der Vleuten, C.P.M. (1996). Quality control: Assessment and examinations. Retrieved June 30, 2008 from http://www.oeghd.or.at/zeitschrift/1996h1-2/06_art.html

Schwiebert, P., & Davis, A. (1993). Increasing inter-rater agreement on a family medicine clerkship oral examination—A pilot study. *Family Medicine*, 25, 182–185.

Simpson, R.G., & Ballard, K.D. (2005). What is being assessed in the MRCGP oral examinations? A qualitative study. *British Journal of General Practice*, 55, 420–422.

Swanson D.B., Norman G.R., & Linn R.L. (1995). Performance-based assessment: Lessons learnt from the health professions. *Educational Researcher*, 24, 5–11.

Thomas, C.S., Mellsop, G., Callender, K., Crawshaw, J., Ellis, P.M., Hall, A., et al. (1992). The oral examination: A study of academic and non-academic factors. *Medical Education*, 27, 433–439.

Turnball, J., Danoff, D., & Norman, G. (1996). Content specificity and oral certification examinations. *Medical Education*, 30, 56–59.

van der Vleuten, C.P.M., & Swanson, D.B. (1990). Assessment of clinical skills with standardized patients: State of the art. *Teaching and Learning in Medicine*, 2, 58–76.

Wakeford, R., Southgate, L., & Wass, V. (1995). Improving oral examinations: Selecting, training, and monitoring examiners for the MRCGP. *British Medical Journal*, 311, 931–935.

Wass, V., Wakeford, R., Neighbour, R., & van der Vleuten, C. (2003). Achieving acceptable reliability on oral examinations: An analysis of the Royal College of General Practitioners membership examination's oral component. *Medical Education*, 37, 126–131.

Weingarten, M.A., Polliack, M.R., Tabenkin, H., & Kahan, E. (2000).

Variations among examiners in family medicine residency board oral examinations. *Medical Education, 34,* 13–17.

Yaphe, J., & Street, S. (2003). How do examiners decide? A qualitative study of the process of decision making in the oral examination component of the MRCGP examination. *Medical Education, 37,* 764–771.

Yudkowsky, R. (2002). Should we use standardized patients for high stakes examinations in psychiatry? *Academic Psychiatry, 26*(3), 187–192.

12

ASSESSMENT PORTFOLIOS

ARA TEKIAN AND RACHEL YUDKOWSKY

The word portfolio comes from the Latin word *portare* (to carry) and *folium* (leaf, sheet). The Webster Dictionary's definition of portfolio is "a flat, portable case for carrying loose papers [and] drawings" (Webster's Encyclopedia, 1996). In health professions education, a portfolio is a collection of evidence documenting progress, accomplishments and achievements over time. Unlike written exams and performance tests, whose scope is limited to behaviors and characteristics that can be observed and measured at a single point of time, portfolios provide a means to assess competencies such as self directed learning, which are demonstrated over the course of months or years. Portfolios also comprise a vehicle for the longitudinal, multi-method, multi-source assessment of learner achievement. While portfolios can be used for both instruction and assessment purposes, our focus will be on the use of portfolios for assessment. In this chapter we will describe both single-competency and multi-source or "omnibus" assessment portfolios, and focus on the challenge of using portfolios to obtain valid and reliable scores.

Portfolios and Reflection

A portfolio in the health professions is not simply a collection of work samples or a record of activities; the distinctive aspect of a portfolio is the reflective component, an opportunity for the learner to provide a commentary on the included items and explicate their meaning to the reader. As such it is a unique and individual creation and a dynamic record of personal and professional growth.

A portfolio can serve as both a *vehicle* to promote reflective learning and as *evidence* of that reflection and of other learning. The use of portfolios to facilitate learning is based on the experiential/reflective learning models of Kolb (1984) and Schön (1987) (Figure 12.1). These models emphasize the need to reflect on an experience, often together with a coach or mentor, in order for the experience to be incorporated effectively as new learning. The process of portfolio development promotes this reflection: writing about experiences is itself a tool that forces thinking, structuring thoughts and reflection, thus supporting professional development (Pitkala & Mantyranta, 2004).

Types of Portfolios and their Contents

The contents of a portfolio depend on its purpose. As a vehicle to promote reflection, a formative or learning portfolio may include private, reflective responses to learning experiences, including reflection on errors and mistakes. These reflections may be reviewed and discussed with a mentor, tutor or peers for the purpose of formative assessment and feedback. Summative or assessment portfolios, on the other hand, consist of a public compilation of evidence of learning and/or work samples, often reflecting a learner's best work, most typical work, or work on a theme (Davis, et al., 2001b; O'Sullivan, et al., 2004; Paulson, Paulson, & Meyer, 1991; Rees, 2005). While an assessment portfolio may include selected entries from the learning portfolio, the different purposes should be explicit, and the selection

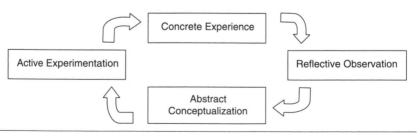

Figure 12.1 Kolb's Experiential Learning Cycle.*

Source: *Adapted from Kolb (1984).

of reflective entries to be made public should be left to the learner (Pinsky & Fryer-Edwards, 2004; Pitts, 2007).

A portfolio can serve to document the accomplishment of a single curricular objective or competency such as self-directed learning. Portfolios are especially suited to providing evidence for the achievement of competencies that are difficult to observe directly in controlled circumstances at a single point in time. By providing an annotated, reflective record of activities over time, portfolios can afford indirect observation of complex competencies such as practice-based learning and improvement or system-based practice. In addition, the process of selecting and justifying "best work" for an assessment portfolio allows the learner to demonstrate aspects of professionalism such as the ability to reflect on and self-assess one's own work, and implies a deep understanding of the characteristics and criteria that determine the quality of the work (Pinsky & Fryer-Edwards, 2004).

Portfolios can also complement single-source, single-competency assessment by providing a rich multidimensional description of the learner's accomplishments over time and verifying the achievement of multiple and complex learning objectives. An "omnibus" assessment portfolio is a compilation of evidence from a variety of methods and sources. The omnibus portfolio can include entries across the spectrum of Miller's pyramid from "knows" to "does" (Downing & Yudkowsky, Chapter 1, this volume and Figure 12.2). Entries can continue to accumulate in the portfolio until the evidence is sufficient for the decision required. As faculty gain experience with assessment portfolios, patterns of exceptional or dysfunctional learning, like "growth charts," can provide an opportunity for early intervention and remediation.

Scoring the Portfolio

The primary challenge of assessment portfolios is how to move from a collection of evidence to a single summative score or decision. As an example, imagine an omnibus portfolio consisting of four components: annual written exam scores, annual performance test (OSCE) scores, monthly end-of-rotation clinical evaluations, and semi-annual reflections by the learner. Some possibilities for scoring the portfolio are:

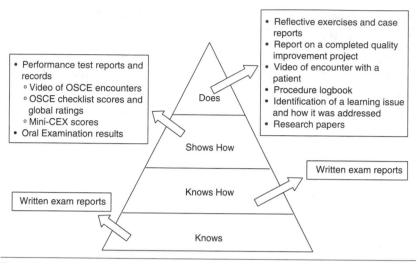

- Performance test reports and records
  - Video of OSCE encounters
  - OSCE checklist scores and global ratings
  - Mini-CEX scores
- Oral Examination results

- Reflective exercises and case reports
- Report on a completed quality improvement project
- Video of encounter with a patient
- Procedure logbook
- Identification of a learning issue and how it was addressed
- Research papers

Does

Shows How

Written exam reports

Knows How

Written exam reports

Knows

Figure 12.2 Miller's Pyramid (Miller, 1990): Sample Elements that can be Included in an Omnibus Assessment Portfolio.

- Score each component separately, and average the scores across components for the final portfolio score (*compensatory scoring*). In such situations, good performance on one or more components will compensate for the poor performance on other components. For example, if a student performs poorly on the monthly end of rotation clinical evaluation, good performance on the other three components will compensate for poor performance on this component. In a compensatory system, it is difficult to give feedback about each component, because the score is an aggregate of several components.
- Score each component separately; the learner must reach a minimum standard in each component in order to pass (*conjunctive scoring*). A student performing poorly on the monthly end of rotation clinical evaluation will not get a passing score irrespective of good performance on the other three components, because the scores for each component do not compensate for each other. (For more on conjunctive vs compensatory scoring see Chapter 6 in this volume.)
- Rate the portfolio-as-a-whole using an analytic or primary trait rating rubric (see Chapters 7 and 9). For example, the portfolio-as

-a-whole could be rated on characteristics such as organization, completeness, or quality of reflection. Alternatively the portfolio-as-a-whole could be rated on the quality of evidence provided for each of several individual competencies such as communication, knowledge, or professionalism.

- Rate the portfolio-as-a-whole using a single global rating rubric—for example, a five-point scale ranging from definite pass to definite fail.

Optional steps include an oral "defense" of the portfolio to allow examiners to probe for additional information and understanding; discussions between examiners to reach a consensus grade; and requesting additional information and/or rating by additional examiners for marginal or borderline students.

Designing a Portfolio System: Addressing Threats to Validity

Portfolios face the same threats to validity as other assessment methods (Downing & Haladyna, Chapter 2, this volume and Table 12.1). Because of these challenges, portfolios are best used as part of a comprehensive assessment system that can triangulate on learner competence (Webb, et al., 2003; Melville, et al., 2004).

The contents of the portfolio should systematically sample the learning objectives to be assessed. A portfolio intended to assess the self-directed learning of nurse practitioners, whose entries include only a log of textbook reading, is an example of a *construct under-representation* (CU) or under-sampling validity challenge (see Chapter 2). CU can be avoided by providing learners with a portfolio structure and guidelines that specify the learning objectives to be documented, the types of desirable evidence, and the amount of evidence required, systematically sampling work *over time* and *over tasks*. For example, guidelines for a portfolio intended for the assessment of self-directed learning might specify including:

- An explanation of five new learning objectives initiated by critical incidents
- Learning plans to achieve these objectives

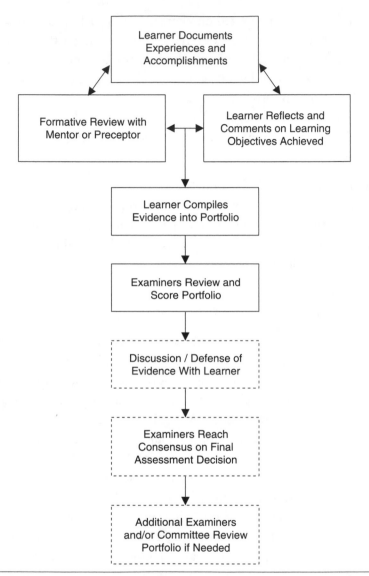

Figure 12.3 Assessment Portfolio Steps.

- A description of the educational activities undertaken
- A reflective self-appraisal of learning showing that growth and professional development is taking place.

Construct irrelevant variance (CIV) occurs when scores inadvertently include elements other than the ability to be assessed. These irrelevant elements ("noise" in the scores) can be due to either learner or rater factors. Learners may contribute to CIV when they are reluctant to reflect honestly on errors or to expose their weaknesses in the context of an assessment. Separating the reflective (formative) and assessment (summative) functions of the portfolio, and allowing learners to select the "best work" or "best evidence" entries to make public in the assessment portfolio can help minimize this problem (Pinsky & Fryer-Edwards, 2004).

Portfolio raters are subject to the same biases and errors as raters for oral exams and performance exams (see Table 12.1) (Roberts, Newble, & O'Rourke, 2002; Ward, Gruppen, & Regehr, 2002). One approach to the rater (dis)agreement challenge is to standardize the contents of the portfolio and to use multiple raters whenever possible – parallel to the approach for standardizing essay, oral and performance exams. An example would be to have various portfolio entries scored by different raters, resulting in multiple "observations" by multiple raters. Another tactic is to include portfolio entries such as OSCE or MCQ results with known high reliability; the portfolio as a whole partakes of the reliability of its component parts. As with other subjective judgments, benchmarks for acceptable entries, frame-of-reference rater training and rater consensus through discussion can improve rater agreement (McGaghie, et al., Chapter 8, this volume; O'Sullivan, et al., 2002, 2004; Pitts, et al., 2002; Rees & Sheard, 2004).

Reliability of Portfolios

Nonetheless, the ability of portfolio ratings to achieve acceptable levels of psychometric reliability is still at issue. Gadbury-Amyot, et al. (2003) had seven faculty raters score 20 portfolios of baccalaureate dental hygiene students using a scoring rubric based on primary trait analysis: faculty rated the portfolio on seven subscales such as "growth and development," "competencies," "lifelong learning," and "communication" using a four-point Likert scale where 1 = no evidence of the trait and 4 = complete evidence of the trait. A generalizability analysis D-study (see Kreiter, Chapter 4, this volume) established that three raters, each scoring the portfolio on ten subscales, would provide an acceptable phi coefficient (reliability) of 0.83. On the other hand, several studies have concluded that low inter-rater reliability precludes the use of portfolios for a high stakes, summative assessment (Melville, et al., 2004; Pitts, Coles, & Thomas, 1999 and 2001). For example, in a series of studies, Pitts et al. trained experienced general practice trainers to rate the portfolios of participants in a Trainers Course and assessed their level of agreement. Using a six-point scale, the portfolio-as-a-whole was rated on six characteristics such as "reflective learning process," "awareness of educational resources" and "recognition of effective teaching behaviors." To assess the reliability of pass/fail decisions the scale was collapsed to a dichotomous score of "pass" or "refer." The study found only slight to fair agreement between raters, with kappas ranging from 0.05 to 0.36 for eight independent assessors. While they were able to achieve "moderate" agreement after discussion between pairs of examiners, they concluded that "despite explicit instructions to compilers [learners], considerable investment in assessor training, and the negotiation, agreement and publication of overt criteria, individual assessments . . . show only fair inter-rater reliability and are untrustworthy in high-stakes assessment" (Pitts, et al., 2002).

Disaggregating the portfolio and scoring the components independently increases psychometric reliability, but at the expense of the holistic, developmental view of the learner that is the portfolio's raison d'etre. An alternative approach to the reliability problem is to use qualitative research methodology to assure the appropriate evaluation of the portfolio-as-a-whole (Driessen, et al., 2005; McMullan, et al., 2003, Webb, et al., 2003). This approach emphasizes establishing the credibility and dependability of the portfolio rating, rather than using traditional psychometric measures of reliability. How credible is the final decision, and how much can I depend on it? The *credibility* of an assessment is improved by employing triangulation (combining different information sources—analogous to multiple raters), prolonged engagement (e.g., multiple formative reviews of the portfolio over time—analogous to multiple observations), and member checking (reviewing and discussing the assessment with the student). *Dependability* is enhanced by audit (quality assurance procedures with external

Table 12.1 Threats to Validity: Portfolios

	Problem	Remedy
Construct under-representation (CU)	Not enough evidence of learning is presented	Provide learners with guidelines for type and quantity of evidence needed; Formative review with preceptor
	Evidence is not presented for all learning objectives	Specify portfolio structure based on blueprint of learning objectives; Formative review with preceptor
Construct-irrelevant variance (CIV)	Examiner bias	Provide scoring rubric Train examiners to use rubric Rater consensus discussion
	Systematic rater error: Halo, Severity, Leniency, Central tendency	Benchmarks, frame of reference training for examiners Rater consensus discussion
	Ability to reflect may be confounded with writing ability	Oral discussion/defense of portfolio Formative review of portfolio for correct writing and presentation before official submission
	Insincere reflective entries because of confidentiality and privacy concerns	Separate formative and summative functions of portfolio Give learners control over which reflective entries to include
Reliability indicators	Generalizability Inter-rater reliability or agreement Reproducibility of pass/fail decisions Credibility Dependability	

auditors) and audit trail (documentation of the assessment process to enable external checks). These qualitative approaches to the assessment and quality assurance of the portfolio-as-a-whole can help avoid reductionism and preserve an integrated, holistic view of the learner as a unique individual developing over time.

Case Examples

The following case studies illustrate three creative adaptations of portfolios for the assessment of learners in the health professions.

Case Example 12.1: A High-Stakes Omnibus Portfolio Assessment to Establish Readiness for Graduation (Davis, et al., 2001a, b)

After moving to outcome-based education in 1996–1997, Dundee medical school redesigned its final examinations to meet the needs of the new curriculum. The final examinations occured in two parts. At the end of Year-4, knowledge, problem solving and clinical skills were assessed by means of written tests and an OSCE. At the end of Year-5, faculty members evaluated overall progress towards all 12 of the desired learning outcomes, including personal and professional development, by means of an omnibus portfolio. All three of the examination components—written tests, OSCE, and portfolio—had to be passed for graduation.

The portfolio included entries such as:

- Pre-marked samples of student work
  - Ten short patient presentations
  - Seven case discussion reports
  - One Year-4 project report
- Procedure log, signed by faculty
- Faculty assessment forms from Special Study Modules and electives
- Learning contracts from medicine and surgery apprentice-ships with grades awarded for each learning outcome
- The student's personal summary of progress towards each of the 12 learning outcomes, reflecting on and justifying his or her accomplishments.

Scoring the Portfolio

Two examiners independently read and graded each of the 12 outcomes, based on the evidence presented in the portfolio. They discussed their ratings and agreed on areas of strength and weakness to be explored with the student during the oral review.

After a 40-minute oral review and defense of the portfolio, the examiners again independently assigned grades for each outcome based on the student's performance during the oral review. They then reached consensus on a final set of grades, on which pass/fail decisions were based.

Students who received consensus grades of "marginal fail" on at least two outcomes, or definite fail on one outcome, proceeded to remediation and/or further examination by OSCE and an additional review of the portfolio.

Year 1 studies demonstrated a 98% pass/referred agreement between two independent pairs of examiners.

Case Example 12.2: Showcase or "Best Work" Portfolios for Psychiatry Residents (O'Sullivan, et al., 2002 and 2004)

Psychiatry residents were asked to exhibit their "best work" in five of 13 essential topic areas each year, including topics such as initial evaluation and diagnosis, treatment course, self directed learning, working with teams, crisis management, legal issues, and presentation/teaching skills. Four of the topics were freely selected by residents; an entry in the area of bio/psycho/social formulation was mandatory. Resident guidelines specified the meaning of each topic, what to include in the entry, and the rubric showing how the entry would be evaluated. For each entry, residents selected a case or experience to showcase their "best work" in that topic. Entries were not developed specifically for the portfolio. Residents submitted copies of (de-identified) patient documentation that they had produced, and wrote a brief reflective self-assessment explaining how this case and the supporting documentation demonstrated their competency.

Scoring the Portfolio

Program faculty developed topic-specific, six-point scoring rubrics in which the low end indicated a lack of knowledge or skill that could place patients at risk and the high end indicated an ability to deal with complex problems effectively and creatively. Two external examiners who were unfamiliar with the residents and their patients scored each of the portfolio entries. Portfolio entries were sorted by topic, and raters scored all entries within a given topic (across residents) before moving to the next topic. Raters were trained by scoring benchmark entries.

Overall portfolio scores tended to increase with year of training. Scores were moderately correlated with a national, in-training written exam, but not with clinical rotation ratings. A generalizability analysis and D-study showed that five entries scored by two raters provided sufficient reliability for norm-referenced (relative) decisions with $G = 0.81$, and that five entries scored by three raters or six entries scored by two raters would provide sufficient reliability for criterion referenced (absolute) decisions.

As an unintended consequence, the portfolios identified poor performance across residents in certain topic areas, resulting in an almost immediate change in the curriculum.

Case Example 12.3: A Clinical Portfolio for Baccalaureate Nursing Students (Lettus, Moessner, & Dooley, 2001)

Regent's College created a portfolio assessment option to meet the needs of experienced registered nurses returning to school to obtain their Baccalaureate degree. The portfolio allowed these senior nurses, who were not always providing traditional hands-on nursing care, to document clinical competencies essential to nursing practice. Students developed their portfolios individually and at their own pace, based on a detailed portfolio development guide provided by the college.

The portfolio included three sections:

- Section 1 consisted of a resume that identified educational and professional experiences such as formal and continuing education and professional committee work, and reflected on the learning gained from these experiences. As a capstone for this section, the student identified an area of professional growth, engaged in a professional activity in this area, and wrote a scholarly paper about the learning attained.
- Section 2 was structured around competency objectives. The student developed a learning statement for each objective, describing and documenting his or her accomplishment of the objective; each statement had to be accompanied by two to four pieces of supportive evidence such as a course description, performance review, or letter from a supervisor.
- Section 3 of the portfolio was a case study that demonstrated the student's ability to care for a patient/client over time, making clinical decisions supported by the nursing literature.

A series of three one-hour telephone conferences for six to eight students and a nurse educator provided a formative, supportive opportunity to discuss the meaning and content of the portfolios.

Scoring the Portfolio

The portfolio development guide included examples of acceptable responses to each objective and acceptable documentation; sample case studies; and the scoring criteria for the learning statements and case study.

To avoid confounding clinical competencies with writing skills, the portfolio was reviewed for grammar, spelling, and errors in structure and format, and returned for revision before being submitted for scoring. A random sample of the documentation was verified to prevent fraud.

Examiners participated in a two-day training session to review the guidelines and to rate and discuss sample portfolios. Three raters scored each portfolio independently; the final pass/fail decision was reached by consensus. If a section was failed students repeated that section only.

Summary

Portfolios can provide a useful structure for gathering multi-method, multi-source, reflection-annotated evidence about the achievements of learners over time, but are open to the same threats to validity as other qualitative or holistic assessments. Portfolios have been used extensively for learning and assessment in nursing education and increasingly in undergraduate, graduate, and continuing medical education; with learners in dentistry, occupational therapy, physical therapy, and other health professions; and for faculty promotion and tenure (Table 12.2). With increases in Internet technology, educators are also experimenting with computer-based, web-based and e-portfolio structures (Carraccio & Englander, 2004; Dornan, Lee, & Stopford, 2001; Parboosingh, 1996; Rosenberg, et al., 2001). Table 12.3 provides a summary of guidelines for the successful implementation of assessment portfolios in the health professions.

Table 12.2 Portfolios in the Health Professions

Nursing	Jasper, 1995
	Wenzel, et al., 1998
	Gallagher, 2001
	Lettus, et al., 2001
Medicine	Challis, 1999
	Mathers, et al., 1999
	Pinsky & Fryer-Edwards, 2001
	Wilkinson, et al., 2002
	O'Sullivan, et al., 2002 and 2004
	Driessen, et al., 2003
	Gordon, 2003
Dentistry	Chambers, 2004
Dental Hygeine	Gadbury-Amyot, et al., 2003
Occupational Therapy	Zubizarreta, 1999
Physical Therapy	Paschal, et al., 2002
Faculty Promotion and Tenure	Hafler & Lovejoy, 2000

Table 12.3 Practical Guidelines for Assessment Portfolios

Introducing the portfolio
- Introduce portfolios slowly with input and feedback from learners and faculty
- Clarify goals
- Separate working (formative) and summative (performance) portfolio functions
- Provide support and training in the use of portfolios for both learners and faculty

Implementing the portfolio
- Provide learners with a standard structure and guidelines for the type and quantity of material to be included in the portfolio
- Sample learners' work over tasks and over time
- Provide frequent formative feedback in a supportive educational climate
- Provide time for creating portfolio entries within the structure of existing activities

Assessing the portfolio
- Provide benchmarks and frame-of-reference training to raters
- Allow raters to discuss scores and reach a consensus
- Use both qualitative and quantitative approaches to assessment and quality assurance
- Triangulate the results of the portfolio assessment with other assessment methods

References

Carraccio, C., & Englander, R. (2004). Evaluating competence using a portfolio: A literature review and web-based application to ACGME competencies. *Teaching and Learning in Medicine*, 16, 381–387.

Challis, M. (1999). AMEE Medical Education Guide No. 11 (revised) Portfolio-based learning and assessment in medical education. *Medical Teacher*, 21, 370–377.

Chambers, D.W. (2004). Portfolios for determining initial licensure competency. *Journal of American Dental Association*, 135(2), 173–184.

Davis, M.H., Friedman Ben-David, M., Harden, R.M., Howie, P., Ker, J., McGhee, C., et al. (2001a). Portfolio assessment in medical students' final examination. *Medical Teacher*, 23: 357–366.

Davis, M.H., Friedman Ben-David, M., Harden, R.M., Howie, P., Ker, J., McGhee, C., et al. (2001b). AMEE Medical Education Guide # 24: Portfolios as a method of student assessment. *Medical Teacher*, 23, 535–551.

Dornan, T., Lee, C., & Stopford, A. (2001). SkillsBase: A web-based electronic learning portfolio for clinical skills. *Academic Medicine*, 76, 542–543.

Driessen, E., Schuwirth, L., Van Tartwijk, Vermont, J., & van der Vleuten, C. (2003). Use of portfolios in early undergraduate medical training. *Medical Teacher*, 25, 18–21.

Driessen, E., van der Vleuten, C., Schuwirth, L., Van Tartwijk, J., & Vermont, J. (2005). The use of qualitative research criteria for portfolio assessment as an alternative to reliability evaluation: A case study. *Medical Education*, 39, 214–220.

Gadbury-Amyot, C.C., Kim, J., Palm, R.L., Mills, G.E., Noble, E., & Overman, P.R. (2003). Validity and reliability of portfolio assessment of competency in a baccalaureate dental hygiene program. *Journal of Dental Education*, 67(9), 991–1002.

Gallagher, P. (2001). An evaluation of a standards based portfolio. *Nurse Education Today*, 21, 409–416.

Gordon, J. (2003). Assessing students' personal and professional development using portfolios and interviews. *Medical Education*, 37, 335–340.

Hafler, J.P., & Lovejoy Jr., F.H. (2000). Scholarly activities recorded in the portfolios of teacher-clinician faculty. *Academic Medicine*, 75, 649–652.

Jasper, M.A. (1995). The potential of the professional portfolio for nursing. *Journal of Clinical Nursing*, 4, 249–255.

Kolb, D. (1984). *Experiential learning: Experience as a source of learning and development*. Englewood Cliffs, NJ: Prentice Hall.

Lettus, M.K., Moessner, P.H., & Dooley, L. (2001). The clinical portfolio as an assessment tool. *Nursing Administration Quarterly*, 25, 74–79.

Mathers, N.J., Challis, M.C., Howe, A.C., & Field, N.J. (1999). Portfolios in continuing medical education—effective and efficient? *Medical Education*, 33, 521–530.

McMullan, M., Endacott, R., Gray, M., Jasper, M., Miller, C., Scholes, J., et al. (2003). Portfolio and assessment of competence: A review of the literature. *Journal of Advanced Nursing*, 41(3), 283–294.

Melville, C., Rees, M., Brookfield, D., & Anderson, J. (2004). Portfolios for assessment of pediatric specialist registrars. *Medical Education*, 38, 1117–1125.

Miller, G. (1990). The assessment of clinical skills/competence/performance. *Academic Medicine*, 65, S63–S67.

O'Sullivan, P.S., Cogbill, K.K., McClain, T., Reckase, M.D., & Clardy, J.A. (2002). Portfolios as a novel approach for residency evaluation. *Academic Psychiatry*, 26, 173–179.

O'Sullivan, P.S., Reckase, M.D., McClain, T., Savidge, M.A., & Clardy, J.A. (2004). Demonstration of portfolios to assess competency of residents. *Advances in Health Sciences Education*, 9, 309–323.

Parboosingh, J. (1996). Learning portfolios: Potential to assist health professional with self-directed learning. *Journal of Continuing Education in the Health Professions*, 16, 75–81.

Paschal, K.A., Jensen, G.M., & Mostrom, E. (2002). Building Portfolios: A means for developing habits of reflective practice in physical therapy education. *Journal of Physical Therapy Education*, 16, 38–53.

Paulson, F.L., Paulson, P.P., & Meyer, C.A. (1991). What makes a portfolio a portfolio? *Educational Leadership*, 48, 60–63.

Pinsky, L.E., & Fryer-Edwards, K. (2004). Diving for PERLS: Working and performance portfolios for evaluation and reflection on learning. *Journal of General Internal Medicine*, 19, 582–587.

Pitkala, K., & Mantyranta, T. (2004). Feelings related to first patient experiences in medical school: A qualitative study on students' personal portfolios. *Patient Education and Counseling*, 54, 171–177.

Pitts, J. (2007). Portfolios, personal development and reflective practice. *Understanding Medical Education Series*. Edinburgh, Scotland: Association for the Study of Medical Education.

Pitts, J., Coles, C., & Thomas, P. (1999). Educational portfolios in the assessment of general practice trainers: Reliability of assessors. *Medical Teacher*, 33, 515–520.

Pitts, J., Coles, C., & Thomas, P. (2001). Enhancing reliability in portfolio assessment: "Shaping" the portfolio. *Medical Teacher*, 23, 351–355.

Pitts, J., Coles, C., Thomas, P., & Smith, F. (2002). Enhancing reliability in portfolio assessment: Discussions between assessors. *Medical Teacher*, 24(2), 197–201.

Rees, C. (2005). The use (and abuse) of the term "portfolio". *Medical Education*, 39, 436–437.

Rees, C., & Sheard, C. (2004). The reliability of assessment criteria for undergraduate medical students' communication skills portfolios: The Nottingham experience. *Medical Education*, 38, 138–144.

Roberts, C., Newble, D., & O'Rourke, A. (2002). Portfolio-based assessments in medical education: Are they valid and reliable for summative purposes? *Medical Education*, 36, 899–900.

Rosenberg, M.E., Watson, K., Paul, J., Miller, W., Harris, I., & Valdivia, T.D. (2001). Development and implementation of a web-based evaluation system for an internal medicine residency program. *Academic Medicine*, 76, 92–95.

Schön, D.A. (1987). *Educating the reflective practitioner: Toward a new design for teaching and learning in the professions.* San Francisco, CA: Jossey-Bass.

Ward, M., Gruppen, L., & Regehr, G. (2002). Measuring self-assessment: Current state of the art. *Advances in Health Sciences Education: Theory and Practice,* 7, 63–80.

Webb, C., Endacott, R., Gray, M.A., Jasper, M.A., McMullan, M., & Scholes, J. (2003). Evaluating portfolio assessment systems: What are the appropriate criteria? *Nursing Education Today,* 23, 600–609.

Webster's Encyclopedic Unabridged Dictionary of the English Language (1996). New York: Gramercy Books, Random House Value Publishing, Inc.

Wenzel, L.S., Briggs, K.L., & Puryear, B.L. (1998). Portfolio: Authentic assessment in the age of the curriculum revolution. *Journal of Nursing Education,* 37, 208–212.

Wilkinson, T.J., Challis, M., Hobma, S.O., Newble, D.I., Parboosingh, J.T., Sibbald, R.G., et al. (2002). The use of portfolios for assessment of the competence and performance of doctors in practice. *Medical Education,* 36, 918–924.

Zubizarreta, J. (1999). Teaching portfolios: An effective strategy for faculty development in occupational therapy. *American Journal of Occupational Therapy,* 53, 51–55.

List of Contributors

Steven M. Downing, PhD, Associate Professor, University of Illinois at Chicago, College of Medicine, Department of Medical Education.

Steven M. Downing received a PhD from Michigan State University (MSU) in Educational Psychology, specializing in educational measurement. He has more than 25 years' experience in working with high-stakes testing programs in medicine and the professions.

In 2001, Dr. Downing joined the faculty of the University of Illinois at Chicago, Department of Medical Education. He teaches courses in all areas of testing and assessment for the Masters of Health Professions Education (MHPE) program and advises students with interests in educational measurement in the health professions. Formerly, he was Director of Health Programs and Deputy Vice President at the National Board of Medical Examiners (NBME), Senior Psychometrician at the American Board of Internal Medicine (ABIM), and Director of Psychometrics and Senior Program Manager for the Institute for Clinical Evaluation (ICE) at the American Board of Internal Medicine. Dr. Downing consults with various national and international testing programs in all areas of test development and psychometrics, with particular interests in selected-response formats, test validity issues, testing program evaluation, and computer-based testing.

Dr. Downing's research interests in educational measurement and assessment in medical education have resulted in more than 100 research papers, book chapters, and presentations at national and international professional conferences. Dr. Downing is the senior editor for a comprehensive book on test development, *Handbook of Test Development*, published by Lawrence Erlbaum in January 2006.

Rachel Yudkowsky, MD, MHPE, Assistant Professor, University of Illinois at Chicago, College of Medicine, Department of Medical Education.

Rachel Yudkowsky received her MD from Northwestern University Medical School in 1979, and is Board Certified in Psychiatry. She served as medical student psychiatry clerkship director, psychiatry residency program director, and director of education for the Evanston Hospital Department of Psychiatry, and as associate director of graduate medical education for the Department of Psychiatry and Behavioral Sciences of Northwestern University Medical School. She received a Masters degree in Health Professions Education (MHPE) in 2000.

Dr. Yudkowsky joined the Department of Medical Education of the University of Illinois at Chicago in 1999. She served as associate director of faculty development from 1999–2005, and has been director of the Dr. Allan L. and Mary L. Graham Clinical Performance Center since 2000, where she develops standardized patient and simulation-based programs for the instruction and assessment of students, residents, and staff. Her areas of research interest include performance assessment using standardized patients and setting passing standards for performance tests.

Dr. Yudkowsky is immediate past Chair of the Research and Grants Committee of the Association of Standardized Patient Educators, and serves on the Editorial Board of the journal Simulation in Healthcare. She teaches in the MHPE program and conducts workshops on HPE topics both nationally and internationally.

Thomas M. Haladyna, PhD—Chapter 2 (Validity)

Thomas M. Haladyna is Professor Emeritus at Arizona State University (ASU). Tom has been an elementary school teacher, a research professor, and a test director at American College Testing Program and faculty member in the College of Teacher Education and Leadership at ASU. He specializes in designing and validating testing programs, and he has worked in more than 50 national, regional, and state testing programs. His research has principally focused on issues affecting the validity of test score interpretations and how to better develop test items. He has authored or co-authored 12 books, more than 60 published journal articles, and hundreds of conference papers and technical reports. Currently, Tom co-edited the *Handbook of Test Development* with Steve Downing, and has several, ongoing research projects on testing.

Rick D. Axelson, PhD—Chapter 3 (Reliability)

Rick D. Axelson is Assistant Professor in the Department of Family Medicine and faculty consultant in the Office of Consultation and Research in Medical Education at the University of Iowa Carver College of Medicine. He received an MS in Statistics and a PhD in Sociology from the University of Arizona. Over the past 15 years, he has been involved with developing and implementing educational assessment systems at colleges and universities. In 2003, he and his colleagues founded the LearningAssessment@Listserv.cccnext.net to facilitate the development of effective assessment practices in the California Community College system. Most recently, he served as the Assistant Vice Provost for Institutional Research, Assessment, & Planning at the University of Missouri-Kansas City, where he worked with academic departments on enhancing their program review and outcomes assessment processes. His research interests include program evaluation (theory, methods, practice), learning outcomes assessment, learning communities, and the role of social and psychological factors in learning environments.

Clarence D. Kreiter, PhD—Chapter 3 (Reliability) and Chapter 4 (Generalizability)

Clarence D. Kreiter is Professor in the Department of Family Medicine and the Office of Consultation and Research in Medical Education at the University of Iowa Carver College of Medicine. Dr. Kreiter received his PhD in quantitative foundations of educational psychology from the University of Iowa. He serves on the editorial boards of two medical education research journals and has published on topics related to innovative cognitive and clinical skill assessments, selection methods for medical school admissions, evaluation of teaching, simulation, OSCE test design, Bayesian reasoning, generalizability analysis, and validity generalization. As a professor with the University of Iowa Carver College of Medicine, he consults on research design and statistics and teaches graduate-level medical education assessment courses.

Ara Tekian, PhD, MHPE—Chapters 6 (Standard Setting), 11 (Oral Exams) and 12 (Portfolios)

Ara Tekian, PhD, MHPE is Associate Professor and Director of International Affairs at the Department of Medical Education (DME), University of Illinois at Chicago. He joined DME in 1992 as Head of the International Programs and participates in teaching in the Master's of Health Professions Education (MHPE) program. Dr. Tekian teaches courses in curriculum development, assessment and instruction, and medical simulations; and has organized and conducted over 140 international workshops in more than 35 countries in different parts of the world. Dr. Tekian was the winner of the 1997 Teaching Recognition Program Award selected by the UIC Council for Excellence in Teaching and Learning. He was the 2006 Program Chair for Education in the Professions' Division of American

Educational Research Association (AERA), and serves on the *Educational Researcher* Editorial Board. He is the President Elect for 2009. He is the primary author of the book *Innovative Simulations for Assessing Professional Competence: From Paper-and-Pencil to Virtual Reality* published in 1999.

William C. McGaghie, PhD—Chapters 8 (Observational Assessment) and 10 (Simulations in Assessment)

William C. McGaghie is currently the Jacob R. Suker, MD, Professor of Medical Education and Professor of Preventive Medicine at the Northwestern University Feinberg School of Medicine. Dr. McGaghie received his PhD degree from Northwestern University. He has previously held faculty positions at the University of Illinois College of Medicine and the University of North Carolina School of Medicine. Dr. McGaghie has been a medical education scholar for 35 years, writing about topics including personnel and program evaluation, research methodology, medical simulation, attitude measurement, and faculty development. He serves on the editorial boards of six scholarly journals and consults with a variety of professional boards, agencies, institutes, and medical schools worldwide.

John Butter, MD—Chapter 8 (Observational Assessment)

John Butter is Assistant Professor of Medicine, Department of Medicine and Augusta Webster Office of Medical Education, Northwestern University Feinberg School of Medicine. Dr. Butter received his MD degree from Northwestern University and completed his residency at Beth Israel Hospital, in Boston. After serving on the faculty at Dartmouth Medical School, he joined the faculty of Northwestern University Feinberg School of Medicine. He co-directs the Clinical Education Center and has leadership positions in the clinical skills program at Northwestern. He has published on topics related to clinical skills development and competency based mastery learning. He also serves as Associate Program Director for the

Internal Medicine Residency and Associate Division Chief for Education in General Internal Medicine.

Marsha Kaye, RN, MSN—Chapter 8 (Observational Assessment)

Marsha Kaye is Director of Standardized Patient Programs at the Clinical Education Center of the Office of Medical Education and Faculty Development, Northwestern University Feinberg School of Medicine. She received her Masters of Science in Nursing at Yale University. She currently serves on the board of the Association of Standardized Patient Educators and has published articles on the use of standardized patients in teaching clinical skills to medical students. For the past ten years and now as Director of Standardized Patient Programs, she is responsible for the development and administration of the use of standardized patients in teaching, assessment and remediation of clinical skills to medical students at the undergraduate level. Before entering in the field of medical education, she was a Pediatric Nurse Practitioner.

S. Barry Issenberg, MD—Chapter 10 (Simulations in Assessment)

S. Barry Issenberg is Professor of Medicine, University of Miami Miller School of Medicine and the Gordon Center for Research in Medical Education. He received his MD degree from the University of Miami. Dr. Issenberg serves as Project Director for the technical and curricular research and development of Harvey, the Cardiopulmonary Patient Simulator and computer-based training and assessment system. In addition, Dr. Issenberg leads a national consortium of clinicians and medical educators from 14 medical centers. The consortium meets quarterly to develop curricula in cardiology, neurology and emergency medicine and to design its outcomes research studies. The consortium has designed, implemented and published the results of several multi-center studies that have shown the effectiveness of simulation technology to teach and assess clinical skills.

Index

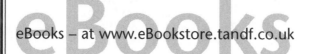